Point-of-Care Assessment in Pregnancy *and* Women's Health

ELECTRONIC FETAL MONITORING AND SONOGRAPHY

Cydney Afriat Menihan, CNM, MSN, RDMS, C-EFM
Nurse Midwife and Perinatal Consultant
Florida and Rhode Island

Ellen Kopel, MS, RNC-OB, C-EFM
Perinatal Consultant
Tampa, Florida

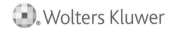 Wolters Kluwer

Philadelphia • Baltimore • New York • London
Buenos Aires • Hong Kong • Sydney • Tokyo

D0905658

Senior Acquisitions Editor: Shannon Magee
Product Development Editor: Ashley Fischer
Senior Production Project Manager: Cynthia Rudy
Manufacturing Manager: Kathleen Brown
Marketing Manager: Mark Wiragh
Design Coordinator: Joan Wendt
Production Service: Aptara, Inc.

© 2014 by Wolters Kluwer Health
Two Commerce Square
2001 Market Street
Philadelphia, PA 19103 USA
LWW.com

Printed in China

Library of Congress Cataloging-in-Publication Data

Menihan, Cydney Afriat, 1951- author.
  Point-of-care assessment in pregnancy and women's health : electronic fetal monitoring and sonography / Cydney Afriat Menihan, Ellen Kopel.
    p. ; cm.
  Includes bibliographical references and index.
    ISBN 978-1-4511-9228-5 (alk. paper)
  I. Kopel, Ellen, author. II. Title.
  [DNLM: 1. Fetal Monitoring–methods. 2. Heart Rate, Fetal–physiology. 3. Point-of-Care Systems. 4. Ultrasonography, Prenatal–methods. WQ 209]
  RG628
  618.3′2075—dc23
                                                                                    2014009120

To purchase additional copies of this book, call our customer service department at (800) 638-3030 or fax orders to (301) 223-2320. International customers should call (301) 223-2300.

10 9 8 7 6 5 4 3 2 1

RRS1406

To my sister Susan, superb mentor, mediator, and all-around maven.

*To Amber Bettez, whose spirit, wisdom, and fortitude have
proven that, from time to time, the young teach and inspire even
the seasoned;*

To the next generation of nurses and midwives who will carry on;

and

*To the University of Pittsburgh School of Nursing (1969–1973)
for getting me off on the right foot.*

Cydney Afriat Menihan

*To Zachary—my reason for everything and who has brought more
depth, wisdom, and love to my life than I ever imagined possible.*

*To my Mom—for, among many other things, her excellent editing
skills that helped me appreciate the art of writing.*

*To Cydney—a wealth of knowledge and a stellar mentor, colleague,
and friend—for sharing this book series journey with me.*

But for Ohio State…

Ellen Kopel-Puretz

ontributors and Reviewers

CONTRIBUTORS

Patricia Robin McCartney, RNC, PhD, FAAN
Director of Nursing Research
Department of Nursing, MedStar Washington
  Hospital Center
Washington, DC

Betty Kay Taylor, CNM, MSN, RDMS
OB/GYN and Fetal Echo Sonography
Rogue Regional Medical Center and Providence
  Medical Center
Medford, Oregon
(Chapter 12, Maternal Cervical Length
  Measurement)

REVIEWERS

Teresa M. Bieker, MBA, RDS, RDCS, RVT
Lead Sonographer, Division of Ultrasound
University of Colorado Hospital
Aurora, Colorado

Dianna Dowdy, CNM, DNP, RDMS
Adjunct Faculty
Vanderbilt University, Nashville, Tennessee
University of Alabama, Huntsville, Alabama
Private Practice, Huntsville, Alabama

Bonnie Flood Chez, MSN, RNC
President
Nursing Education Resources
Tampa, Florida

Serguei Kabakov, PhD
Principal Engineer
Maternal-Fetal Care
GE Healthcare
Laurel, Maryland

Ira Kantrowitz-Gordon, CNM, PhD
Assistant Professor
Department of Family and Child Nursing
University of Washington School of Nursing
Seattle, Washington
Providence Medical Group
Everett, Washington

Anthony Lathrop, PhD, CNM, RDMS
HealthNet
Indiana University Health
Adjunct Faculty
University of Indianapolis School of Nursing
Indianapolis, Indiana

Suzan J. Menihan, CNM, MSN
Assistant Professor of Nursing
New England Institute of Technology
East Greenwich, RI

Jeffrey L. Puretz, MD, FACOG
Obstetrician/Gynecologist
Women's Care Florida/Lakeland Obstetrics
  and Gynecology
Lakeland, Florida

Marilyn (Baba) Wilhm, BA, BS, BSN, MA, RDMS
Fetal Echo Sonographer
Noninvasive Cardiology
The Johns Hopkins All Children Heart Institute
St. Petersburg, Florida

CONTRIBUTORS/REVIEWERS/CONSULTANTS
to the Predicate Text, *Electronic Fetal Monitoring:
Concepts and Applications* (2001, 2008)

Cynthia Belew, CNN, MS
Rebecca Cady, RNC, BSN, JD
Bonnie Flood Chez, MSN, RNC
Wendy E. Colgan, RNC, BSN
Linda Goodwin, RNC, MEd
Wendy Heibel, RN, BSN
Washington C. Hill, MD, FACOG
John F. Huddleston, MD
Catherine H. Ivory, PhD, RNC-OB
Brian Jack, MD
Mona Brown Ketner, RN, MSN
Susan Griffiths Knowles, RNC, BSN, CCAP
Marilyn R. Lapidus, RNC, BSN, JD
Patricia McCartney, RNC, PHD, FAAN
Lisa A. Miller, CNM, JD
Lettie J. Primeaux, RNC, BSN
Kathleen Rice Simpson, RNC, PhD, FAAN
Jami Star, MD
Susan K. Weimer, RN
Linda Given Welch, CNM, MS
Chris Wood

Foreword

"Point-of-care" solutions represent our "new normal" with respect to both fetal heart rate monitoring (EFM) and sonography.

Advances in technology, enhanced portability, streamlined electronic documentation and order entry systems have made a significant difference in the ability of clinicians to provide care across all specialties and from diverse vantage points—particularly at the point of care. Author Thomas Friedman in his best-selling book, *The World Is Flat: A Brief History of the Twenty-First Century,* captures it well. The title is his metaphor for viewing the global world as a "level playing field" in terms of commerce, where all competitors have an equal opportunity to remain competitive in a global market in which historical and geographical divisions are becoming increasingly irrelevant. Similarly, our "commerce," as clinicians caring for women in obstetrics and gynecology, is the opportunity to level our playing field by offering open access to best practice resources available, to all specialties associated with our practice, irrespective of venue. Whether care takes place in the office, in the hospital, or in the field (trauma/transport), we now have the technical capability and communication tools to provide reasonably seamless care. Our technologies provide us with unlimited equal opportunity to improve patient care and safety via electronic fetal monitoring and ultrasonography.

Enter, *Point-of-Care Assessment in Pregnancy and Women's Health: Electronic Fetal Monitoring and Sonography,* as our most current resource available to perinatal clinicians to address the complementary relationship between these technologies and their optimal utilization in practice. This innovative text by Cydney Afriat Menihan and Ellen Kopel is divided into two sections for discussion: Electronic fetal heart rate monitoring (EFM) followed by sonography.

EFM for antepartum and intrapartum evaluation of fetal status has been preserved as an integral part of perinatal practice for the last 40 years. Since inception, however, it has been subjected to years of critical evaluation, which has included randomized clinical trials and a meta-analysis questioning the efficacy, specificity, and validity of the technique; development of nomenclature systems intended to improve upon clinical interpretation, communication, and documentation of EFM data; and, most recently, research related to management algorithms that have been proposed to further identify the fetus who has a greater likelihood for the development of significant acidemia.

Along the way, the concepts of standardization of information and consensus development became increasingly important targets for further study in an effort to enhance communication and collaboration among physicians, nurse–midwives, and nurses responsible for the interpretation of EFM data. In 2008, The Eunice Kennedy Shriver National Institute of Child Health and Human Development (NICHD) consensus panel proposed the universal adoption of a uniform system of terminology for classifying any FHR pattern as Category I, II, or III based on specific criteria. This three-tiered nomenclature system categorized tracings that range from "normal" (Category I), which is thought to rule out fetal metabolic acidemia; to the opposite end of the spectrum (Category III), with tracings considered to be "abnormal" and most consistently associated with fetal acidemia. Category II, the largest of the three categories, represents those patterns whose characteristics meet neither Category I nor Category III criteria. It is referred to as "indeterminate" because it is inconsistently associated with fetal acidemia. It also represents approximately >80% of the FHR patterns encountered in labor. As such, this category poses a significant challenge for clinicians because there has been no recommended, standardized national approach to management for this heterogeneous group. However, current research is underway with a proposed algorithm for management of these patterns as one evidenced-based approach for clinicians to consider (Clark et al. Intrapartum management of Category II FHR tracings: towards standardization of care. *Am J Obstet Gynecol*, 2013).

Yes, we began a 40-year journey with great expectations for this new technology. And yes, we probably have raised more questions about it than we have found answers. However, it is only through this path of scientific inquiry that we now have evolved EFM professional practice resources, educational programs, and competence validation tools.

This 40-year EFM journey witnessed a parallel evolution in ultrasound technology and its application in clinical practice. It represented a shift from the physician/sonographer's domain to the point-of-care nurse in triage, labor and delivery, and other important areas of women's health care. A first point of entry for sonographic assessment into the nursing main most likely was in association with the bio-ysical profile. While performing the NST, a logical ext step was to incorporate the assessment of amniotic fluid volume (modified BPP), and then to move forward to performing the complete biophysical profile (BPP). In practice, many nurses began to utilize sonography "ad hoc" to determine fetal presentation or confirm fetal cardiac activity (with or without formal training or certification to do so). This suggested the need to further evaluate overall the competencies necessary to provide point-of-care fetal assessment using two pieces of modern technology: EFM and ultrasound.

This new book, ***Point-of-Care Assessment in Pregnancy and Women's Health: Electronic Fetal Monitoring and Sonography,*** is the latest in the series of textbooks authored by Cydney Afriat Menihan and Ellen Kopel, who also authored the first two editions of *Electronic Fetal Monitoring: Concepts and Applications*. All three are excellent examples of valuable, comprehensive practice resources written by clinicians for clinicians. What makes this new text unique is that it highlights the clinical interdependence of complementary point-of-care technologies, EFM and sonography.

The first section, EFM, begins with basic information about the physiology of the fetal heart rate and fetal monitoring technology, and also addresses elements of informational technology. Chapters on fetal heart rate interpretation focus on current definitions and their application through extensive "practice exercises" related to application of NICHD nomenclature as well as principles of standardized interpretation. The chapter on competence validation speaks to the numerous tools available, such as checklists, audits, tracing reviews, case studies, simulation, credentialing/certification, and unit-specific safety initiatives that can be standardized and cross all disciplines.

The second section, sonography, highlights the clinical interdependence of point-of-care sonography as a complementary technology in conjunction with EFM. For instance, if a Category II tracing is evident during labor, a biophysical profile (BPP) may be performed to provide further information concerning fetal metabolic status. Similarly, with a Category II tracing, fetal sonographic imaging targeting fetal growth may suggest intrauterine growth restriction and potential placental compromise, which could generate greater concern about fetal oxygenation than a Category II tracing in a normally growing fetus.

Overall, the best discussion of point-of-care sonography should answer the questions of who, what, when, and why: Who should or can be incorporating sonography into clinical practice, what type of imaging is indicated, when is the appropriate timing for evaluation, and why is the plan of care indicated?

This innovative resource provides comprehensive answers to these queries with an overview of the requisite principles that should be in place prior to incorporating point-of-care sonography into clinical practice. The chapter on maternal and fetal assessment includes professional organization guidelines, indications for diagnostic ultrasound, and recommendations for clinical competence development and assessment. This section of the book also includes an in-depth explanation as to how the ultrasound equipment functions, with particular emphasis on the knowledge necessary to obtain the best images. Subsequent chapters focus on point-of-care sonographic assessment divided into first-, second-, and third-trimester evaluations. A final chapter is devoted specifically to point-of-care evaluation of fetal well-being, including a comprehensive discussion of biophysical profile parameters. Also, as increasing numbers of nurses, midwives, and nurse practitioners provide women's health care, attention is also directed to practice-specific sonography, such as gynecologic and reproductive medicine imaging.

Guidelines for appropriate integration of these skills into clinical practice is supported by AWHONN (2010) and ACNM (2012), as both professional organizations appreciate that didactic and clinical education are essential and that point-of-care ultrasound imaging should only be performed by individuals who have acquired the necessary knowledge, skill, and training.

This new textbook stands out from any others currently available in the marketplace. It provides precisely what our professional organizations recommend as well as what is clinically essential to provide safe and effective point-of-care assessment to fetuses and women: a solid didactic base of knowledge in both electronic fetal monitoring and sonography.

Bonnie Flood Chez, MSN, RNC
President
Nursing Education Resources
Tampa, Florida

Preface

Although it is used as a matter of course today, quite a bit of history surrounds the evolution of electronic fetal monitoring (EFM) and its integration into routine clinical practice. As the authors have great respect for and affinity toward historical context, the reader will note that a number of references throughout this book predate those ordinarily cited in scholarly work. This is not an oversight; rather, it is a nod to some of the landmark findings, original source material, and "gold standard" publications on both EFM and sonography. To lend some perspective to a younger generation of clinicians, the electronic fetal monitor predated the integration of the personal computer into popular use by a quarter of a century and preceded advances such as laptops, mobile phones, and tablets by even longer; yet, EFM technology has not undergone many substantial changes (with the exception of what can be considered "bells and whistles") since it was introduced into the marketplace in the late 1960s.

After more than 40 years in the clinical setting and utilization in the vast majority of births in the United States, EFM's benefits to perinatal outcome are still debated. Nonetheless, electronic fetal monitors have become a fixture in the majority of delivery rooms in the United States, and this screening technique has become firmly ensconced in obstetric practice as a first-line method of fetal assessment. It is important to remember that the intent in developing an electronic means of evaluating fetal well-being was to prevent intrapartum asphyxia; the incidence of intrapartum death and neurologic injury were specifically targeted. Although evidence-based practice has become fundamental in contemporary health care delivery, neither the public nor the clinical community in the 1960s and 1970s was as cognizant of prospective, randomized, controlled trials. EFM became commercially available before sufficient testing defined its capabilities (as did other medical devices, pharmaceuticals, and practices).

Critics maintain that there has been no significant change in neonatal morbidity since the introduction of EFM. With regard to the rate of neurologic injury, however, we now understand that other causes of cerebral palsy exist and that <10% of cases are attributable to intrapartum events.[1-3] It has been suggested that perhaps the wrong end point was chosen for determining the value of EFM.[4,5] If the majority of cerebral palsy cases are attributable to

causes other than fetal hypoxia, how can EFM be measured for success against its incidence?

Factors that contributed to fetal and neonatal mortality and morbidity in the late 1960s and early 1970s were different than the challenges faced today. Neonatology was just emerging as a subspecialty, and neonatal intensive care units were a rarity. In most cases, little or no attempt was made at saving the extremely premature fetus or neonate, as there was little means of support available postnatally. It wasn't until progress in mechanical ventilation of the neonate in the 1970s and the advent of surfactant in the 1980s that great advances in neonatal outcomes began to occur. Neonatal care has steadily improved and continues to do so, and premature infants who didn't survive 30 years ago now do. Unfortunately, a certain percent do sustain permanent damage. These factors set the scenario for the current manifestation of neonatal morbidity and mortality.

Cesarean birth rates are another issue when evaluating the impact of EFM. In 1970, cesarean birth rates were 5.5%.[6] By 1988, 20 years after the introduction of EFM, cesarean birth rates escalated to a previously unprecedented 24.7%.[7] At the time, many opponents of EFM attributed the sharp rise in cesarean birth rate to increased use of this technology. In evaluating cesarean birth rates, it is necessary to understand that it wasn't until the late 1980s that a movement toward attempting vaginal birth after cesarean (VBAC) arose. Prior to that time, nearly all women who had cesarean births were relegated to repeat cesarean delivery. The trend toward VBAC was driven by multiple sources—many women wanted the opportunity to deliver vaginally, an alternative that was believed by many care providers to be safer and preferable to cesarean birth. Also, the reduced cost of a vaginal delivery versus a cesarean birth was appealing to insurance providers. The change in obstetric practice to promoting VBAC led to a steady decline in repeat cesarean birth rates from 1989 to 1996. By 1996, cesarean rates had declined to what is now known as a historic low of 20.7%, as the VBAC rate increased by 50%.[8] Concern over the rate of uterine rupture and corresponding rise in poor neonatal outcome,[9,10] however, mandated greater attentiveness from providers[11,12] and led to a sharp decline in the rate of VBAC.

According to the latest available data, the cesarean birth rate rose nearly 60% from 1996 to 2009,[13] l then stabilized between 2009 and 2012.[14] The use of this dramatic increase is multifactorial and o longer attributed to the use of EFM but, rather, to other obstetric trends, such as the popularity of labor induction, the advent of cesarean delivery on maternal request, decline in the use of forceps and vacuum extraction to 3.50% of births,[13] cessation of vaginal breech delivery,[15,16] and increased numbers of multiple and preterm births. Today, rather than focusing on EFM as the primary cause of increased cesarean birth rates, it is more reasonable to recognize the multifactorial composition of this problem. Many more pregnancies that once would have been considered ill advised due to their high-risk nature are now attempted and even encouraged by other medical specialties, including assisted reproductive specialists. Advances in general medicine and the subspecialty of perinatology have furthered care of patients with diabetes, hypertension, cardiac defects and insufficiencies, HIV/AIDS, and autoimmune diseases. Societal changes have also affected the patient population in obstetrics. More women of a later maternal age are having children. The popularity of various ever-changing recreational drugs affects fetuses in ways we recognize and in those we likely will not fully understand for years to come. Alcohol and tobacco also continue to challenge perinatal health. While progress has been made in providing access to perinatal care, there are still financial and cultural barriers to overcome.

Clearly, the most positive effect of EFM acknowledged since the 1990s is that the fetus is accepted as a patient "to whom the perinatal team has a definitive duty."[4] The most significant and direct contribution of EFM is the reduction in the rate of intrapartum stillbirth.[17] Rarely does a fetus die unexpectedly during the labor process, as occurred in decades past. Unfortunately, it is true that some practitioners rush to verdict at the first hint of fetal compromise, performing assisted or operative delivery before exhausting all means of assessing fetal well-being. However, adjunct methods of assessment, such as sonography, are increasingly available to be utilized to more accurately diagnose fetal compromise and guide intervention. Used appropriately, EFM is a very effective screening tool.

The greatest misconception about EFM is the belief that it is a diagnostic tool. EFM is useful only as a screening tool, comparable in utility to a sphygmomanometer. If a patient's blood pressure were to exceed normal limits, we would never presume to know, based solely on that reading, whether she has hypertensive disease or is just having a stressful day. As with all good screening tests, the fetal monitor is highly predictive of negative results (~98%). What the fetal monitor does not do well is predict fetal distress. When the FHR pattern is suggestive of hypoxia, it is falsely positive nearly 90% of the time.[18] Even with its imperfections, in all of the years since the development of EFM, it has yet to be replaced with another methodology.

The 21st century very quietly added a new symbiotic relationship to health care: point-of-care sonography and EFM. It would be difficult to find a labor and delivery unit or obstetric triage unit without both fetal monitors and at least one ultrasound machine that can be quickly accessed to image, for example, the fetal presenting part, measure amniotic fluid, or visualize fetal cardiac activity. The biophysical profile is a perfect example of this symbiotic relationship: It cannot be performed without both pieces of electronics. Additionally, a biophysical profile may be used during labor to gather more data pertaining to fetal status in light of a Category II tracing.

With this increased complementary use of sonography in both fetal assessment and women's health care, increasing numbers of nurses, advanced nurse practitioners, and midwives trained for such are performing point-of-care obstetric and/or gynecologic ultrasound examinations. This added skill is supported by the Association of Women's Health, Obstetric and Neonatal Nurses[19] and the American College of Nurse Midwives.[20] As it is now essential for all members of the health care team to have comprehensive knowledge of this technology, we determined that this book would be incomplete without providing the basics of point-of-care sonography along with EFM. Our aim is to educate clinicians who use EFM or sonography to any degree in their practice to acquire and employ data appropriately and effectively.

Cydney Afriat Menihan
Ellen Kopel

REFERENCES TO FOREWORD

1. Macones G, Hankin G, Spong CY, et al. The 2008 National Institute of Child Health and Human Development Workshop Report on Electronic Fetal Monitoring Update on Definitions, Interpretation, and Research Guidelines. *Obstet Gynecol.* 2008;112(3).
2. Clark SL1, Nageotte MP, Garite TJ, Freeman RK, Miller DA, Simpson KR, Belfort MA, Dildy GA, Parer JT, Berkowitz RL, D'Alton M, Rouse DJ, Gilstrap LC, Vintzileos AM, van Dorsten JP, Boehm FH, Miller LA, Hankins GD. Intrapartum management of category fetal heart rate tracings: towards standardization care. *Am J Obstet Gynecol.* 2013 Aug;209(2):89–97.
3. Association of Women's Health, Obstetric, and Neonatal Nurses (AWHONN). *Ultrasound examinations performed by nurses in obstetric, gynecologic, and reproductive medicine settings: clinical competencies and education guide,* 3rd ed. Washington, DC: AWHONN; 2010.
4. American College of Nurse Midwives (ACNM). *Position statement: midwives' performance of ultrasound in clinical practice.* Silver Spring, MD: Author; 2012.

REFERENCES TO PREFACE

1. Nelson KB, Ellenberg JH. Antecedents of cerebral palsy: multivariate analysis of risk. *N Engl J Med.* 1986;315:81–86.
2. Blair E, Stanley FJ. Intrapartum asphyxia: a rare cause of cerebral palsy. *J Pediatrics.* 1988;12(4):515–519.
3. American College of Obstetricians and Gynecologists (ACOG), American Academy of Pediatrics (AAP). *Neonatal encephalopathy and cerebral palsy: Defining the pathogenesis and pathophysiology.* Washington, DC: ACOG; 2003.
4. Paul R. Electronic fetal monitoring and later outcome: a thirty-year overview. *J Perinatol.* 1994;14(5): 393–395.
5. Parer J, King T. Fetal heart rate monitoring: is it salvageable? *Am J Obstet Gynecol.* 2000;182:282–287.
6. Placek PJ, Taffel SM. Trends in cesarean section rates for the United States, 1970–78. *Public Health Rep.* 1980;95(6):540–548.
7. U.S. Department of Health and Human Services. (2000). Healthy People 2010, Priority Area 14. Available from http://www.cdc.gov/nchs/data/hp2000/childhlt/14cpt.pdf. Accessed February 10, 2014.
8. Menacker F, Curtin SC. Trends in cesarean birth and vaginal birth after previous cesarean, 1991–99. *Natl Vital Stat Rep.* 2001;49(13):1–16.
9. McMahon MJ, Luther ER, Bowes WA, et al. Comparison of a trial of labor with an elective second cesarean section. *N Engl J Med.* 1996;335:689–695.
10. Sachs,BP, Kobelin C, Castro MA, et al. Risks of lowering cesarean-delivery rate. *N Engl J Med.* 1999; 340(1):54–57.
11. American College of Obstetricians and Gynecologists (ACOG). *Vaginal birth after previous cesarean delivery.* ACOG Practice Bulletin, 54. Washington, DC: Author; 1999.
12. American College of Obstetricians and Gynecologists (ACOG). *Vaginal birth after previous cesarean delivery.* ACOG Practice Bulletin, 54. Washington, DC: Author; 2004.
13. Martin JA, Hamilton BE, Ventura SJ, et al. Births: Final data for 2011. *National vital statistics reports, (62)1.* Hyattsville, MD: National Center for Health Statistics; 2013.
14. Hamilton BE, Martin JA, Ventura SJ, Division of Vital Statistics. Births: Preliminary data for 2012. *Natl Vital Stat Rep.* 2013;62(3):1–20.
15. Hannah ME, Hannah WJ, Hewson SA, et al. (2000). Planned caesarean section versus planned vaginal birth for breech presentation at term: a randomised multicentre trial. Term Breech Trial Collaborative Group. *Lancet.* 2000;356(9239):1375–1383.
16. Martin JA, Hamilton BE, Sutton PD. Births: final data for 2004. *National vital statistics reports, (55)1.* Hyattsville, MD: National Center for Health Statistics; 2006.
17. Vintzileos AM, Nochimson DJ, Guzman ER, et al. Intrapartum electronic fetal monitoring versus intermittent auscultation: a meta-analysis. *Obstet Gynecol* 1995;85(1):149–155.
18. Low JA, Victory R, Derrick EJ. Predictive value of electronic fetal monitoring for intrapartum fetal asphyxia with metabolic acidosis. *Obstet Gynecol.* 1999;93: 285–291.
19. Association of Women's Health, Obstetric, and Neonatal Nurses (AWHONN). *Ultrasound examinations performed by nurses in obstetric, gynecologic, and reproductive medicine settings: clinical competencies and education guide,* 3rd ed. Washington, DC: AWHONN; 2010.
20. American College of Nurse Midwives (ACNM). *Position statement: midwives' performance of ultrasound in clinical practice.* Silver Spring, MD: Author; 2012.

Acknowledgments

The authors wish to extend heartfelt appreciation for the time and expertise generously offered by the contributors and reviewers. One set of eyes is never sufficient to ensure thorough coverage of the material and accuracy in its presentation. Special thanks are extended to Kathleen Rice Simpson, RNC, PhD, FAAN, whose work on Electronic Fetal Monitoring Competence Validation in our previous text, *Electronic Fetal Monitoring: Concepts and Applications*, provided a strong basis for Chapter 7 in this work.

CAM
EK

Also, a retroactive thank you to prior contributors to other works in sonography that I edited: Judith Adams, RN, DN, DMU; Paula Cardillo, MS, RVT, RDMS; Sylvia Closson Ross, PhD, CNM; Marty Deviney, RT, RDMS; Diane Hodgman, CNM, MSN; Ann Hodredge, FNP, CNM, MSN; Carolyn Hopkins, BS, RNP, RDMS; Gale M. Kennedy, BS, RDMS, RT; Catharine M. Treanor, MS, RNC; and Wayne Persutte, BS, RDMS.

CAM

Contents

SECTION 2
Ultrasound in Women's Health Care and Pregnancy   215
Introduction to Section 2   216

APPENDICES

Electronic Fetal Monitoring

CHAPTER 1

Maternal–Fetal Physiology of Fetal Heart Rate Patterns

The rationale for electronic fetal monitoring (EFM) is based on the knowledge that when normal metabolic processes are interrupted, either by a lack of oxygen (O_2) or an inability to expel end-products, the subsequent accumulation of acids may damage all or part of the living system.

Fetal well-being depends on adequate functioning of sources and suppliers of oxygen and waste removal mechanisms. These include the maternal system, the placenta, the uterus, and the umbilical cord. At this time, the relationship between specific fetal heart rate (FHR) patterns and fetal acidemia is supported by observational studies only. However, the relationship appears to be strong.[1] It has been well established that a reassuring fetal heart rate tracing is an excellent predictor of the absence of fetal metabolic acidemia.[2] A functional understanding of FHR pattern interpretation inherently and necessarily requires a clear understanding of the relationship between the maternal and fetal chemical and neurologic interactions and exchanges. This chapter explains the physiology of the maternal–fetal unit and relates its functioning to FHR patterns. The specific FHR patterns are discussed in detail in Chapter 3.

MATERNAL OXYGENATION

The maternal respiratory system is the only source of oxygen for the fetus. The fetus cannot survive without it (Figure 1–1). If the maternal oxygen supply or oxygen-carrying capacity is diminished at any level of the process, fetal oxygenation is certain to decrease at some point. This can occur in conjunction with any maternal respiratory, circulatory, hemolytic, or cardiac condition that affects maternal oxygenation. Examples of these include, but are certainly not limited to, asthma, pulmonary embolus, pulmonary edema, pneumonia, hypertension, hypotension, anemia, sickle cell disease, and various forms of cardiac decompensation or insufficiency. To maintain optimal or even sufficient fetal oxygenation, maternal oxygenation must be adequately maintained and supported.

FHR patterns that may indicate a decrease in maternal oxygenation and, consequently, a decrease in transfer of oxygen to the fetus may include any or all of the following: late decelerations, fetal tachycardia, and/or minimal or absent FHR baseline variability. Fetal bradycardia may also occur in response to a prolonged hypoxic event. The physiologic basis of the late deceleration pattern is believed to originate with a decrease in oxygen available to the fetus, most commonly due to a decrease in the amount of oxygen perfused to the fetus through the placenta. The hypoxic fetus may respond to the decrease in oxygen transfer across the placenta that normally occurs during uterine contractions by slowing its heart rate. The FHR then continues at a decreased pace until after the contraction has ended and uterine perfusion returns, re-oxygenating the fetal–placental unit. It is only after blood flow to the fetus has fully resumed (when the uterus has relaxed) that the FHR returns to its baseline rate. The occurrence of this process is demonstrated by the presence of late decelerations in the FHR tracing.

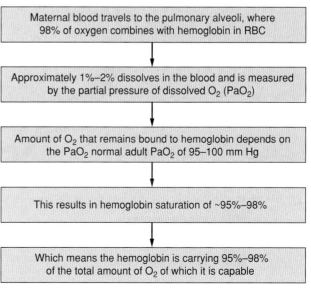

Maternal blood travels to the pulmonary alveoli, where 98% of oxygen combines with hemoglobin in RBC

↓

Approximately 1%–2% dissolves in the blood and is measured by the partial pressure of dissolved O_2 (PaO_2)

↓

Amount of O_2 that remains bound to hemoglobin depends on the PaO_2 normal adult PaO_2 of 95–100 mm Hg

↓

This results in hemoglobin saturation of ~95%–98%

↓

Which means the hemoglobin is carrying 95%–98% of the total amount of O_2 of which it is capable

FIGURE 1–1. Maternal blood flow.

If the fetus becomes hypoxic, rising levels of carbon dioxide (CO_2) stimulate the chemoreceptors and increase sympathetic activity, causing the FHR baseline to rise. Due to the effects of these same compensatory mechanisms, loss of variability in the FHR baseline usually accompanies fetal tachycardia.

Stork Byte

I feel blue without you, O_2 . . .
If my oxygen content is already low, any extra stress (like contractions) may cause me to deoxygenate.

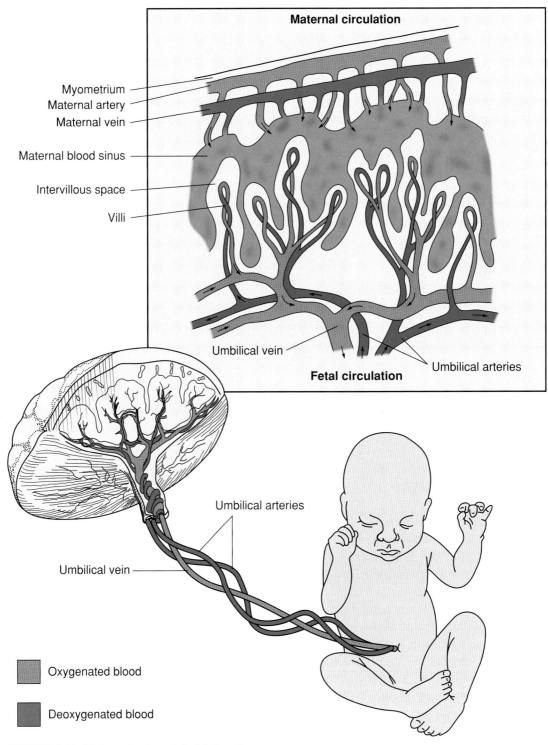

FIGURE 1–2. Maternal–placental–fetal exchange.

PLACENTAL CIRCULATION

The placenta is the organ that connects the maternal and fetal systems and performs many of the same functions for the fetus that its lungs assume in extrauterine life. The fetus relies on the placenta for transfer of oxygen and nutrients and removal of waste products. The placenta accomplishes this through the villi, which are fetal tissue that project into the maternal blood that is circulating in the intervillous space. It is through these projections that transfer of oxygen, carbon dioxide, and nutrients occurs. Oxygenated blood from the mother is carried to the placenta by the uterine arteries. Blood enters the intervillous space under positive arterial pressure, bathes the fetal villi, and then drains back to the maternal veins (Figure 1–2).

A microscopic layer of fetal trophoblasts in the placenta serves as a filter, permitting the exchange of nutrients and waste products between the maternal and fetal systems without fetal and maternal blood cells coming into contact with one another. The passage of nutrients and waste products across this membrane occurs due to six mechanisms: facilitated diffusion, passive diffusion, active transport, bulk flow, pinocytosis, and breaks in the system (Table 1–1). Deoxygenated blood is carried from the fetus to the placenta through the two umbilical arteries. These umbilical arteries split off into smaller capillaries that traverse the fetal villi. The villi project into the intervillous space, where maternal and fetal blood supplies exchange necessary gases (e.g., oxygen and carbon dioxide) and nutrients. Following this transaction, oxygenated blood is carried back into fetal circulation by way of a single umbilical vein.

Stork Byte

Thanks to my placental trophoblasts, my blood stays separate from Mom's blood…unless there's a break-in!

As the maternal hemoglobin travels to the fetus, there are factors that cause oxygen to be released from the hemoglobin, so that the fetal hemoglobin cells can pick up the oxygen. Some of the factors that cause this release and transfer are:

1. Increased fetal need for oxygen
2. Anaerobic glycolysis
3. Production of hydrogen ions (decreased pH)
4. Heat
5. Decreased oxygen transfer from environment to fetus
6. Severe fetal anemia
7. Hemoglobinopathies

Due to vasoconstriction, blood flow across the intervillous space is diminished during uterine contractions. This temporary reduction in perfusion forces the fetus to rely on any oxygen that might be available in its system until the contraction ends and normal blood flow resumes. It is similar to the

TABLE 1–1 MECHANISMS OF TRANSPORT

Mechanism	Description	Substances Exchanged
Passive diffusion	No energy required; substances pass from one area to another; transport based on concentration gradient from areas of high to low concentration	Oxygen, carbon dioxide, sodium, chloride, lipids, fat-soluble vitamins, some medications
Facilitated diffusion	Energy may be required; transport is faster than that based on concentration gradient; "pump"	Glucose, other carbohydrates
Active transport	Energy required; transport occurs against the concentration gradient; carrier molecules involved	Amino acids, water-soluble vitamins, large ions (calcium, iron)
Bulk flow	Transport based on hydrostatic or osmotic gradient	Water, dissolved electrolytes
Pinocytosis	Molecules are enclosed in small vesicles that are pinched off on one side of the placenta and traverse to the other side; contents are then released	Immunoglobulins, serum proteins
Breaks	Villi may break off within intervillous space, and contents may be extruded into maternal circulation; maternal intravascular contents may be taken up by fetal circulation	Fetal Rh-positive cells

Adapted from Afriat CI. *Electronic Fetal Monitoring.* Rockland, MD: Aspen; 1989, and Chaffee E, Greisheimer E. *Basic Physiology and Anatomy.* Philadelphia, PA: Lippincott; 1969.

mechanisms engaged when holding one's breath to go under water. The vast majority of fetuses show no change in their heart rate or acid–base status during contractions. When placental vasculature and circulation are compromised, however, the fetus is likely to be affected by these episodes of diminished placental blood flow. Examples of maternal health factors that contribute to diminished placental function include, but are not limited to type 1 diabetes, hypertension, and smoking. Other conditions that may compromise the oxygen–carbon dioxide transfer through the placenta include placental dysfunctions, such as those that occur with placenta previa, abruptio placentae, chorioamnionitis, postterm gestation, and intrauterine growth restriction.

Events that may occur transiently, such as uterine tachysystole (six or more contractions in 10 minutes, averaged over a 30-minute window[2,3]) or maternal hypotension, may diminish placental blood flow and lead to the occurrence of late decelerations. Tachysystole has been associated with significant oxygen desaturation.[4] Alleviating transitory causes of uteroplacental insufficiency usually allows the fetus to recover and subsequently remediates the FHR pattern. If the events that are initiating the late deceleration pattern occur repetitively or over a prolonged period of time, oxygen is quickly depleted and the late decelerations become accompanied by other nonreassuring signs, such as tachycardia, decreased variability, bradycardia, and loss of accelerations.

Stork Byte

Hey, it's getting a little cramped in here! Six or more contractions in 10 minutes, averaged over a 30-minute window, may be too much for me to handle! Please, let me come up for air!

Since maternal and fetal blood supplies are maintained independently, it may be consequential when fetal cells enter the maternal system. A break in the system, such as that which occurs during abruptio placentae, is a common means by which fetal and maternal blood mix. If blood incompatibilities such as Rh, ABO, or other antigen factors are present, isoimmunization can result, and the resulting hemolytic effects on the fetus can be devastating. Since 1976, it has been known that sinusoidal FHR patterns (explained in Chapter 3) are most often attributable to Rh sensitization or other forms of fetal anemia.[5]

UTERINE BLOOD FLOW

The blood flow to and through the uterus is a key determinant in placental function. Approximately 10–15% of maternal cardiac output (~500–750 mL/min) flows through the uterus of the term gestation. Unlike the rest of the human vascular system, which can constrict and dilate under central nervous system (CNS) control, the uterine vascular bed is believed to constantly maintain maximum dilation. Only an increase in maternal cardiac output can improve uterine blood flow.

Because uterine blood flow is known to decrease during contractions, a diminished amount of oxygen, carbon dioxide, and nutrients is exchanged between fetal and maternal blood during this time. This causes a loss of oxygen to the fetus and a buildup of carbon dioxide within the fetal circulation. Although a healthy, well-oxygenated fetus will have a small reserve of oxygen from which to draw, this will be depleted quickly with repeated episodes of hypoxia. With each uterine contraction and subsequent decrease in perfusion, the fetus without reserve is placed in life-threatening circumstances.

Factors that contribute to decreased uterine blood flow are both iatrogenic and noniatrogenic (Table 1–2). The noniatrogenic causes include fetal hemorrhage secondary to abruptio placentae, placental deterioration, hypertension, hypotension, autoimmune disease, smoking, tachysystole, and uterine tachysystole. Those that are of iatrogenic etiology commonly occur secondary to treatments and interventions by the perinatal team. For example, administration of oxytocin and other uterotonic agents can lead to excessively long and/or too frequent contractions. Uterine tachysystole may cause late or prolonged decelerations even in the well-oxygenated fetus as a result of the extended period during which uteroplacental blood flow is diminished. In most of these situations, the fetus will have enough oxygen in reserve to recover from the loss of blood flow. A fetus with chronic placental deterioration, however, may not have the ability to recover from an iatrogenic insult such as tachysystole. Tocolytic agents, such as terbutaline, may be used to treat FHR decelerations in the presence of uterine hypertonus or tachysystole. They may also be used in the absence of uterine tachysystole when an abnormal FHR pattern occurs in response to uterine activity. The neonate's condition may benefit from the improvement in uterine blood flow.[6]

TABLE 1-2   POSSIBLE ETIOLOGIES OF DECREASED UTERINE BLOOD FLOW

Etiology	Physiologic Effect
Iatrogenic	
Maternal supine position	Inferior vena cava compression, possible aortic compression, decreased venous return; decreased uteroplacental blood flow
Tachysystole (induced)	Decreased uteroplacental blood flow
Regional anesthesia	Maternal hypotension and decreased uteroplacental blood flow
Valsalva maneuver (closed-glottis "pushing")	Decreased fetal oxygenation[8]
Noniatrogenic	
Placental abruption Pregnancy-induced hypertension Chronic hypertension Tachysystole (spontaneous) Smoking Substance abuse Malnutrition	Alteration of placental vasculature, chronic placental change, decreased uteroplacental blood flow
Pregnancy-induced hypertension Chronic hypertension Smoking Substance abuse Collagen-vascular disease	Maternal vasoconstriction, decreased uteroplacental blood flow
Placental abruption Type 1 diabetes Postdate pregnancy Smoking	Decreased functional placenta surface area due to calcifications, infarctions

The administration and management of regional anesthesia can contribute to diminished uteroplacental blood flow. It is of fundamental importance to support maternal circulation and prevent hypotension before, during, and after the administration of medications. Maternal hypotension can cause late decelerations due to the resulting decrease in blood flow to the uterus. The reduction in uterine blood flow potentiates a decrease in blood flow through the uterine arteries, subsequently decreasing blood flow across the placenta. Positioning the patient in the maternal supine position is a common yet avoidable cause of hypotension. The Valsalva maneuver (i.e., maternal breath holding with expulsive efforts during second-stage labor) is another practice to be considered. Various studies have indicated that the resulting maternal hemodynamic effects from breath holding may decrease fetal oxygenation.[7,8]

THE UMBILICAL CORD

Oxygen-rich blood is carried to the fetus from the placenta through the umbilical vein. Deoxygenated blood is carried away from the fetus by two umbilical arteries. Changes in the blood flow through the umbilical cord can impact FHR. Pressure exerted on the umbilical cord can compress the umbilical vein and the umbilical arteries.[9]

If the umbilical cord is only partially compressed, as occasionally happens during uterine contractions, it is possible for the umbilical vein to be occluded while the arteries remain patent because the walls of the umbilical vein are thinner and more easily compressed than the walls of the arteries. When the umbilical vein is occluded, the flow of oxygen-rich blood to the fetus is diminished. This results in a sympathetic response in the fetus because the change in oxygenation stimulates the chemoreceptors to effect a transient increase in the FHR. It also causes the fetus to become hypotensive, secondary to hypovolemia, which also stimulates the fetal baroreceptors to trigger an increase in the FHR.

If the umbilical cord becomes further compressed, the umbilical arteries may also become occluded. At this time, as the fetal heart is attempting to pump against a blockade, the FHR slows in order to pump more forcibly. This causes an increase in the fetal blood pressure, and that increased pressure stimulates the fetal baroreceptors. Stimulation of the baroreceptors causes a parasympathetic response; the FHR drops abruptly, resulting in a variable deceleration of the FHR (explained further in Chapter 3).

As the contraction wanes, cord compression may be progressively alleviated, first relieving pressure on the arteries and leaving only the umbilical vein occluded. The fetal chemoreceptors and baroreceptors again produce a sympathetic response to that change in compression and may transiently accelerate the FHR. These brief accelerations, which can precede, follow, or occur on both sides of a variable deceleration, are an inherent part of the variable deceleration pattern and are referred to as *shoulders*. This is a benign finding usually associated with moderate FHR baseline variability.

If the fetus is already experiencing compromise, the response to cord compression may be quite different. There may be no acceleration present as the cord is compressed, only the occurrence of a variable deceleration. The variable deceleration is likely to fall far below the FHR baseline in this instance. Additionally, the FHR baseline will likely be tachycardic and have little variability. In an attempt to recover from the variable deceleration to its baseline rate, the compromised fetus first raises its heart rate above the baseline and then effects a very gradual return to baseline rate. These particular types of increases in the FHR that occur as part of the variable deceleration pattern are referred to as *overshoots*. When overshoots are present, there is usually minimal or absent FHR baseline variability. Overshoots are considered to be a nonreassuring sign in the term fetus because this pattern is associated with autonomic nervous system (ANS) impairment.[10]

CHEMORECEPTORS AND BARORECEPTORS

Chemoreceptors and baroreceptors factor significantly in CNS control over the autonomic activities of heart rate and respiratory effort.[11] Stimulation of either type of receptor can effect a change in the FHR in response to gas or pressure changes in the fetal circulation.

Chemoreceptors

Chemoreceptors are nerve receptors found in both peripheral and CNS blood vessels that sense the chemical makeup of the surrounding environment. A change in the pH of the blood causes the chemoreceptors to initiate afferent nerve impulses to either speed up or slow down respiratory activity or heart rate. Stimulation of the carotid body chemoreceptors may cause a tachycardia with increased blood pressure or an occasional bradycardia with hypotension. Stimulation of the peripheral aortic chemoreceptors may result in parasympathetic stimulation and bradycardia. However, it is the central chemoreceptors that are located in the medulla oblongata that respond to changes in oxygen and carbon dioxide tension in the blood and spinal fluid. Acid–base balance is further explained later in this chapter.

Stork Byte

My heart is beating faster—either something really exciting is happening in here, or my chemoreceptors just kicked in!

Baroreceptors

Baroreceptors are sensors that are highly sensitive to changes in the pressure of the blood against vessel walls. Arterial baroreceptors are located in the walls of the aortic arch and the carotid bodies. If the arterial pressure rises above normal levels, the baroreceptors signal the cardiac system to slow the FHR. Stimulation of the baroreceptors causes vasodilation and a lowering of the arterial blood pressure. If the arterial pressure begins to fall below normal levels, the baroreceptors receive less stimulation and a reflex increase in the FHR results. At the same time, a vasoconstriction in the peripheral blood vessels occurs, causing arterial blood pressure to rise.

The venous system also has baroreceptors. These are located in the walls of the terminal portions of the venae cavae and the right atrium, with afferent fibers traveling to the vagus nerve. When baroreceptors located in the veins are activated by high venous blood pressure, an increase in the FHR results.

Stork Byte

I can't take all this pressure!
When arterial pressure increases, the baroreceptors slow my heart rate and cause vasodilation in order to decrease arterial pressure.

CENTRAL NERVOUS SYSTEM

The anatomic portion of the CNS includes the brain and the spinal cord. The physiologic part includes the somatic (voluntary) nervous system and the autonomic (involuntary) nervous system. The somatic nervous system consists of nerve fibers that connect the CNS with structures of the body wall, such as the skin and skeletal muscles. The ANS consists of fibers that connect the CNS with smooth muscle, cardiac muscle, and the glands. It is the ANS that is directly responsible for changes in the FHR (Figure 1–3).[11]

The Autonomic Nervous System

Both structurally and functionally, the ANS may be divided into two parts: the sympathetic and parasympathetic nervous systems. The word *sympathetic* indicates a relationship between two parts whereby a change in one part affects the other. The parasympathetic nervous system functions to inhibit or oppose the effects of the sympathetic nervous system on specific organs (Figure 1–4).

Parasympathetic Nervous System

The primary function of the parasympathetic nervous system is to coordinate activities related to the restoration and conservation of body energy and the elimination of bodily waste. Its major component, the vagus nerve, networks the brain and the heart (Figure 1–3). When the parasympathetic nervous system is activated, the vagus nerve carries the message from the cardioinhibitory center of the brain to the sinoatrial and atrioventricular nodes of the heart, telling them to decrease the rate of firing and transmission, thereby slowing the FHR. This communication commonly occurs, for example, when the fetal head is compressed—the resulting increase in intracranial pressure causes a decrease in cerebral blood flow, stimulating the parasympathetic nervous system to activate the vagus nerve and subsequently decrease the FHR. Potential initiators of this chain of events in which the fetal head is compressed include (1) cephalopelvic disproportion (pressure of

the fetal head against the maternal bony pelvis), (2) fetal descent (fetal head compression by the vaginal musculature), (3) cervical examination (direct pressure of the clinician's fingers), (4) forceps or vacuum application directly to the head, and/or (5) the fetal head being pressed against the cervix during contractions.

When the parasympathetic nervous system is stimulated in the adult, several responses occur. Motor responses include stimulation of the sphincter muscle of the iris, causing the pupils to contract; constriction of the bronchioles, causing difficulty with breathing; and stimulation of the intestines, stomach, and urinary bladder. Inhibitory responses also occur due to smooth muscle relaxation. This results in the dilation of the blood vessels of the salivary glands and external genitalia. The parasympathetic nervous system also controls secretory function by causing the stomach and pancreas to increase secretory activity and generate thin, watery saliva.

In short, stimulation of the parasympathetic nervous system in the adult causes the pupils to constrict (protecting the eyes from excessive light), gastrointestinal function to be promoted (so food energy can be taken into the body and stored for future use), heart rate to be slowed (so cardiac muscle has the opportunity to rest), and bladder and bowel function to be regulated (so waste products are properly removed from the body). Similarly in the fetus, stimulation of the parasympathetic nervous system will cause a decrease in the FHR and may trigger release of meconium. Release of meconium can be a normal physiologic response and does not necessarily indicate fetal compromise.

Stork Byte

Easy on my cranium, please!
Pressure on my head makes the parasympathetic nervous system lower my heart rate.

A comparison of maternal and fetal heart rate changes is particularly interesting during labor. As discussed earlier, it is not uncommon for the fetal heart rate to slow during contractions as a result of fetal head compression and stimulation of the vagus. However, when maternal heart rate (MHR) is recorded during labor, decelerations of MHR do not occur. Generally, what will be seen will be increases or accelerations of the MHR during contractions.[12]

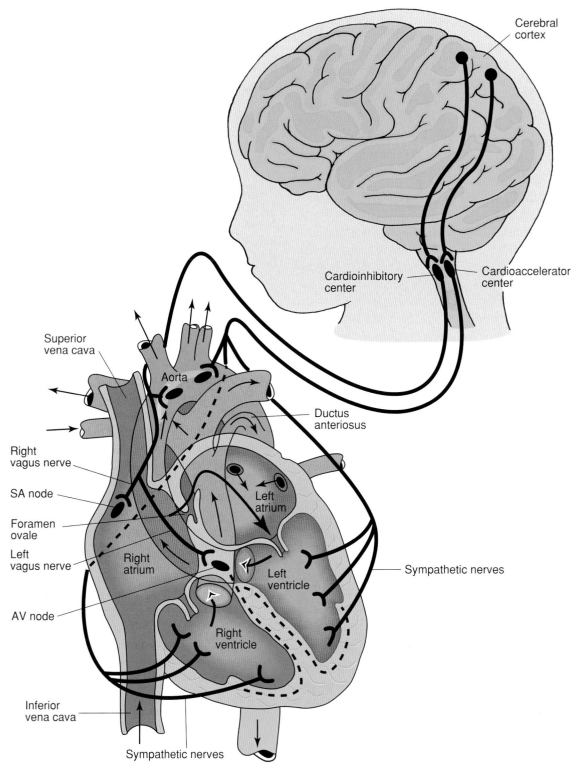

FIGURE 1–3. Central nervous system's control over heart rate. Note the baroreceptors, chemoreceptors, and pacemaker sites of the heart. Abbreviations: AV, atrioventricular; SA, sinoatrial.

Sympathetic Nervous System

Changes in the external environment are responsible for stimulation of the sympathetic nervous system. The most commonly known effect that external factors have on the body is the sympathetic nervous system's "fight or flight" response to any situation perceived as an emergency. The sympathetic nervous system prepares the body for the intense muscular activity that may be involved in meeting the challenges of a stressful situation. When such motor

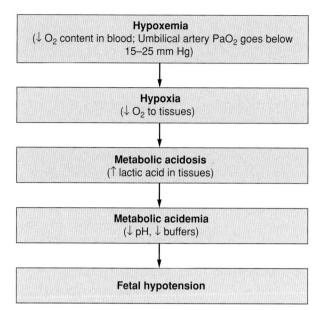

| Hypoxemia |
| ($\downarrow$ O$_2$ content in blood; Umbilical artery PaO$_2$ goes below 15–25 mm Hg) |

↓

| Hypoxia |
| ($\downarrow$ O$_2$ to tissues) |

↓

| Metabolic acidosis |
| ($\uparrow$ lactic acid in tissues) |

↓

| Metabolic acidemia |
| ($\downarrow$ pH, $\downarrow$ buffers) |

↓

| Fetal hypotension |

FIGURE 1–4. Fetal physiologic response to changes in blood flow and compensatory mechanisms.

functions in the adult are stimulated, the radial muscle of the iris contracts (dilating the pupils), the pilomotor muscles contract (causing goose-bumps), and the smooth muscle in the sphincters of the gastrointestinal tract and the urinary bladder contract to retain their contents. The heart beats faster and more forcibly, and vasoconstriction of blood vessels occurs in the viscera and skin.

Relaxation of smooth skeletal and cardiac muscles causes blood vessels to dilate. In addition, the muscle in the walls of the gastrointestinal tract and urinary bladder relax and the bronchioles dilate, making breathing easier. Stimulation of secretory functions increases the activity of the sweat glands and the secretion of epinephrine by the adrenal glands. Viscid saliva is produced, causing a feeling of dryness in the mouth. Stimulation of glycogenolysis facilitates the breakdown of glycogen to glucose, which is then released into the bloodstream to augment the available fuel source.

In summary, when the sympathetic nervous system is stimulated in the adult, the pupils dilate, saliva production decreases, adrenaline and glucose are produced, the gastrointestinal tract slows down, and cardiac and respiratory rates increase. Visceral and skin blood vessels constrict, whereas those in skeletal muscle, heart muscle, lungs, and brain dilate. These actions shunt blood to the vital organs. The fetus responds similarly when stimulated by loud noise, vibration, maternal abdominal palpation, scalp stimulation, or application of the fetal spiral electrode (FSE).

Stork Byte

Two thumbs up!
If I'm awake, not medicated, and well-oxygenated, then stimulating my sympathetic nervous system with a fetal acoustic stimulator should cause my heart rate to accelerate—and accelerations are a good sign from me!

Maintaining Balance

The actions and effects of the sympathetic nervous system counterbalance those of the parasympathetic nervous system. They function collaboratively to maintain a balance, unless one is sufficiently stimulated to override the other. This interaction is visually apparent in the maintenance of and changes in FHR baseline rate and variability, which is explained further in Chapters 2 and 3.

Development and Functioning of the Autonomic Nervous System

By approximately 32 weeks' gestation, the fetal ANS is expected to be fully developed and capable of effecting predictable responses to various stimuli as demonstrated by changes in its heart rate. Many fetuses accomplish such development at an even earlier gestational age. The mature ANS is demonstrated by the presence of variations in the duration between each cardiac cycle. This normal occurrence of sinus arrhythmia is recognized as FHR baseline variability. The presence of variability in the FHR tracing is a visual display of the synergistic workings of the sympathetic and parasympathetic nervous systems. The fetal CNS is sensitive to changes in oxygen exchange with the maternal system and to its own carbon dioxide production, and it uses the ANS to effect actions intended to maintain a normal environment. The presence or absence of variability in the FHR, therefore, is the primary indicator of fetal oxygenation.[13,14]

Stork Byte

An expression of gratitude…
The presence of variability in my baseline heart rate indicates that I am well-oxygenated, thank you very much!

Prior to 32 weeks' gestation, the fetal ANS is not yet fully mature. Sufficient evidence exists showing that fetuses between 28 and 32 weeks' gestation do demonstrate FHR accelerations in response to movement or stimulation, but those accelerations do not rise in height nor remain accelerated for as long as a more mature fetus. Nonetheless, those smaller accelerations (10 bpm × 10 seconds) in this subgroup of preterm fetuses indicate that the fetus is well-oxygenated.[2]

ACID–BALANCE BALANCE

The maintenance of proper acid–base balance within the human body is essential to well-being. When the maternal–uterine–placental exchange system is interrupted, the potential exists for fetal acidosis, which can lead to permanent damage or death. When fetal blood is analyzed, it is the blood from the fetal umbilical vein that reflects uteroplacental status. This is largely dependent on maternal condition. The composition of the blood from the umbilical arteries reflects uteroplacental status, as well as fetal oxygenation.[15]

The purpose of EFM is to screen for the development of hypoxia, although the fetal monitor is not a good measure of fetal deoxygenation. For this reason, there are direct measures of fetal oxygenation that may be utilized in conjunction with EFM to help in determining those truly hypoxic fetuses from those with FHR tracings that are suspicious for hypoxia. Two such valuable adjuncts to EFM for determining fetal status include fetal scalp stimulation (which, for reasons discussed later in this chapter, has replaced the use of fetal scalp blood sampling) and vibra-acoustic stimulation, a technique that is discussed in detail in Chapter 4.

All chemical processes in the living cell involve the balance of hydrogen (H^+) and hydroxyl (OH^-) ions. The concentration of each of these elements in the body fluids determines the degree of acidity or alkalinity (pH) (Table 1–3). If there are more hydrogen ions, the fluid is acidic; if there are more hydroxyl ions, the fluid is alkaline. The pH value is the means by which the measurement of hydrogen ion concentration is expressed. The amount of H^+ ions retained determines acid–base status: the greater the concentration of H^+ ions, the higher the acidity. The measurement of hydrogen ion concentration is inversely expressed as the pH (e.g., the higher the hydrogen ion concentration, the lower the pH).

The body and all living cells are sensitive to changes in acidity and alkalinity. An alteration in the pH of blood affects the functioning of many cells. In the blood, there are buffer salts that keep the pH relatively constant. As a clinical example of

TABLE 1–3 THE AUTONOMIC NERVOUS SYSTEM

Parasympathetic	Sympathetic
Pupillary constriction	Pupillary dilation
Production of watery saliva	Dry mouth
Bronchiole constriction	Increased lung capacity
Increased gastrointestinal activity	Decreased gastrointestinal activity
Increased bladder activity	Retention of bladder contents
Dry skin	Increased sweating, pilomotor muscle contraction (goose-bumps)
Slowed heart rate	Increased heart rate
	Increased adrenal gland secretions
	Increased glycogenolytic function

Data from Chaffee E, Greisheimer E. *Basic Physiology and Anatomy.* Philadelphia, PA: Lippincott; 1969.

alterations in pH status, consider the person who has experienced prolonged vomiting. Because there is significant loss of gastric fluid, which contains the acid *hydrogen chloride,* the blood becomes more alkaline and the person enters a state of alkalosis. Conversely, a person with lung disease who cannot exhale carbon dioxide as rapidly as it is produced accumulates this acid within the blood. As the pH value lowers, this person enters a state of acidosis. Alkalosis and acidosis can cause permanent damage to organs or progress to a fatal condition if the acid–base balance is not quickly restored.[15]

Acids

The body produces two groups of acids: volatile acids (such as carbonic acid) and nonvolatile acids (such as lactic acid). Carbonic acid is formed by hydration of carbon dioxide. Alveolar ventilation regulates carbon dioxide levels in the adult and normally maintains a carbon dioxide partial pressure in the alveoli and arterial blood of 40 mm Hg. As a normal adaptive change, these pressures are altered during pregnancy. Because of her increased ventilation, a pregnant woman's carbon dioxide partial pressure is typically 30–32 mm Hg (Table 1–4). This allows the fetus to readily dispose of carbon dioxide by diffusion across the placenta, providing there is adequate intervillous and umbilical blood flow.

TABLE 1-4 ADULT ACID–BASE PARAMETERS

pH	pO$_2$	pCO$_2$	Base Deficit
Nonpregnant Woman			
7.40	90–100 mm Hg	40 mm Hg	0
Pregnant Woman			
7.40	90–100 mm Hg	30–32 mm Hg	0

Nonvolatile acids are produced by anaerobic metabolism.[13] Lactic acid is a major end product of anaerobic metabolism and is produced when the demand of muscles for oxygen during work exceeds the supply. When lactic acid accumulates, the need for oxygen is increased. This is usually experienced as feeling "out of breath," and the person in whom this is occurring responds by increasing her rate and depth of respiration. These increased respiratory efforts bring a greater amount of oxygen into the system, allowing for lactic acid to change into pyruvic acid and carbon dioxide through the process of aerobic metabolism. If the body is unable to effectively accomplish this and lactic acid continues to accumulate, muscle fatigue results. Excessive amounts of lactic acid depress the activity in muscle cells, leading to decreased muscle responsiveness.

In the adult, nonvolatile acids are excreted through the renal system. This process is slower than the rate of excretion of carbon dioxide, requiring hours rather than seconds to accomplish. The fetus disposes of nonvolatile acids by diffusion across the placenta. As in the adult, the process is slower than the diffusion of carbon dioxide.[15]

Fetal Metabolism

Knowledge of acid–base balance should be applied to care of the fetus. The normal fetal metabolic process begins as glucose is broken down into lactic acid. Oxygen is required to facilitate the next step, which is to convert lactic acid into carbon dioxide and water. Carbon dioxide is a waste product of this process and is disposed of by the fetus through diffusion across the placenta into the maternal system. This is how the fetus produces energy (Table 1–5).

Buffers

If there is any interruption in blood flow to the uterus, across the placenta, or through the umbilical cord, fetal acid–base imbalance may result. Oxygen is necessary to complete the metabolic process by changing lactic acid into excretable end-products. If fetal hypoxemia (decreased oxygen content in the blood) develops and is allowed to continue, hypoxia (decreased oxygen in the tissues) will result. Without oxygen, lactic acid is not broken down and begins to accumulate in the blood and the tissues. This buildup of lactic acid causes retention of hydrogen ions, an increase in their presence in the blood (acidemia), and an increase in their concentration in the tissues (acidosis). The fetus responds by activating its buffer system. Buffers are chemical substances that resist changes in the pH of a solution when an acid

TABLE 1-5 FETAL ACID–BASE PARAMETERS*

pH	pO$_2$	pCO$_2$	Base Excess
Fetal Blood Sample			
7.25–7.40	18–22 mm Hg	40–50 mm Hg	0–11 mEq/L
Venous Cord Sample**			
7.25–7.45	17.2–40.8 mm Hg	26.8–49.2 mm Hg	0–11 mEq/L
Arterial Cord Sample**			
7.18–7.38	5.6–30.8 mm Hg	32.2–65.8 mm Hg	0–11 mEq/L

*Clinically significant fetal acidemia is defined as pH <7.00 for umbilical artery pH and <7.20 for scalp blood.[20,21] Normal fetal base deficit is 0 to 11 mEq/L. A base deficit >11 is considered potential metabolic acidosis.[20,22,23]

**The umbilical venous blood gas always has a higher pH, a lower pCO$_2$, and a higher pO$_2$ than the umbilical arterial blood gas.[15]

or base is added to it. Most buffers are comprised of a substance that is both weakly acidic and the salt of that substance. These pairs can react with relatively strong acids or bases and replace them with less harmful substances. These less volatile substances can then be eliminated from the body. Buffers are of primary importance in maintaining the proper ratio of hydrogen and hydroxyl ions in the body. Bicarbonate (HCO_3) is the most important buffer used by the fetus to normalize its environment.

When a fetal or cord blood gas sample is analyzed, information about how much HCO_3 was used by the fetus is expressed directly as a numeric value and also indirectly by the base deficit. Base deficit (referred to as base excess when reported as a positive integer) indicates the degree of metabolic acidosis. The higher the base deficit (or the lower the base excess), the greater the amount of buffer used. Because bicarbonate is a buffer used to control metabolically produced acids, a high base deficit points to significant acidosis. Calculation of base deficit or base excess is based on pH and pCO_2; if pH and pCO_2 are within normal limits, the base deficit or base excess must also be.[15]

In metabolic acidosis, the oxygen supply to the fetus is diminished over a period of time, causing an increase in the concentration of lactic acid. Bicarbonate is consumed in an effort to neutralize the buildup of acid. As this buffer base becomes depleted, the pH value continues to fall as the fetus becomes hypoxic. This can lead to permanent damage to tissue and organs. When the fetus is unable to excrete nonvolatile acids, its behavior is affected. This is demonstrated by a decrease in or lack of fetal movement, an absence of fetal tone, and a loss of fetal breathing movements. A reduction in the amount of amniotic fluid may also occur if there is a prolonged period of lactic acid accumulation. Changes in the FHR tracing that may be observed include minimal or absent FHR baseline variability, tachycardia, a loss of accelerations, and, ultimately, terminal bradycardia (Table 1–6).

With respiratory acidosis, there is no production or accumulation of lactic acid. Respiratory acidosis occurs quickly and has the potential for rapid recovery. An example of this is the swimmer who holds his or her breath for a prolonged underwater swim. With breath holding, carbon dioxide accumulates and pH subsequently decreases. After resurfacing, the swimmer takes a big gasp of air. This causes heart rate and respirations to increase, promoting oxygen supply and consumption, and stabilizing the pH. In the

TABLE 1–6 METABOLIC ACIDOSIS

Parameter	Value	Reason
pH	Low; <7.20	Acidosis is present.
pCO_2	Normal; <60	No oxygen is present to allow conversion of lactic acid to CO_2.
pO_2	Low; <20	Lack of O_2 is the problem instigating the metabolic acidosis.
HCO_3	Low; <22	This buffer is used to neutralize metabolically produced acids.
Base excess	High; >8–11	Reflects amount of buffer used to neutralize acids.

fetus, respiratory acidosis may be reflected in the FHR pattern as a rise in the baseline FHR, a decrease in or loss of baseline variability, and a loss or diminution of accelerations. Usually, when the cause of the respiratory acidosis is corrected, the FHR experiences a relatively quick recovery. At delivery, a fetus with respiratory acidosis may have a low 1-minute Apgar score, but will usually respond to stimulation and oxygen administration and have a normal 5-minute Apgar score (Table 1–7).

It is possible for the fetus to experience respiratory and metabolic acidosis simultaneously. This

TABLE 1–7 RESPIRATORY ACIDOSIS

Parameter	Value	Reason
pH	Low; <7.20	Acidosis is present.
pCO_2	High; >60	Process continued through to production of this end product, which can't be excreted and is accumulating in the fetus.
pO_2	Normal; >20	Supply of O_2 is not the problem.
HCO_3	Normal; >22	Works against metabolically produced acids—not needed in this instance.
Base excess	Normal; <8–11	Measures buffers that work against metabolically produced acids—value is normal because buffers are not being used.

TABLE 1–8 MIXED ACIDOSIS

Parameter	Value	Reason
pH	Low; <7.20	Acidosis is present.
pCO_2	High; >60	What is converted to CO_2 can't be excreted and is accumulating in the fetus (respiratory acidosis).
pO_2	Low; <20	Lack of O_2 is instigating the metabolic part of the acidosis.
HCO_3	Low; <22	This buffer is being used to neutralize metabolically produced acids.
Base excess	High; >8–11	Reflects amount of buffer used to neutralize acids.

condition is referred to as *mixed acidosis* and combines the worst values of each (Table 1–8).

Stork Byte

Respiratory acidosis is acute…but metabolic acidosis isn't cute at all!

A variety of events can cause decreased perfusion to and through the uterus, placenta, and umbilical cord, negatively affecting fetal acid–base status. If the fetus is already compromised, even marginally, the onset of metabolic acidosis will be faster and, therefore, the risk of metabolic acidosis is even greater. It is of fundamental importance to continuously assess and support the maternal system's maintenance of optimal uteroplacental perfusion.

Assessment of Fetal Acid–Base Balance

EFM is used in both antepartum and intrapartum settings to assist the provider in determining whether the uterus is the optimal environment for the fetus. EFM may be the sole means of assessing fetal status, or it may be used in conjunction with other techniques. Regardless of the reason for its initiation or the setting in which it is used, EFM's most beneficial feature is its capacity to display early signs of fetal compromise to the alert and discerning clinician.

Fetal Scalp Blood Sampling (Scalp pH)

In 90% of fetuses that demonstrate nonreassuring FHR patterns, no actual hypoxia/acidosis exists. Therefore, alternate methods of assessing acid–base

status are needed to prevent unnecessary intervention.[3,16] Utilization of fetal scalp blood sampling in combination with EFM had been shown to decrease the number of cesarean births for fetal distress.[17] Sampling of the fetal blood during labor was a technique that was utilized up until relatively recently and provided a snapshot analysis of the acid–base status of the fetus with a Category 2 type FHR pattern. This procedure was invasive to both the mother and the fetus; it involved puncturing the fetal scalp to obtain a small sampling of blood that was collected in a capillary tube and then analyzed for pH value. There were a number of limitations to this method of fetal assessment. Technical difficulties to be negotiated included mastery of the procedure, completion of the procedure on the laboring patient (who may not have wished to remain still or who may have experienced discomfort), and positioning of the patient (what was optimal for the practitioner was often not the same in regard to promotion of maternal–fetal perfusion).

Other problems existed in regard to processing of the fetal scalp blood sample. The laboratory may have reported the pH of the blood sample, which prevented the clinicians from distinguishing between respiratory and metabolic acidosis. A complete blood gas result contains determination of the base deficit/base excess. Additionally, the timing of sampling affected the pH value. For example, a sample obtained during a deceleration or bradycardia produced a lower value not accurately reflective of fetal status. Contamination of the sample with blood, meconium, or amniotic fluid also affected results. Finally, blood obtained from caput had potential to yield falsely low results.

As a result, fetal scalp blood sampling is rarely, if ever, performed today. Knowledge of this technique is helpful, as it did leave a lasting contribution to EFM. Correlations made between particular FHR patterns and pH values led to improved understanding and interpretation of fetal status.[18–20]

Scalp Stimulation

Based mainly on the work of Clark, Gimovsky, and Miller, manual stimulation of the fetal scalp has eliminated the use of fetal scalp blood sampling.[18,19] Initially, these researchers performed a retrospective study (N = 200) that revealed that no fetus responding to a scalp pH sampling procedure by producing an acceleration (≥15 bpm × ≥15 seconds) had a scalp pH <7.21. In their 1984 prospective study (N = 100), they sampled fetuses with FHR patterns suggestive of acidosis by applying 15 seconds of gentle digital pressure to the fetal scalp followed by 15 seconds of pressure applied with an Allis clamp. Their results are summarized here:

36/100 Acceleration with digital pressure	pH 7.19–7.40
15/100 No response to digital pressure, acceleration with Allis clamp	pH 7.23–7.33
49/100 No response to either stimulus	pH <7.20 (19) pH <7.23 (30)

The researchers reported the following impressions as conclusions of their study:

• Induced accelerations reflect a fetus with an intact ANS.
• A fetus with the ability to demonstrate spontaneous or induced accelerations is not acidotic.

Scalp stimulation is performed only when the FHR has recovered to baseline. The incidence of misleading results is greater if these procedures are done during a deceleration or bradycardia, when a state of hypoxia may exist. Fetal scalp stimulation is a test of how well the fetus is maintaining its oxygenation and reflects its ability to recover from an insult[18]; therefore, it is only performed during periods of FHR baseline.

Umbilical Cord Blood Gas

Guidelines published by the American College of Obstetrics and Gynecology (ACOG) recommend umbilical cord arterial blood gases as the most objective method of assessing fetal metabolic condition at birth.[18] In the neonate, the umbilical venous blood gas always has a higher pH, a lower pCO_2, and a higher pO_2 than the umbilical arterial blood gas.[15] The recommendation is to obtain cord samples in certain circumstances (e.g., newborns with low 5-minute Apgar scores or with abnormal FHR tracings). Umbilical cord gases with a pH <7.0 and a base deficit ≥12 mmol/L indicate a fetal metabolic acidosis possibly due to an intrapartum event and has an increased association with poor outcome.[18]

In conclusion, the entire clinical picture needs to be taken into account to accurately interpret the meaning of the FHR tracing. If the FHR tracing is a Category 1, there is evidence of the absence of fetal metabolic acidemia.[2] If the FHR tracing is a Category 2, or has nonreassuring components, then steps must be taken to further evaluate fetal acid–base status.

REFERENCES

1. Parer JT, King T, Flanders S, et al. Fetal acidemia and electronic fetal heart rate patterns: Is there evidence of an association? *J Matern Fetal Neonatal Med.* 2006;19(5):289–294.
2. Macones G, Hankin G, Spong CY, et al. The 2008 National Institute of Child Health and Human Development Workshop report on electronic fetal monitoring update on definitions, interpretation, and research guidelines. *Obstet Gynecol.* 2008;112(3):510–515.
3. American College of Obstetricians and Gynecologists. *Management of Intrapartum Fetal Heart Rate Tracings.* ACOG Practice Bulletin Number 116. Washington, DC: Author; 2010.
4. Simpson KR, James DC. Effects of oxytocin-induced uterine hyperstimulation during labor on fetal oxygen status and fetal heart rate patterns. *Am J Obstet Gynecol.* 2008;199:34.e1-5.
5. Rochard F, Schifrin B, Goupil F, et al. (1976). Nonstress fetal heart monitoring in the antepartum period. *Am J Obstet Gynecol.* 1976;126(6):699–706.
6. American College of Obstetricians and Gynecologists. *Intrapartum Fetal Heart Rate Monitoring: Nomenclature, Interpretation, and General Management Principles.* ACOG Practice Bulletin 106. Washington, DC: Author; 2009.
7. Association of Women's Health, Obstetric and Neonatal Nurses. *Nursing Care and Management of the Second Stage of Labor.* 2nd ed. Washington, DC: Author; 2008.
8. Simpson KR, James DC. Effects of immediate versus delayed pushing during second-stage labor on fetal well-being: A randomized clinical trial. *Nurs Res.* 2005;54(3):149–157.
9. Ikeda T, Murata Y, Quilligan E, et al. Histologic and biochemical study of the brain, heart, kidney and liver in asphyxia caused by occlusion of the umbilical cord in near-term fetal lambs. *Am J Obstet Gynecol.* 2000;182(2):449–457.
10. Schifrin B, Hamilton-Rubenstein T, Shields JR. Fetal heart rate patterns and the timing of fetal injury. *J Perinatol.* 1994;14:174–181.
11. Chaffee E, Greisheimer E. *Basic Physiology and Anatomy.* Philadelphia, PA: Lippincott; 1969.
12. Sherman DJ, Frenkel E, Kurzweil Y, et al. Characteristics of maternal heart rate patterns during labor and delivery. *Am J Obstet Gynecol.* 2002;99(4):542–547.
13. Parer JT. *Handbook of Fetal Heart Rate Monitoring.* 2nd ed. Philadelphia: W. B. Saunders; 1997.
14. Parer JT. (1998). Effects of fetal asphyxia on brain cell structure and function: Limits of tolerance. *Comp Biochem Physiol A Mol Integr Physiol.* 1998;119(3):711–716.
15. Pomerance J. *Interpreting Umbilical Cord Blood Gases.* 2nd ed. Glendora, CA: BNMG; 2012.
16. Low JA, Victory R, Derrick EJ. Predictive value of electronic fetal monitoring for intrapartum fetal asphyxia with metabolic acidosis. *Obstet Gynecol.* 1999;93:285–291.
17. Macones G, Depp R. Fetal monitoring. In: H Wildschut, C Weiner, T Peters, eds. *When to Screen in Obstetrics*

and Gynecology. Philadelphia: W. B. Saunders; 1996: 202–218.

18. Clark S. Fetal heart rate response to scalp blood sampling. *Am J Obstet Gynecol.* 1982;144:706.

19. Clark SL, Gimovsky ML, Miller FC. The scalp stimulation test: A clinical alternative to fetal scalp blood sampling. *Am J Obstet Gynecol.* 1984;148(3):274–277.

20. American College of Obstetricians and Gynecologists. *Umbilical Artery Blood Acid–Base Analysis.* ACOG Committee option 348. (2006, Reaffirmed 2010). Washington, DC: Author; 2006.

21. Gilstrap L. (1999). Fetal acid–base balance. In: RK Creasy, R Resnik, eds. *Maternal–Fetal Medicine.* 4th ed. Philadelphia, PA: W. B. Saunders; 1999:331–340.

22. Helwig J, Parer J, Kilpatrick S, Laros R. Umbilical cord blood acid–base state: What is normal? *Am J Obstet Gynecol.* 1996;174(6):1807–1812.

23. Reis E, Gabbe S, Petrie R. Intrapartum evaluation. In: S Gabbe, J Niebyl, JL Simpson, eds. *Obstetrics: Normal & Problem Pregnancies.* New York: Churchill Livingston; 1999:387–421.

CHAPTER 2

Electronic Fetal Heart Rate Monitoring Equipment and Technology

To accurately interpret the data presented by the electronic fetal monitor, it is necessary to have a basic understanding of both the workings and the limitations of the equipment. A generic description of instrumentation is provided in this chapter; however, it is essential for the clinician to be knowledgeable regarding the specific operations of the actual equipment at the bedside. The greatest effect on the data is produced by the mode of monitoring employed. Information about both the fetal heart rate (FHR) and uterine activity (UA) may be gathered using sensors that are placed either internally or externally.

ACQUISITION OF FETAL HEART RATE DATA

Fetal Electrocardiogram

Signal Processing

The most accurate means for assessing the FHR is through internal monitoring, currently accomplished by using the fetal spiral electrode (FSE). The lead wires of the spiral electrode conduct the electrical signal of the fetal QRS waveform complex (fetal electrocardiogram; FECG) to the electronic fetal monitor. From the FECG data, the electronic fetal monitor determines the FHR. The cardiotachometer is a component within the electronic fetal monitor that converts the FECG signal into the FHR. This processing is accomplished through the application of a mathematical equation:

$$FHR = \frac{60}{t}$$

| $60 \leftarrow$ | Representing 60 seconds occurring per 1 minute |
| $t \leftarrow$ | Representing the interval between successive QRS complexes |

To determine the unknown factor of t to enter into this equation, the cardiotachometer measures the time elapsed between the R peaks of successive QRS complexes (Figure 2–1).

Trending of Data

Once the factor of t is determined, it is then entered into the equation, FHR = 60/t. The product of this equation is the FHR, expressed in beats per minute (bpm). The FHR is then plotted on the FHR channel of the strip chart in bpm. Sinus arrhythmias are normal in the fetus and present as varying R–R intervals (t). Longer R–R intervals are represented by a slower FHR, whereas shorter R–R intervals are exhibited as a faster FHR. These fluctuations of the FHR from one beat to the next are recognized in the FHR tracing as *baseline variability*.

(*Note:* Prior to the adoption of the initial National Institute of Child Health and Human Development guidelines for electronic fetal monitoring terminology in 1997,[1-3] this R–R interval data [obtained only via internal monitoring] was further distinguished by use of the term *short-term variability*. Observation of the continuous recording of this data over a period of time allowed for even further determination of variations in the FHR baseline, previously known as *long-term variability*. For a variety of practical reasons delineated in the 1997 publication, such analysis and dissection of the baseline variability is no longer a clinical practice.)

Ultrasound

The FHR may also be determined from the signal acquired through use of external sensors. When properly placed on the maternal abdomen, the ultrasound transducer detects the movements of the fetal heart that occur with each beat. The ultrasound transducer contains crystals that transmit and receive high-frequency sound waves using the piezoelectric effect. The piezoelectric effect is the conversion of electrical energy into mechanical sound wave energy and vice versa. This is accomplished in the ultrasound transducer by the application of voltage to the crystals, which causes them to vibrate at a predetermined frequency. When this sound wave

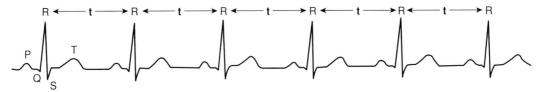

FIGURE 2–1. Fetal electrocardiogram.

meets the fetal heart, its frequency becomes either compressed or stretched by the beating motion of the fetal heart and is reflected back to the crystals. The reflected sound wave is converted back into electrical energy at a frequency altered from the original transmitted frequency. The difference between the frequency of the sound wave that is transmitted and that which is reflected back is referred to as the *Doppler shift*. The Doppler shift frequency can be used to produce the audible sound that is recognized as the fetal heart beat and also provides the raw data from which the FHR can be determined by using the equation, FHR $= 60/t$.

Continual transmission and reception of sound waves to and from the ultrasound transducer is known as "continuous wave" ultrasound. This is accomplished by having certain crystals dedicated to emitting sound waves, whereas others only receive the reflected signal. Continuous wave ultrasound was used in early versions of the ultrasound transducer until it was replaced by pulse Doppler technology. Pulse Doppler ultrasound allows all of the crystals in the transducer to both send and receive sound waves. Each of the crystals inside the transducer is timed to transmit sound waves and then "stand by" for a predetermined period (the amount of time it takes for the signal to be transmitted and reflected). The crystals are then reactivated as receivers for the ultrasound signal as it is returned for processing. Pulse Doppler ultrasound makes it possible to monitor more than one fetus simultaneously. Because of the timing or frequency built into each crystal, the signal emitted by the ultrasound transducer for the purpose of evaluating one fetus will not be received by the ultrasound transducer that is tracking the second fetus.

Signal Processing

The external mode of monitoring requires different processes for identifying the factor of t for use in the equation, FHR $= 60/t$, than that which is used with internal monitoring. Determining the factor of t is very straightforward with internal monitoring—it is the time elapsed between the clearly identifiable, successive R peaks of the QRS complex. The raw data gathered by the ultrasound transducer do not contain such distinct reference points from which the factor of t may be figured. These data are created by electronically comparing the reflected ultrasound signal to the transmitted signal. The original signal is "subtracted" from the reflected signal, and the resulting waveform is representative of the motion of the fetal heart (Figure 2–2). To facilitate determination of the factor t, the waveform is filtered to reduce the amount of high-frequency component. These filtered waveforms are irregularly shaped and lack an obvious common distinguishing element from which the timing of the occurrence of one waveform could be compared to that of the next (Figure 2–3). To assist in converting these raw data into useful information, the monitor employs a method referred to as *autocorrelation*. Autocorrelation is a process of successively comparing waveforms to identify their similarities. Once such features are recognized, a template of the waveforms is created and is used as a comparison to incoming waveform data (Figure 2–4). As correlations in the data are determined, the factor of t can be calculated from the peaks of the correlation function.

Trending of Data

Another difference of external versus internal monitoring is that information concerning the individual intervals between each successive fetal heart beat is

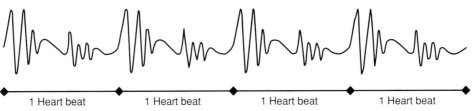

1 Heart beat   1 Heart beat   1 Heart beat   1 Heart beat

FIGURE 2–2. Raw waveform.

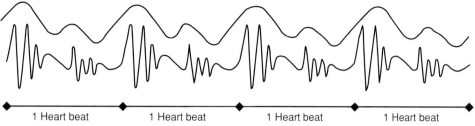

FIGURE 2–3. Waveform with filter applied.

not represented in the FHR tracing. Instead, once the factor of t is determined, it is applied in the equation FHR = 60/t and then averaged over several successive beats. It is only after this multiple beat average has been calculated that the FHR is determined and plotted on the strip chart. This averaging process is repeated continuously as data become available. Fluctuations in the FHR will be represented by variations in these averaged figures as the trend of the FHR is traced over a period of time. These variations are recognized by the clinician as *FHR baseline variability.* Due to these averaging processes, use of internal monitoring via an FSE provides a more accurate evaluation of FHR baseline variability.

(*Note:* Prior to the adoption of 1997 NICHD terminology into clinical practice, fluctuations in the FHR obtained via external monitoring were further distinguished by use of the term *long-term variability.* Today, in accordance with current recommendations,[2–4] the distinction between long- and short-term variability is no longer made. The visibly apparent fluctuations in the recorded trend of the FHR baseline [whether obtained internally or externally] are now simply referred to collectively as *baseline variability.*)

Limitations of Technology

Half-Counting and Double-Counting
Capabilities vary between types and brands of electronic fetal monitors, and it is necessary to understand the features of the equipment in use. Typically, the ultrasound transducer has the ability to recognize the FHR that is occurring within the range of approximately 50 to 210 bpm. As the FHR approaches the outer limits of this range, it may be difficult to obtain a clear signal by external means. Occasionally, when the FHR nears the lower limits of the capacities of

the ultrasound transducer, the electronic fetal monitor may begin to erroneously consider the motion data resulting from one heart beat to instead be that of two separate beats. This is exhibited by the intermittent trending of the FHR on the strip chart at twice the actual rate. Such an event is referred to as *double-counting* (Figure 2-5). As the FHR approaches the upper limits of the capability of external monitoring, *half-counting* may occur. The monitor may only recognize every other section of motion data as a heart beat, thereby intermittently presenting the FHR at half the actual rate on the strip chart (Figure 2-6). During the occurrence of both double-counting and half-counting, the audible signal will likely remain the most accurate indicator of the actual FHR. Internal monitoring may be selected to remedy to either event, as its range is wider (30–240 bpm). At rates above 240 bpm, the FHR will likely record on the tracing at half the actual rate (half-counting); however, the audible signal will often continue as high as 300 bpm. With an FHR below 30 bpm that is acquired via internal monitoring, the FHR may not record on the tracing but will likely remain audible. In any instance when something unusual is occurring and there is data available that is only evident to those present and that is not being captured for archiving (in this case, the audible FHR signal), it is essential to document this information.

Maternal Signal
The maternal pulse should be assessed and compared against the electronic fetal monitor's audible signal each time electronic fetal monitoring (EFM) is initiated or the mode of monitoring is changed.[5,6] The maternal heart rate may be transmitted by either mode of monitoring. The spiral electrode conducts

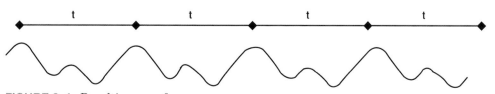

FIGURE 2–4. Resulting waveform.

1) 08/12/00 12:20
   COMMENTS: DIFFICULT TO MONITOR FH DURING UCS. MD
   CONSULTED.
2) 08/12/00 12:23
   12:38 BP 131/71 M 94 P 70
   COMMENTS: FH AUDIBLE 90'S/100'S DURING UC.

3) 08/12/00 12:24
   116/118 EXTERNAL INOP
   COMMENTS: MD PRESENT TO PLACE INTERNAL MONITORS.
4) 08/12/00 12:25
   116/118 FECG EXTERNAL IUP
5) 08/12/00 12:26
   COMMENTS: SPIRAL ELECTRODE PLACED. 6 CMS NOW.

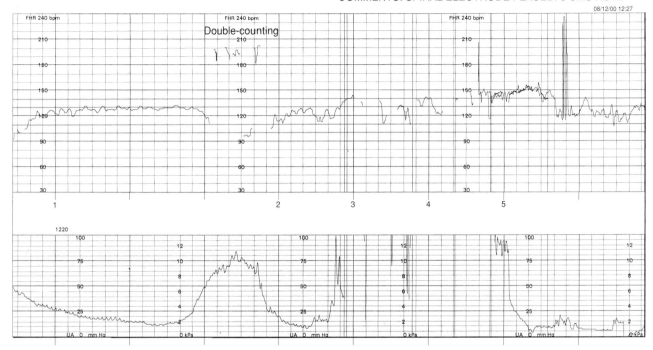

FHR = 130 bpm

FIGURE 2–5. Double-counting.

1) 05/23/99 11:25
   COMMENTS: PT REMAINS L SIDE WITH O2 ON.

2) 05/23/99 11:25
   BP 130/80 M 96 P118
   COMMENTS: T 101² ORAL.

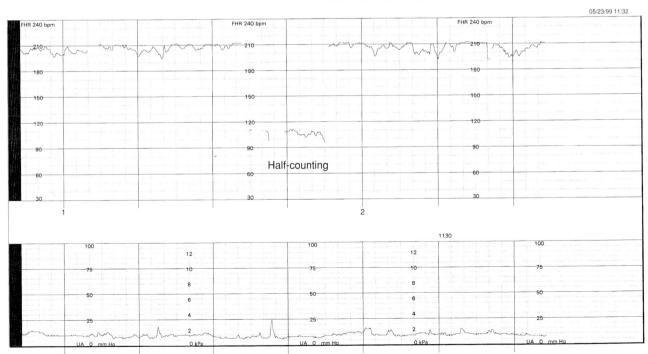

FHR = 210 bpm

FIGURE 2–6. Half-counting.

1) 03/24/01 15:20
   FM POWER ON 116 EXTERNAL INOP TOCO
2) 03/24/01 15:22
   COMMENTS: PT TRANSFERRED FROM TRIAGE TO LDR
   WITH DR PRESENT, SPIRAL ELECTRODE ON. U/S IN
   PROGRESS. P88. NO FHR, PT INFORMED. PT DISTRAUGHT,
   SOCIAL SVC. CONSULT ORDERED.

3) 03/24/01 15:25
   PT STATES HAVING FELT NO MOVEMENT SINCE LAST PM.
4) 03/24/01 15:27
   EFM DC'D NOW. OPTIONS FOR CARE EXPLAINED.

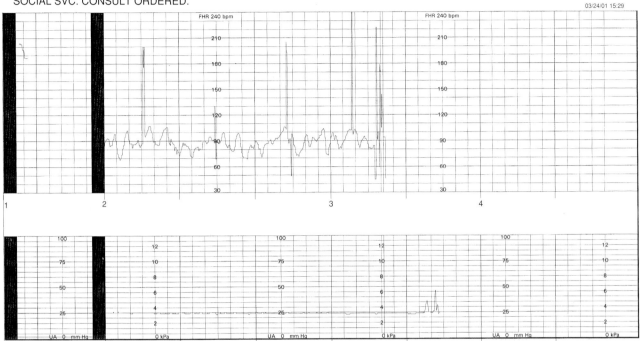

MHR = 90 bpm

FIGURE 2–7. Maternal heart rate acquired via a fetal spiral electrode applied to the vertex in a case of fetal demise.

ECG information to the electronic fetal monitor. In most cases, there are two sets of ECG data available—fetal and maternal. The electronic fetal monitor recognizes the stronger of these two signals. As the spiral electrode is applied directly to the fetus, the FECG is expected to provide the stronger signal. If the spiral electrode is inadvertently applied to maternal tissue or to a fetus that is not alive, the maternal signal will appear stronger and, therefore, be the one transmitted (Figure 2–7). The maternal signal may also be erroneously obtained when using the ultrasound transducer.[7] When the transducer is placed over the maternal vessels, it will sense and record the movement data caused by pulsation (Figure 2–8). The tracing of maternal heart rate is easily discerned by comparison of the maternal pulse to the monitor's audible signal. For documentation purposes, it is useful if the maternal heart rate can also be automatically obtained and printed or trended directly on the fetal strip chart. Additionally, electronic fetal monitors are often equipped with technology to differentiate between heart rates and/or alert to duplicate rates when simultaneous acquisition of more than one set of heart rates (e.g.,

FHR and MHR or twins) is in progress. Understanding the functioning of the equipment at the bedside is an essential competency.

Regardless of the mode of monitoring utilized, critical thinking and employment of knowledge of FHR patterns and maternal physiology is essential in recognizing such occurrences. For example, because it is known that the maternal heart rate is likely to accelerate during second-stage labor and that fetuses rarely demonstrate such a pattern at this time,[8] it is reasonable to suspect erroneous acquisition of maternal heart rate if a pattern resembling FHR accelerations is displayed on the strip chart while the patient is actively pushing. It is always necessary to interpret the FHR within the context of the current and specific clinical situation.

Stork Byte

Pump up the volume! If there is a discrepancy between what you see on the strip chart and what you are hearing from the electronic fetal monitor, listen up! The **sound** of my heart beat is the definitive indicator of my actual heart rate.

1) 10/31/00 03:27
   COMMENTS: MATERNAL PULSE AUDIBLE, U/S TRANSDUCER ADJUSTED.
   BP 109/58 M 73 P 95

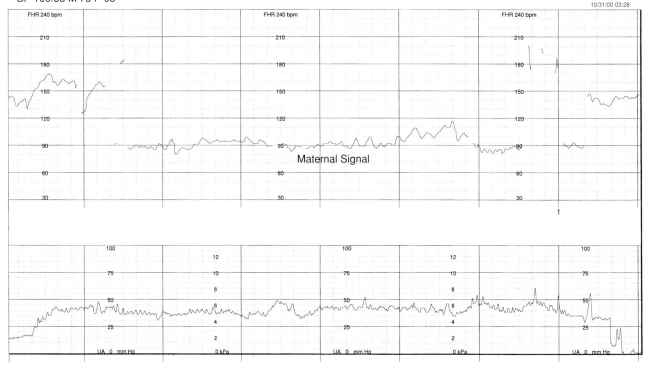

MHR = 90 bpm

FIGURE 2–8. Maternal heart rate obtained with ultrasound transducer.

Stork Byte

The ABC's of EFM

A = Absence of my heart rate allows the electronic fetal
monitor to record my mom's heart rate

B = Beware and stay alert! Take my mom's pulse and
compare it to the audible signal from the electronic
fetal monitor

C = Confirm the presence of my FHR by looking for
cardiac activity with an ultrasound machine if you
are in doubt

Dysrhythmia versus Artifact

The presence of a fetal dysrhythmia also poses a
challenge to EFM. The rapid fluctuations in the FHR
during a dysrhythmia make it extremely difficult to
capture the FHR signal using an ultrasound transducer. A fetoscope, stethoscope, or M (motion)-mode
sonography would provide better data. Internal monitoring may also be an option, although, with some
types of dysrhythmias, it may be difficult to continuously observe the FHR baseline. If internal monitoring is being used, the electronic fetal monitor may
be connected to a standard ECG recorder to observe
the FECG and assist in diagnosis of the type of dysrhythmia. This connection requires the fetal monitor

to have an output connector to retrieve an analog
FECG signal, and the standard ECG recorder to
have a compatible input connector to feed the signal.

It is important to recognize the difference between
the presence of a dysrhythmia and the occurrence of
artifact. Artifact occurs when there is interference
in the FECG signal being transmitted by the spiral
electrode. This can occur at the application site, in
instances of incomplete application, or when there is
a large amount of hair on the fetal head. Such interference of signal transmission commonly occurs when
the spiral electrode is applied without first rupturing
membranes. Artifact can also occur when the connection points of the spiral electrode to the monitor
are disturbed. This can occur in relation to maternal
activity. For instance, artifact may be noted to occur
simultaneously with events such as contractions,
as the patient seeks comfort and moves her body in
ways that interrupt the signal. Unlike dysrhythmias,
artifact appears in the FHR tracing as disorganized
deflections of varying lengths above or below the FHR
signal. Although dysrhythmias may appear either
continuously or intermittently on the strip chart,
depending on their etiology, they maintain unifor-
mity in their appearance. Dysrhythmias present as
organized deflections of equal or similar lengths that

occur at regular intervals to form a pattern. Also, the conspicuously irregular sounding beat of a dysrhythmia usually serves as an audible indicator to the clinician that this condition is present. More than one type of dysrhythmia may be present. Dysrhythmias are explored in further detail in Chapter 3.

Common Challenges to Signal Acquisition

Although frequent assessment and adjustment of the ultrasound transducer should be considered standard practice, there are some additional variables to consider that may necessitate an increase in the frequency of these activities. These include maternal size, shape, positioning, and activity level, as well as fetal position, fetal activity, gestational age, and multiple gestation. It may prove difficult, for instance, in some cases of increased maternal body habitus to obtain the FHR externally and may, therefore, be necessary for the nurse to be available at the bedside to manually direct the positioning of the ultrasound transducer. This type of attention may also be required with variations in maternal and fetal activity and positioning to obtain an adequate signal.

Stork Byte

Tag, you're "it"! I like to move around a lot and so does my mom. That means you have to come and find me by adjusting the transducers!

Gestational age must also be considered when performing EFM. Not only does the preterm fetus pose a challenge to monitoring, but the clinician must also evaluate the type, value, and utility of the information being obtained. In cases of extreme prematurity, when the objective is simply to affirm presence of a FHR and the rate itself, it may be more prudent to assess the fetus with a fetoscope, hand-held Doppler, or by sonographic examination. An awareness and understanding of fetal physiology and growth are necessary to assist the clinician to evaluate the FHR using methods and parameters that are appropriate to gestational age.

Monitoring of the multiple gestation incorporates many of the considerations discussed previously. Unique to this situation, however, is the necessity to ensure that each of the fetuses is actually being monitored. Most electronic fetal monitors that are capable of monitoring multiple fetuses simultaneously are also equipped with the technology to allow the clinician to visually distinguish between two or more fetal heart rates or to alert the clinician to investigate when the FHR tracings have marked similarities. An overview of the utility of internal and external FHR monitoring can be found in Table 2–1.

Stork Byte

Who's who? With multiples, we all need to be heard! Do you know how to work your equipment to distinguish between each of our FHR tracings?

ACQUISITION OF UTERINE ACTIVITY DATA

The significance of the FHR data as presented on the strip chart is interpreted with respect to concurrent uterine activity. Uterine activity data also carry import as a parameter in various clinical situations. Uterine activity may be determined with either internal or external sensors.

During the active phase of labor, adequate uterine activity is considered to be contractions that occur approximately every 2 to 4.5 minutes and measure 25 to 75 mm Hg in intensity.[3] Proper spacing of contractions (at least 1 minute rest between) allows the uterus to achieve a state of relaxation, thus supporting optimal uteroplacental perfusion between contractions. Resting tone of the uterus between contractions should be 15 to 20 mm Hg, and the uterus should palpate as soft. The duration of contractions should be approximately 60 to 90 seconds.

It is important to take steps to avoid and/or remedy the occurrence of tachysystole (defined as six or more contractions in a 10-minute time frame, averaged over a 30-minute window[2]) and hypertonus (contractions lasting more than 2 minutes), regardless of whether the FHR has begun to show signs of adverse affect. If tachysystole and/or hypertonus are allowed to persist, complications are likely to occur that affect the mother and/or the fetus. Tachysystole and hypertonus may occur in response to induction/augmentation agents or may happen spontaneously. In the event of hypertonus, it is necessary to provide resuscitative measures such as maternal position changes, fluid bolus, and discontinuing or decreasing induction/augmentation medications, regardless of whether changes in the FHR have yet begun to occur in response.[9–11] Administration of tocolytics to decrease uterine activity may also be necessary. Such interventions are certainly indicated if changes in the FHR are noted.[2]

TABLE 2–1 OVERVIEW: MODES OF MONITORING FHR

	Internal (FECG) Signal Source: Electrical	External (Ultrasound) Signal Source: Motion

Indications	Unsatisfactory external tracing
	Abnormal/suspicious external tracing
	Patient/practitioner preference
		Screening/fetal assessment
		Antepartum/early labor, can be placed regardless
		    of status of:
		      Membranes
		      Dilation
		      Station/presentation
		Patient/practitioner preference

Advantages	More accurate Continuous Variability Patient comfort Dysrhythmias	Noninvasive Easy to apply Antepartum/early in labor

Limitations	Requires:
	    Ruptured membranes
	    Adequate dilatation
	    Favorable station/presentation
	Invasive to both patient and fetus
		Variability
		Halving
		Doubling
		Maternal signal
		Arrhythmias
		Readjustment
		    Maternal/fetal activity
		    Maternal size/shape

Contraindications (relative)	Presentation: Face, fontanelles, genitalia Placenta previa; undiagnosed bleeding Transmittable maternal infection Need for maintenance of intact membranes Patient refusal	Patient refusal

Intrauterine Pressure Catheter

The most accurate measure of uterine activity is accomplished internally through the use of an intra-uterine pressure catheter (IUPC). The IUPC provides information regarding the strength, frequency, and duration of contractions. It also measures the uterine resting tone, the tension of the uterine muscle between contractions. The IUPC may be of either the fluid-filled or sensor-tipped varieties. Both types of catheters measure hydrostatic pressure within the uterus and display the reading on the strip chart on a scale of 0 to 100 mm Hg (United States) and 0 to 13 kPa (used in some international settings). Because the IUPC is referenced to atmospheric pressure ("zeroed"), it provides an absolute measurement of intra-amniotic pressure. The techniques by which this zeroing is accomplished can vary significantly among types and brands of catheters. As with any technical equipment, information provided by the IUPC must be analyzed for accuracy and the catheter adjusted accordingly. Palpation of contractions and uterine resting tone is a simple technique that can be helpful in affirming that the data provided by the IUPC are consistent with actual uterine activity.

Tocotransducer

Uterine activity may also be measured externally, with the use of a tocotransducer. The tocotransducer houses a sensor that detects changes in myometrial tone, such as that which occurs during a contraction. Although the tocotransducer is referenced and a baseline is established when this device is applied to the maternal abdomen, these are arbitrary settings because the tocotransducer is not equilibrated to atmospheric pressure. The tocotransducer, therefore, provides a relative rather than an absolute measurement of pressure. The clinical significance of this is that the height of the contractions as presented on the strip chart is not indicative of the strength of contractions nor is uterine resting tone accurately represented. Although the tocotransducer is a useful tool for determining the approximate frequency and duration of contractions, it is necessary to palpate the maternal abdomen and query the patient

TABLE 2–2 OVERVIEW: MODES OF MONITORING UTERINE ACTIVITY

	Internal Intrauterine Pressure Catheter	External Tocotransducer

Indications	Unsatisfactory external tracing
	Dysfunctional labor
	VBAC
	Patient/practitioner preference
		Screening/fetal assessment
		Antepartum/early labor, can be applied regardless
		   of status of:
		     Membranes
		     Dilation
		     Station/presentation
		Patient/practitioner preference

Advantages	Provides absolute measurement in mm/Hg
	Provides information about:
	   Strength, duration, and length of contraction
	   Uterine resting tone
	Amnioinfusion
		Noninvasive
		Easy to place
		Antepartum/early in labor
		Indicates frequency and length of contractions

Limitations	Requires:
	   Ruptured membranes
	   Adequate dilation
	   Favorable station/presentation
	Invasive to patient
		Readjustment:
		   Maternal/fetal activity
		   Maternal size/shape
		Does not provide information about:
		   Strength or exact duration of contractions
		   Uterine resting tone

Contraindications	Placenta previa, undiagnosed bleeding, suspected abruption	Patient refusal

to determine the strength of contractions and the uterine resting tone.

Stork Byte

Don't forget about my main squeeze! If you don't know what Mom's uterus is doing, then you can't really tell what's happening with me.

Challenges to Signal Acquisition

Challenges to monitoring uterine activity externally include placement technique and maternal activity, positioning, and body mass. The performance and subsequent utility of the tocotransducer are highly dependent on placement technique. The tocotransducer should be applied to the maternal abdomen in the area of the uterine fundus and where the contractions are most strongly palpated. It is important to ensure that the tocotransducer is secured tightly enough to acquire a signal but not so much as to interfere with it or cause discomfort to the patient. Placement of the sensor portion of the tocotransducer over the umbilicus may also interfere with the signal. Frequent re-referencing and reapplication of the tocotransducer will likely be necessary if the patient is physically active during the monitoring session. The thickness of the patient's subcutaneous layer will

also affect the uterine activity reading. Less maternal tissue between the uterus and the tocotransducer allows uterine activity to register more prominently on the strip chart. A greater amount of maternal tissue buffers the myometrial contraction from the tocotransducer and may blunt the appearance of uterine activity on the strip chart. Depending on the amount of tissue present, the effect may range from producing a less impressive looking trend of uterine activity on the strip chart to completely preventing the information from being presented. Information about uterine activity is integral in the interpretation of FHR patterns and assessment of maternal and fetal well-being. The acquisition and maintenance of these data are responsibilities inherent to the performance of EFM. An overview of the utility of internal and external monitoring of uterine activity can be found in Table 2–2.

PRESENTATION OF DATA

Chart Paper Speed

Once the FHR and uterine activity data have been acquired, a trend of the information is then presented on the strip chart. Factors that affect the appearance of these data include the paper speed and paper scaling. The paper speed affects the rate at which the paper moves through the recorder of the electronic fetal monitor but does not alter the rate at which FHR and uterine activity information is acquired and presented. Throughout the United States, the majority of institutions run their electronic fetal monitors at a paper speed of 3 cm/min. In other countries outside the United States, however, the practice is to have the paper speed set at 1 or sometimes 2 cm/min. At this slower rate, the information presented on the strip chart takes on a compressed appearance. It is important to realize that although the data look different at varying speeds, the significance of the information remains the same.

Stork Byte

Don't judge simply by appearance! If you don't like the look of my heart rate, do something to help me. Changing the way my heart rate *appears* on the strip chart does not change what I am trying to tell you about my condition.

Chart Paper Scaling

In the United States, most institutions use chart paper that trends the FHR on a 30- to 240-bpm scale, partitioned into 10-bpm vertical increments. Some countries use chart paper that trends the FHR on a 50- to 210-bpm scale. This type of chart paper apportions the vertical scaling into 20-bpm blocks. As with the selection of paper speed, these differences in paper scaling are a matter of preference. It is important, however, that an institution remain standardized once particular practices are established. When a clinician is familiar with interpreting data at a certain paper speed or scaling, education and a period of adjustment are required to perform analysis on a strip chart that is presented differently (Figure 2–9). There is room for error in interpretation when one is not aware of or accustomed to different paper speed or scaling parameters. Part of the application technique for the electronic fetal monitor should, therefore, include ensuring that both the paper speed and paper scaling meet institutional standards.

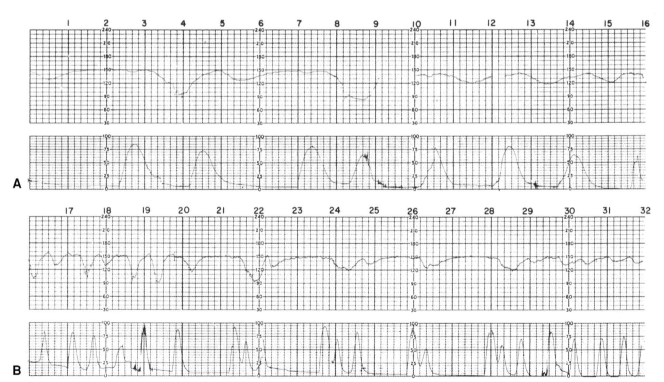

FIGURE 2–9. Fetal heart rate (FHR) tracings at different paper speeds. **(A)** Paper speed, 3 cm/min; spiral electrode. Late decelerations with no baseline variability are seen. **(B)** Paper speed, 1 cm/min; same tracing as in **A**. Note the differences in the shape of the decelerations and in the appearance of the variability. At this paper speed, the FHR pattern may appear to be "better" than it actually is, to a clinician accustomed to 3 cm/min paper speed.

Central Monitor Display

Another issue pertaining to visual interpretation is the discrepancy that may exist between the appearance of the strip chart at the bedside and its presentation on a central monitor system display. The dimensions of the strip chart may vary from the original when displayed on a computer screen, presenting a challenge to clinical interpretation. Additionally, the FHR tracing only has meaning when evaluated within the context of the entire clinical scenario. For this (and other patient care) reasons, it is necessary to perform regular assessments of the strip chart at the bedside. More information on electronic record keeping can be found in Chapter 6.

SUMMARY

A number of issues surround the use of EFM equipment. As with any technology, the accuracy and utility of the information obtained through EFM rely on the skill and competency of the clinicians who operate the equipment and interpret the data. Means for evaluating such competency are addressed in Chapter 7.

REFERENCES

1. National Institute of Child Health and Human Development Research Planning Workshop. Electronic fetal heart monitoring: Research guidelines for interpretation. *J Obstet Gynecol Neonat Nurs.* 1997;26(6):635–640.
2. American Congress of Obstetricians and Gynecologists. *Intrapartum fetal heart rate monitoring.* ACOG Practice Bulletin 106. Washington, DC: Author; 2009.
3. Association of Women's Health, Obstetric and Neonatal Nurses. *Antepartum and Intrapartum Fetal Heart Rate Monitoring: Clinical Competencies and Education Guide.* 5th ed. Washington, DC: Author; 2011.
4. National Institute of Child Health and Human Development Research Planning Workshop; Macones GA, et al. The 2008 National Institute of Child Health Human Development workshop report on electronic fetal monitoring: Update on definitions, interpretations, and research guidelines. *Obstet Gynecol.* 2008;112:661–666; *J Obstet Gynecol Neonat Nurs.* 2008;37:510–515.
5. Murray M. Maternal or fetal heart rate: Avoiding intrapartum misidentification. *J Obstet Gynecol Neonat Nurs.* 2004;33(1):93–104.
6. Doyle C, Angelotti T. Diagnosis of an unsuspected maternal hemorrhage via fetal heart rate tracing. *J Clin Anesthesiol.* 2004;16(6):456–458.
7. Neilson DR, Freeman RK, Mangan S. Signal Ambiguity Resulting in Unexpected Outcome with External Fetal Monnitoring. *Am J Obstet Gynecol.* 2008;198(6):717–724. Obtained from: http://mail.ny.acog.org/website/efm/signalambiguity.pdf
8. Sherman DJ, Frenkel E, Kurzweil Y, Padua A, Arieli S, Bahar M. Characteristics of maternal heart rate patterns during labor and delivery. *Obstet Gynecol.* 2002;99:542–547.
9. Simpson KR, Miller L. Assessment and optimization of uterine activity during labor. *Clin Obstet Gynecol.* 2011;54(1):40–49.
10. Garite TJ, Simpson KR. Intrauterine resuscitation during labor. *Clin Obstet Gynecol.* 2011;54(1):28–29.
11. Simpson KR. (2013). *Cervical Ripening and Induction and Augmentation of Labor.* Practice monograph. Washington, DC: Association of Women's Health, Obstetric and Neonatal Nurses; 2013.

SUGGESTED READINGS

American Congress of Obstetricians and Gynecologists. *Dystocia and the augmentation of labor.* ACOG Practice Bulletin 49. (2003, reaffirmed 2011.) Washington, DC: Author; 2003.

Boehm FH, Fields LM, Hutchison JM, et al. The indirectly obtained fetal heart rate: Comparison of first and second generation electronic fetal monitors. *Am J Obstet Gynecol.* 1986;155(1):10–14.

Carter MC. Signal processing and display—cardiotocographs. *Br J Obstet Gynecol.* 1993;100(Suppl. 9):21–23.

Divon MY, Torres FP, Paul RH, Yeh S. Autocorrelation techniques in fetal monitoring. *Am J Obstet Gynecol.* 1985;151(1):2–6.

Fukushima T, Flores CA, Hon EH, Davidson EC, Jr. Limitations of autocorrelation in fetal heart rate monitoring. *Am J Obstet Gynecol.* 1985;153(6):685–692.

Herbert W, Stuart NN, Butler LS. Electronic fetal heart rate monitoring with intrauterine fetal demise. *J Obstet Gynecol Neonat Nurs.* 1987;(July/August)16:249–252.

Rabello YA, Lapidus MR, Paul RH. *Fundamentals of Electronic Fetal Monitoring.* Wallingford, CT: Corometrics Medical Systems; 1988.

CHAPTER 3

Fetal Heart Rate Pattern Interpretation

Most screening techniques used within the field of medicine produce results to which a numeric value or descriptive name can be definitively assigned in an objective manner. The interpretation of fetal heart rate (FHR) patterns, however, bears the unusual distinction of being subjective and contextual in nature. This is due, in part, to the fact that interpretation of the FHR is based on visual assessment performed by individuals who possess varying degrees of experience and education. Interpretation has been further clouded by differing and, at times, conflicting opinion among experts in the practice of electronic fetal monitoring (EFM). Conflict of opinion exists over nomenclature, classification, and significance of EFM patterns. Such dissent exists on the most insular level as is frequently demonstrated between practitioners at the bedside and also on a global level, as is evident by discrepancies in research and reports. For the purpose of clarity, the authors have chosen to utilize the terminology and classification system suggested by The 2008 National Institute of Child Health and Human Development (NICHD) Workshop Report on Electronic Fetal Monitoring Update on Definitions, Interpretation, and Research Guidelines[1] and later adopted by the American College of Obstetricians and Gynecologists[2] and the Association of Women's Health, Obstetric and Neonatal Nurses.[3] Additional FHR patterns and descriptions not addressed by the NICHD Workshop are otherwise referenced. The purpose of this chapter is to improve the reader's recognition of various FHR patterns.

FETAL HEART RATE BASELINE

Baseline Rate

The normal fetus exhibits an overall constancy in its heart rate that can be considered comparable in nature to the resting heart rate of an adult. Most people maintain a certain average heart rate at rest. Although that rate changes with activity or excitement, it is expected to return to its usual rate when such stimuli are not present. This is also true of the fetus.

As explained in detail in Chapter 1, the FHR is controlled by a number of mechanisms. These include the central nervous system (CNS), the autonomic nervous system (ANS), baroreceptors, chemoreceptors, and the endocrine system. As was also explained previously (see Chapter 2), the recorded trend of the FHR is calculated from the time intervals that elapse between successive beats of the fetal heart. Normally, this interval varies slightly from one beat to the next, causing a certain degree of fluctuation to appear in the recorded trend of the baseline FHR. The bulk of these fluctuations are normally consolidated within a relatively constant and discernible plotting of data that is recognized as the *FHR baseline*. Normal FHR baseline falls within the range of 110 to 160 beats per minute (Figure 3–1). According to the NICHD[4] definition, FHR baseline is "determined by approximating the mean FHR rounded to increments of 5 beats per minute (bpm) during a 10-minute window, excluding accelerations and decelerations and periods of marked FHR variability (>25 bpm)." Often, this integer is quickly determined by visual assessment. If the FHR baseline is plotted over a visually wider range, it may be helpful to actually calculate the mean and then round off; for example, if the bulk of the FHR baseline data is visualized as plotted on the fetal strip chart between 125 to 147 bpm, the mean FHR would be arrived at by adding these two integers (125 + 147) and dividing the result by 2 (272 ÷ 2). The mean (in this case, 136) would then be rounded to the nearest increment of 5 (in this case, 135), if necessary. This method of rounding-off is not meant to prompt an intricate process of mathematical calculation; to the contrary, it was intended to encourage simple and practical visual assessment and interpretation.

To discern a trend in the FHR that can be interpreted as the baseline, it is necessary to observe the recording of the FHR over a period of time. The FHR is usually assessed over a minimum of 10 minutes.

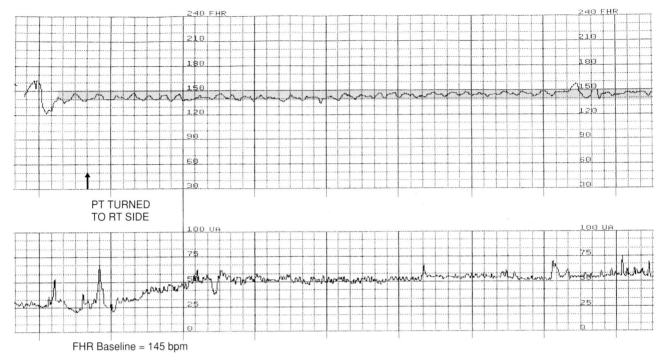

FHR Baseline = 145 bpm

FIGURE 3–1. FHR baseline.

It is important to know that there may be periods during which the FHR baseline cannot be assessed and/or interpreted. As the NICHD[4] definition of FHR baseline states, "excluding accelerations and decelerations and periods of marked FHR variability (>25 bpm)." Accelerations and decelerations are waveform-shaped, transient excursions of the FHR that rise above (accelerations) or fall below (decelerations) the determined FHR baseline and are visually apparent on analysis of the FHR tracing. These waveforms may occur directly in response to contractions (referred to as a *periodic changes*), and some may result from interventions performed by the care team, fetal movement, or maternal positioning, or arise spontaneously (referred to as an *episodic changes*). Accelerations, decelerations, and variability are addressed in detail later in this chapter.

Over the course of any 10-minute portion of the FHR tracing, there must be at least 2 minutes of identifiable baseline data; otherwise, the baseline for that period would be considered *indeterminate*. These 2 minutes of data do not need to occur contiguously to be valid for consideration. If the 10-minute snapshot of FHR data being considered does not contain 2 appreciable minutes of FHR baseline data, the clinician is to refer to the previous 10-minute segment(s) to determine the baseline.[4]

The baseline is the first characteristic of the FHR to be evaluated because it is the parameter against which all other facets of EFM interpretation are based. As mentioned earlier, the baseline is assessed when the FHR is not exhibiting signs of periodic/episodic changes or marked variability. Thus, from a practical standpoint, an optimal time to look for FHR baseline in the laboring patient is in the period immediately prior to the onset of a contraction. Assuming a normal uterine activity pattern, it would be expected that this would be the most likely time when any periodic changes in the FHR, particularly decelerations, would have resolved and the baseline is apt to be most clearly discernible.

Finding the FHR baseline is more than just looking at a segment of the tracing and noting the lowest and highest points where the FHR was recorded. It requires critically evaluating the trend of the FHR at appropriate times to determine the integers between which the bulk of the relevant data are contained. Once the baseline FHR is initially identified for the particular portion of the tracing that is being evaluated, it is useful to reconfirm that finding at other points within the relevant segment of the tracing to ensure accuracy. It is also a good practice to regularly compare observations of the FHR tracing to previously collected data. This process may highlight parameters that may have changed in the interim and help to identify developing trends that may be of concern.

Stork Byte

Worth more than a passing glance . . . correctly interpreting my baseline heart rate keeps you from missing other important characteristics of my heart rate pattern.

Variability

FHR data is collected in a systematic manner. The first parameter to be assessed is the FHR baseline; the next is FHR baseline variability. As mentioned in Chapters 1 and 2, there are normal physiologic variations in the time intervals that elapse between each successive beat of the fetal heart. When the FHR is displayed on the strip chart, these variations are visually apparent in the recorded trend of the FHR (see Appendix C). Fluctuation of the FHR baseline is referred to as *variability*. Variability is an inherent component of the FHR baseline data and, therefore, can only be assessed during the same periods when it is appropriate to assess the baseline FHR.

Stork Byte

Get to know the real me . . . FHR variability is a characteristic of my baseline heart rate. You can only assess it at times when my baseline can be assessed — and that's not during accelerations, decelerations, or contractions!

Moderate Variability

A moderate amount of FHR baseline variability is considered to be fluctuation in the FHR baseline of as little as 6 bpm to as much as 25 bpm (Figure 3–2).[1,2] The presence of *moderate variability* indicates that the autonomic and central nervous systems of the fetus are well developed and well oxygenated. Moderate variability is also a reassuring indication that the fetus is maintaining a measure of tolerance to the changes in blood flow that occur during labor. For the period during which it is observed, moderate variability is highly correlated with the absence of significant metabolic acidemia.[2,5] Attention to and accurate assessment of variability are essential components in the practice of EFM because moderate variability is one of the most important and predictive aspects of the FHR tracing.

Minimal Variability

It may be cause for concern if the FHR baseline appears to have a *minimal variability* (≤5 bpm) or *absent variability* (amplitude range undetectable)[4] because this finding may signify the presence of fetal hypoxia/acidosis. With minimal or absent variability, there is little or no (respectively) discernible fluctuation in the FHR baseline. It is important to consider this finding within the context of the entire clinical picture to more accurately infer its significance in a particular clinical situation.

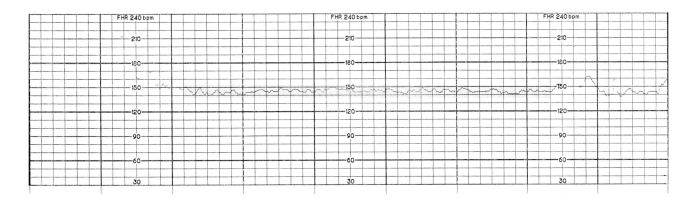

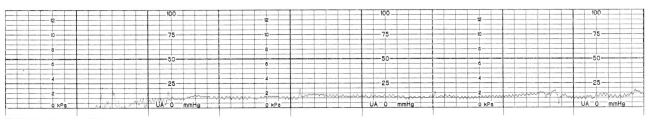

FHR Baseline = 145 bpm

FIGURE 3–2. FHR baseline with moderate variability.

1) 02/22/98 17:05
  17:16 BP 133/58 M 85 P 84

2) 02/22/98 17:06
  COMMENTS: PT INDICATES UNDERSTANDING FOR NEED
  FOR P C/S, ANESTH IN FOR TOP OFF, PREP DONE

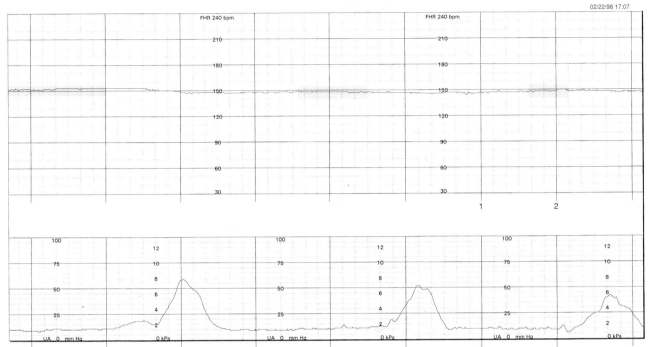

FHR Baseline = 150 bpm

FIGURE 3–3. FHR baseline with minimal variability.

As discussed in Chapter 1, any condition or event that diminishes blood flow to the placenta may deprive the fetus of adequate oxygenation and, if the resulting hypoxemia is sufficient to cause tissue hypoxia and metabolic acidosis, can create a loss of FHR baseline variability. Hypoxic causes of minimal or absent variability are related to diminished blood flow across the placenta or through the umbilical cord. Initially, when such an insult occurs, moderate variability may remain present, indicating that the fetus is effectively compensating for the diminished influx of oxygenated blood. If the cause of decreased perfusion is not corrected; however, variability eventually decreases. This is a warning sign, indicating that the fetus is losing its ability to tolerate or compensate for the stressors placed on it and is becoming hypoxic (Figure 3–3).

The overall correlation between fetal acidemia and minimal or undetectable FHR baseline variability in the presence of decelerations is only 23%. However, deepening of decelerations (periodic/episodic changes in the FHR, discussed later in this chapter) over time, in association with minimal or undetectable FHR baseline variability, may serve as an indicator for intervention.[2,5]

In addition to hypoxia/acidosis, there are other more common reasons for the fetus to exhibit minimal baseline variability. These include fetal sleep, the effects of medications, an immature CNS, fetal dysrhythmias, and cardiac or CNS anomalies. Although fetal sleep is a common cause of minimal variability, it is necessary to remember that this is a transient state that should alternate with periods of moderate variability approximately every 20 to 40 minutes and represents normal fetal physiologic function.[6]

Medications that depress the maternal CNS are likely to produce similar effects on the fetal CNS. Although it is to be expected that variability will decrease after the administration of such medications, this effect on the fetus is temporary. Once the medication is metabolized and excreted, under normal circumstances, variability will return. It is therefore prudent to administer such medications only after fetal well-being has been established. Also, when decreased variability is noted, it is important to review the patient's medication history with her because she may have knowingly or unknowingly exposed the fetus to a sedative or narcotic agent. Loss of variability secondary solely to medication effect does not require intervention.

1) 01/15/01 05:09
   BP 103/58 M 75 P 67
   COMMENTS: ADMIT LABS DRAWN/SENT. PT RESTING
   COMFORTABLY L SIDE.

2) 01/15/01 05:15
   MD CALLED TO EVALUATE PT AND TO BEDSIDE

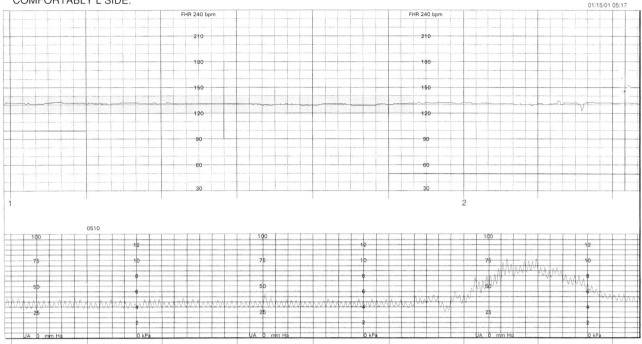

FHR Baseline = 130 bpm

FIGURE 3–4. FHR baseline with absent variability (secondary to fetal anomaly).

The fetus of less than 32 weeks' gestation may exhibit less variability because the ANS may not yet be fully developed (see Chapter 1). It is important to note that, regardless of gestational age, once a fetus has exhibited a certain amount of variability, it has set a standard to which it should be held from that point forward.

Minimal or absent variability is often noted in association with patterns of fetal dysrhythmia. It is also found in the FHR tracings of fetuses with anomalies that affect cardiac, CNS, or ANS functioning. If minimal or absent variability is persistent from the commencement of monitoring and its cause is not known, further investigation is needed (Figure 3–4). If cardiac or CNS anomalies have not previously been ruled out by sonographic examination, it is advisable to have such testing performed.

Steps should be taken to remediate condition(s) suspected of causing minimal or absent variability. These include increasing fetal oxygenation by optimizing blood flow to and through the uterus, placenta, and umbilical cord. This is accomplished by promoting maternal cardiac and hemodynamic functioning (assess maternal vital signs and history; initiate therapies such as position changes and administration of medications, hydration, and oxygen as needed), uteroplacental perfusion (through maternal positioning and eliminating stress of uterine contractions), and blood flow through the umbilical cord (alleviate pressure through maternal positioning). Research utilizing fetal arterial oxygen saturation monitoring (a method of measuring fetal oxygenation directly) scientifically supported that simultaneous use of IV fluid bolus of 1,000 mL, maternal lateral position, and oxygen administration of 10 L/min with a nonrebreather face mask for 15 minutes improves fetal oxygenation.[7] Not all instances of potential hypoxia can be alleviated with such interventions, but it is optimal to perform them in an attempt to support oxygenation of the fetus. If minimal or absent variability is noted at the outset of the monitoring session and there are no other components of the FHR that can be considered reassuring (such as accelerations, explained later in this chapter), then hypoxia should be promptly ruled out. It is possible that a prior hypoxic insult has occurred (Table 3–1).[8,9]

Marked Variability

The presence of more than 25 beats of fluctuation in the FHR baseline is known as *marked variability*

TABLE 3–1 MINIMAL OR ABSENT VARIABILITY

Hypoxic Causes	• Cord prolapse/compression • Maternal hypotension • Tachysystole	• Abruptio placentae • Tachycardia • Dysrhythmia
Nonhypoxic Causes	• Prematurity • Fetal sleep • Medication effect	• Fetal anomaly • Tachycardia • Dysrhythmia

Goal of Intervention	Rationale
Improve uteroplacental blood flow and perfusion through the umbilical cord	Improving the amount and quality of blood flow to the fetus will assist with attempts at recovery

Specific Interventions	Rationale
• Attempt to determine cause	Recognition of causative factors increases efficiency and validates necessity of response.
• If minimal or absent variability is associated with dysrhythmia, obtain sonographic evaluation	Structural examination of fetal heart, heart rate and rhythm, and observation for hydrops, ascites, and other abnormalities should be performed.
• Lateral positioning	Improve maternal circulation and perfusion to placenta; improve blood flow through the umbilical cord.
• Increase IV fluid rate (1,000 mL bolus) unless otherwise contraindicated	Improve maternal circulation and perfusion to placenta; improve maternal hydration to potentiate greater amniotic fluid volume.
• Administer oxygen 10 L/min by nonrebreather mask	Hyperoxygenate maternal blood to increase fetal oxygenation.
• Discontinue oxytocin infusion; remove uterotonic agents; consider tocolytics	Eliminate additional stress of decreased blood flow during contractions until further assessment proves the fetus is not acidotic.
• Assess maternal vital signs	Maternal status directly influences FHR pattern.
• Palpate uterus	Palpation may be the most effective means of determining tachysystole or inadequate uterine resting tone.
• Observe tracing for previously reassuring signs such as accelerations and moderate variability	Accelerations and moderate variability immediately preceding the event suggest that the fetus was not sufficiently hypoxic to produce acidosis prior to entering this episode.
• Initiate procedures to assist in determining fetal acid–base status, such as scalp stimulation. Biophysical profile may also be indicated, depending upon the clinical situation	EFM is only a screening device. Adjunct means of assessment may be helpful in affirming suspicions and making a diagnosis.
• Consider internal monitoring	Internal monitoring with a spiral electrode may provide more accurate assessment.
• Observe for other nonreassuring signs such as rising baseline FHR; marked variability; presence of variable, late, or prolonged decelerations; or bradycardia	These are indicators that the fetal condition may be worsening; operative intervention may be necessary.
• Communicate FHR/UA pattern and interventions to care provider and personnel in charge, and document in medical record	Care provider should assess patient/fetal condition; charge personnel need to plan staffing accordingly and may provide expertise and assistance; medical record should reflect assessments and interventions.
• Prepare for delivery	If minimal or absent variability is found to be of hypoxic etiology and interventions are not effective, expeditious delivery of the fetus is likely indicated.

1) 03/13/00 10:04
  COMMENTS: VE DONE AT THIS TIME BY DR. #1 WHO
  REMAINS IN RM AND IS VIEWING TRACING
  COMMENTS: PT REPOS FROM L TO R SIDE 03/13/00 10:04

2) 03/13/00 10:06
  COMMENTS: DR. #2 IN RM AT THIS TIME TRACING BEING
  VIEWED
  COMMENTS: TERB CALLED FOR IN RM 03/13/00 10:07

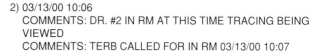

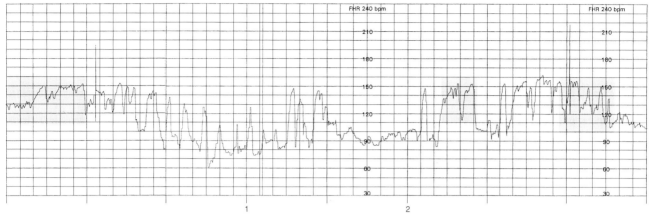

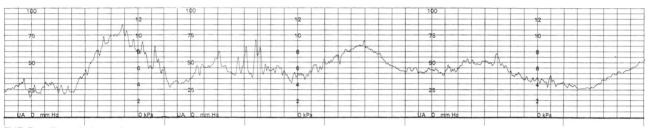

FHR Baseline = indeterminate

FIGURE 3–5. FHR baseline with marked variability.

(Figure 3–5).[4] This pattern is only usually seen intrapartum. Although marked variability is sometimes caused by fetal activity or stimulation, it can also be a sign that the fetus is hemodynamically compromised or mildly hypoxemic.[10] Once again, to put any finding in perspective, it is necessary to consider the entire clinical picture. Query the patient on her perception of fetal activity and attempt to objectively affirm and identify the same. Ensure optimal blood flow to and through the uterus, placenta, and umbilical cord by promoting maternal cardiac and hemodynamic functioning (assess maternal vital signs and history; initiate therapies such as position changes and administration of medications, hydration, and oxygen, as needed). Promote uteroplacental perfusion through maternal positioning and eliminating stress of uterine contractions, and blood flow through the umbilical cord (alleviate pressure through maternal position changes) (Table 3–2).

Tachycardia

If the baseline FHR is maintained above 160 bpm[4] for 10 minutes or longer, this is considered to be a fetal *tachycardia*. A fetal tachycardia may be maternal or fetal in origin. Common conditions that increase maternal heart rate (subsequently raising the FHR) include fever, dehydration, and medication effect. Remediation of the cause of the maternal tachycardia will usually assist the FHR in returning to normal range if the tachycardia is solely of maternal etiology.

Stork Byte

An ounce of prevention . . . Please pay attention to my baseline heart rate! If you see that it's rising, do something to help me—even if my heart rate is still technically within normal limits!

Tachycardia may also result from a fetal compensatory response to hypoxia/acidosis, infection, and tachydysrhythmias. The onset of fetal tachycardia or a rising FHR baseline should be considered serious because it is one of the first signs that the fetus is becoming hypoxic/acidotic. As described previously (see Chapter 1), when there is decreased maternal–fetal perfusion, baroreceptors and chemoreceptors in the

TABLE 3–2 MARKED VARIABILITY

Hypoxic Causes	• Cord prolapse/compression • Maternal hypotension • Tachysystole • Abruptio placentae
Nonhypoxic Causes	• Fetal activity • Fetal stimulation

Goal of Intervention	Rationale
Improve uteroplacental blood flow and perfusion through the umbilical cord	Improving the amount and quality of blood flow to the fetus will assist with attempts at recovery

Specific Interventions	Rationale
• Attempt to determine cause	Recognition of causative factors increases efficiency and validates necessity of response.
• Lateral positioning	Improve maternal circulation and perfusion to placenta; improve blood flow through the umbilical cord.
• Increase IV fluid rate (1,000 mL bolus) unless otherwise contraindicated	Improve maternal circulation and perfusion to placenta; improve maternal hydration to potentiate greater amniotic fluid volume.
• Administer oxygen 10 L/min by nonrebreather mask	Hyperoxygenate maternal blood to increase fetal oxygenation.
• Discontinue oxytocin infusion; remove uterotonic agents; consider tocolytics	Eliminate additional stress of decreased blood flow during contractions until further assessment proves the fetus is not acidotic.
• Assess maternal vital signs	Maternal status directly influences FHR pattern.
• Palpate uterus	or inadequate uterine resting tone may be the most effective means of determining tachysystole.
• Observe tracing for previously reassuring signs such as accelerations and moderate variability	Accelerations and moderate variability suggest that the fetus was not sufficiently hypoxic to produce acidosis upon entering this episode.
• Initiate procedures to assist in determining fetal acid–base status, such as scalp stimulation. Biophysical profile may also be indicated, depending upon the clinical situation	EFM is only a screening device. Adjunct means of assessment may be helpful in affirming suspicions and making a diagnosis.
• Consider internal monitoring	Internal monitoring with a spiral electrode may provide more accurate assessment.
• Observe for other nonreassuring signs, such as rising baseline FHR; minimal or absent variability; presence of variable, late, or prolonged decelerations; or bradycardia	These are indicators that the fetal condition may be worsening; operative intervention may be necessary.
• Communicate FHR/UA pattern and interventions to care provider and personnel in charge, and document in medical record	Care provider should assess patient/fetal condition; charge personnel need to plan staffing accordingly and may provide expertise and assistance; medical record should reflect assessments and interventions.
• Prepare for delivery	If marked variability is found to be of hypoxic etiology and interventions are not effective, expeditious delivery of the fetus is likely indicated.

fetus trigger an increase in the FHR. Clinical opportunities to maximize maternal–fetal exchange include avoiding and remediating problems such as tachysystole (Figure 3–6) and maternal hypotension. In either of these cases, correcting the cause (e.g., discontinuing oxytocin, removal/reversal of uterotonic agents, changing the maternal position) may improve fetal oxygenation and assist the FHR in recovery to its normal range. In the event of infection or tachydysrhythmia, the usual means of intrauterine resuscitation should be employed (i.e., position changes, increased maternal hydration and oxygenation, and decreasing stressors

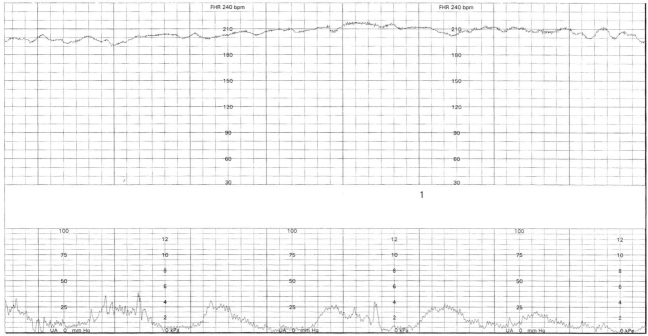

FHR Baseline = 205 bpm

FIGURE 3–6. FHR baseline tachycardia (with tachysystole).

on the fetus such as contractions) in addition to any other medical or pharmaceutical remedies ordered (Table 3–3). Although the normal processes of physiologic development (discussed in Chapter 1) influence the FHR baseline and may cause it to be toward the higher ranges of normal in the preterm fetus, it is important to know that the 110 to 160 bpm baseline FHR range also applies to the preterm fetus. Tachycardia of the FHR baseline in a preterm fetus should be investigated.

Bradycardia

An FHR baseline that is below 110 bpm[4] for a period of 10 minutes or longer is termed a *bradycardia*. This can occur in response to a variety of acute and chronic conditions that may be of hypoxic or non-hypoxic etiology. Also, just as it is understood that adults have varying degrees of normal, the same concept applies to the fetus. On occasion, an FHR baseline may be less than 110 bpm but also have reassuring signs present that demonstrate that the fetus is not acidemic (such as moderate variability and/or accelerations), and that rate may be accepted as normal for a particular fetus.

Hypoxic Etiology

The fetus suffering from untreated chronic deprivation of oxygen has a distinct, suspicious-looking tracing.[11] Typically, either variable or late decelera-

tions are present, denoting a decrease of blood flow through either the umbilical cord or the placenta. As the fetus becomes increasingly hypoxic, carbon dioxide accumulates in the fetal blood. This stimulates the chemoreceptors and causes a compensatory elevation in the FHR. As the increase in the FHR baseline continues, FHR baseline variability decreases and any periodic/episodic changes of the FHR that are present may become less visually apparent. The final phase in this process is bradycardia, a terminal event in the case of prolonged fetal hypoxia or asphyxia.

This chain of events is rarely seen in its entirety because surgical intervention usually preempts its completion. It is also possible for the early phases of progressive fetal compromise to be concealed from the clinician because it may have occurred before admission. This clouds assessment of the FHR tracing because there is no normal pattern to which comparison can be made and deviations identified. For instance, the patient may present for fetal monitoring with an FHR that is technically within normal limits and is without decelerations but lacks both accelerations and variability. Interpretation of such a tracing may be confounding and, therefore, it is imperative to promptly determine the status of fetal oxygenation. A biophysical profile may be useful for this purpose. Scalp stimulation, discussed in Chapter 1, can be

TABLE 3–3 TACHYCARDIA

Related to Maternal Conditions	• Fever • Dehydration • Medication effect	• Anxiety • Thyroid disease
Related to Fetal/Intrauterine Conditions	• Chorioamnionitis • Hypoxia/acidosis • Dysrhythmia	

Goal of Intervention	Rationale
Improve uteroplacental blood flow and perfusion through the umbilical cord	Improving the amount and quality of blood flow to the fetus will assist with attempts at recovery

Specific Interventions	Rationale
• Attempt to determine cause; assess patient history	Recognition of causative factors increases efficiency of response, allows prompt rule out and/or treatment of nonhypoxic causes (fever, dehydration, medication effects, anxiety).
• If tachycardia is associated with dysrhythmia, obtain sonographic evaluation	Structural examination of fetal heart, heart rate and rhythm, and observation for hydrops, ascites, and other abnormalities should be performed.
• Provide explanation, education, support, and comfort measures to patient and her support persons as needed	Maternal anxiety may cause catecholamine release, shunting blood away from the uterus.
• Ensure thyroid disease is under control	Thyroid-stimulating hormone can cross the placenta to the fetus and cause tachycardia.
• Lateral positioning	Improve maternal circulation and perfusion to placenta; improve blood flow through the umbilical cord.
• Assess maternal vital signs, especially temperature and pulse. Periodically reassess for maternal fever.	Maternal fever causes the fetus to become tachycardic. In cases of chorioamnionitis, the fetus often becomes tachycardic before maternal temperature rises. Maternal temperature should be reassessed frequently and treated.
• Increase IV fluid rate (1,000 mL bolus) unless otherwise contraindicated	Improve maternal circulation and perfusion to placenta; improve maternal hydration to potentiate greater amniotic fluid volume.
• Administer oxygen 10 L/min by nonrebreather mask	Hyperoxygenate maternal blood to increase fetal oxygenation.
• Discontinue oxytocin infusion, uterotonic agents; consider tocolytics	Eliminate additional stress of decreased blood flow during contractions until further assessment proves the fetus is not acidotic.
• Observe tracing for reassuring signs such as accelerations and moderate variability	Accelerations and moderate variability suggest that the fetus is not sufficiently hypoxic to produce acidosis.
• Initiate procedures to assist in determining fetal acid–base status, such as scalp stimulation. Biophysical profile may also be indicated, depending upon the clinical situation	EFM is only a screening device. Adjunct means of assessment may be helpful in affirming suspicions and making a diagnosis.
• Consider internal monitoring	Internal monitoring with a spiral electrode may provide more accurate assessment (rule out erroneous signals).
• Observe for other nonreassuring signs such as continuously rising baseline FHR; minimal, absent, or marked variability; presence of variable, late, or prolonged decelerations; bradycardia	These are indicators that the fetal condition may be worsening; operative intervention may be necessary.
• Communicate FHR/UA pattern and interventions to care provider and personnel in charge, and document in medical record	Care provider should assess patient/fetal condition; charge personnel need to plan staffing accordingly and may provide expertise and assistance; medical record should reflect assessments and interventions.
• Prepare for delivery	Emergent delivery is likely if FHR continues to rise or if other nonreassuring signs are present and interventions are not effective.

very useful in such an instance, as long as a deceleration or bradycardia is not in progress at the time this method is employed. Fetal scalp stimulation is a simple procedure and may be helpful in determining whether the fetus is presenting to the clinical setting having already sustained neurologic impairment.

Examples of hypoxic events related to bradycardia include cord prolapse/compression, maternal hypotension, tachysystole, abruptio placentae, or uterine rupture. If the insult that initiated the bradycardia is acute and remediable in nature (such as cord compression, maternal hypotension, and tachysystole) and is identified and treated expeditiously, it is possible that the FHR will return to its normal range. If it does not, a promptly executed cesarean or assisted birth may be indicated.

Cord compression/occlusion can be precipitated by the actions or positioning of the fetus or by such conditions as nuchal cord, cord entanglement, short or knotted cord, occult or overt prolapse, or oligohydramnios. Transient compression of the cord due to fetal position or movement is usually corrected by altering maternal–fetal position. Cord entanglements are not as easily reversible, and hypoxia/acidosis can result. Although position changes may help in the instance of partial or occult prolapse, an overt prolapse requires emergent intervention.

Prolonged or persistent cord compression can result in fetal bradycardia with minimal or absent variability. This type of FHR pattern may precede death in utero and is therefore extremely concerning (Figure 3–7).

Although decreased oxygenation of the fetus is associated with acute episodes of bradycardia (as may result from transitory events of tachysystole or maternal hypotension), variability will usually remain present, provided such occurrences are short-lived. Once the event is corrected and fetal oxygenation resumes, the FHR will usually recover to its prior baseline rate. Chronically decreased blood flow across the uteroplacental unit is also likely to result in FHR bradycardia. This ongoing instance of hypoxia is more concerning however, as demonstrated by minimal or absent variability of the FHR baseline and the inability to recover with interventions (Figure 3–8).

Bradycardia is the most common FHR change when uterine rupture occurs during a trial of labor after a previous cesarean birth. Before the onset of the bradycardia, FHR patterns have been reported to range from reassuring to those with variable or late decelerations and fetal tachycardia.[12,13] This type of bradycardia is representative of fetal hypoxia and requires immediate intervention. In Leung's study, it was noted that fetal intolerance was the

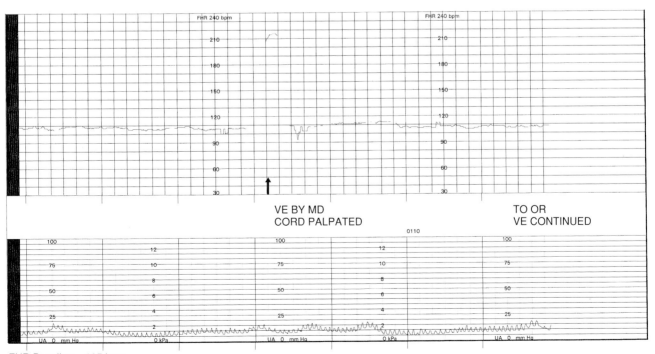

FHR Baseline = 105 bpm

FIGURE 3–7. FHR baseline bradycardia (with cord compression).

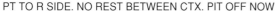

1) 05/25/99 04:24
   MD CALLED TO VIEW TRACING
2) 05/25/99 04:25
   PT TO L SIDE
3) 05/25/99 04:27
   PT TO R SIDE. NO REST BETWEEN CTX. PIT OFF NOW

4) 05/25/99 04:28
   PT TO KNEE CHEST. IV OPEN. O2 ON.
5) 05/25/99 04:29
   MD PRESENT. VE. NO CORD FELT
6) VE CONTINUES. C/S EXPL TO PT

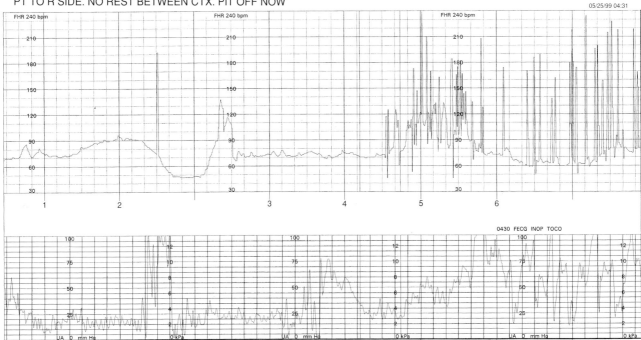

FHR Baseline = Indeterminate

FIGURE 3–8. FHR baseline bradycardia (with tachysystole).

most common signal and that significant neonatal morbidity occurred if a fetal bradycardia lasted 18 minutes or longer before surgical intervention.[12] The rate of perinatal asphyxia after uterine rupture is reported to be 5.1%.[14]

If a trial of labor is attempted after a previous cesarean birth, the onset of bradycardia should be seen as a red flag until proven otherwise. Although it is possible for bradycardia to result from other causes (such as those discussed previously in this chapter), the consequences of uterine rupture are severe enough to warrant preparation for operative delivery if the bradycardia cannot be promptly reversed. In the event that the FHR does not recover with primary interventions (maternal position change, administration of intravenous fluids and oxygen, discontinuation of oxytocin, or removal of uterotonic agents and/or the administration of tocolytics[2,15]), expeditious cesarean delivery is indicated (Figure 3–9).

Nonhypoxic Etiology

If the bradycardia is due to a nonhypoxic cause, such as vagal stimulation during the second stage of labor,[10] it is possible that the fetus can recover. In the second stage of labor, intense intracranial pressure occurs as the fetal head descends through the maternal pelvis and vagina. A second-stage bradycardia may be seen in the adequately oxygenated fetus as a normal response to stimulation of the vagus nerve. The key factor in recognizing the difference between hypoxic and nonhypoxic bradycardia is FHR baseline variability. In hypoxic cases of bradycardia, FHR baseline variability is minimal or absent, whereas, in nonhypoxic instances, it will usually remain moderate (Table 3–4).

PERIODIC/EPISODIC CHANGES OF THE FETAL HEART RATE

Once FHR baseline and FHR baseline variability have been determined, the next step in a systematic review of the FHR is to assess for changes in the FHR that may occur in response to contractions (periodic changes) or that may occur intermittently, resulting from other, noncyclic events (episodic changes). Periodic and episodic changes include various types of

1) 02/06/01 03:30
  COMMENTS: VE BY MD, NO PROLAPSE, UNABLE TO
  ASSESS DILATION. PT C/O PAIN, ANESTHESIA CALLED
  FOR TOP UP.

2) 02/06/01 03:34
  STRIP REVIEWED BY RN; COMMENTS: MD ASSESSING
  TRACING. PT REPOSITIONED LEFT TO RT SIDE, O2
  REMAINS ON 10L VIA FACE MASK, IV FLUIDS REMAIN
  INFUSING, OR TEAM NOTIFIED

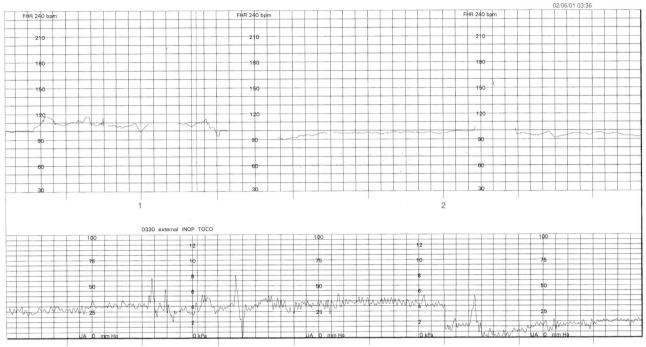

FHR Baseline = 105 bpm

FIGURE 3–9. FHR baseline bradycardia (with uterine rupture).

accelerations and decelerations of the FHR detailed below.

Accelerations

Spontaneous and Induced Accelerations

The term *acceleration* describes the occurrence of a transient increase in the FHR of an amplitude of 15 beats or greater above the FHR baseline, continuing for 15 seconds or longer.[2,4] The duration of the acceleration is assessed from the time the FHR departs from the baseline until its return. Most accelerations return to baseline within 2 minutes (Figure 3–10).

As discussed previously, the premature fetus may not yet have developed full physiologic maturity, particularly in relation to ANS functioning. At less than 32 weeks' gestation, it cannot be assumed that the fetus has the capacity to produce accelerations of ≥15 bpm × ≥15 seconds. Therefore, in the fetus of less than 32 weeks' gestation, accelerations may be satisfactory if there is a transient increase above the FHR baseline by ≥10 bpm that is sustained for ≥10 seconds duration.[2,4] This finding may be significant as an indicator of well-being in the preterm fetus that has not previously demonstrated the ability to accelerate its

heart rate according to the 15 bpm × 15 seconds criterion. Even if it occurs at less than the gestational age expected, once a fetus has demonstrated a certain level of functioning, it should be expected to reproduce those findings or achieve better in all subsequent testing.

Accelerations are an important finding because they indicate that the fetus has a functioning ANS and is not experiencing acidosis.[16] Accelerations are an expected and reassuring event on the tracing of the fetus that is older than 32 weeks' gestation. Accelerations often occur spontaneously, in relation to fetal movement or contractions (Figures 3–11 and 3–12). They also may be induced during the antepartum by the application of a fetal acoustic stimulator to the maternal abdomen (discussed in Chapter 4). Accelerations may also be induced by fetal scalp stimulation.

Although the absence of accelerations can be a nonreassuring finding, this may also occur for relatively brief periods of time due to fetal sleep (expected to last no longer than 40 minutes). Accelerations may be absent for longer periods due to the effects of medication, as can occur with narcotics, propranolol, and magnesium sulfate.[17,18]

TABLE 3–4 BRADYCARDIA

Hypoxic Causes	• Cord prolapse/compression • Abruptio placentae • Maternal hypotension • Uterine rupture • Tachysystole
Nonhypoxic Causes	• Bradydysrhythmia • Vagal stimulation during the second stage of labor • Hypothermia (fetal dive reflex)

Goal of Intervention	Rationale
Improve uteroplacental blood flow and perfusion through the umbilical cord Specific Interventions	Improving the amount and quality of blood flow to the fetus will assist with attempts at recovery Rationale

Specific Interventions	Rationale
• Attempt to determine cause	Recognition of causative factors increases efficiency of response.
• Be cognizant of patient history, particularly previous uterine surgery and/or cesarean birth	Patient with such history is at increased risk of uterine rupture.
• Maintain normal intrauterine temperature by assuring fluid used during amnioinfusion or for flushing fluid-filled intrauterine pressure catheter is at least room temperature. A blood warmer is an acceptable means of warming fluid to assure temperature	Infusion of cold fluid into the uterus may cause a parasympathetic response in the fetus (also known as a "dive reflex") that results in bradycardia.
• Vaginal examination	Check for cord prolapse. If prolapse is detected, lift presenting part off the umbilical cord and continue to do so until delivery of the fetus.
• Discontinue oxytocin infusion; remove uterotonic agents; consider tocolytics	Eliminate additional stress of decreased blood flow during contractions until further assessment proves the fetus is not acidotic.
• Positioning—left lateral, right lateral, knee–chest	Reposition until successful, giving each position a chance to take effect. Improve maternal circulation and perfusion to placenta; improve blood flow through the umbilical cord.
• Increase IV fluid rate (1,000 mL bolus) unless otherwise contraindicated	Improve maternal circulation and perfusion to placenta; improve maternal hydration to potentiate greater amniotic fluid volume.
• Administer oxygen 10 L/min by nonrebreather mask	Hyperoxygenate maternal blood to increase fetal oxygenation.
• Assess maternal vital signs	Maternal status directly influences FHR pattern.
• Palpate uterus	Palpation may be the most effective means of determining tachysystole or inadequate uterine resting tone.
• Observe tracing for previously reassuring signs such as accelerations, moderate variability	Accelerations and moderate variability immediate preceding the event suggest that the fetus was not sufficiently hypoxic to produce acidosis prior to entering this episode.
• When FHR returns to baseline, initiate procedures to assist in determining fetal acid–base status, such as scalp stimulation.	EFM is only a screening device. Adjunct means of assessment may be helpful in affirming suspicions and making a diagnosis.
• Consider internal monitoring	Internal monitoring with a spiral electrode may provide more accurate assessment of the FHR (rule out erroneous signals).
• Consider sonographic evaluation	Direct visualization of the fetal heart may be helpful in ruling out artifactual signals (such as maternal heart rate, half- or double-counting) or fetal dysrhythmias. A biophysical examination may be done after the FHR has recovered to the baseline to assess fetal condition for signs of asphyxia/hypoxia.
• Observe for other previously nonreassuring signs such as rising baseline FHR; minimal, absent, or marked variability; presence of variable, late, or prolonged decelerations	These are indicators that the fetal condition had been progressively worsening before the bradycardia; operative intervention is likely.
• Communicate FHR/UA pattern and interventions to care provider and personnel in charge, and document in medical record	Care provider should assess patient/fetal condition immediately; charge personnel need to plan staffing accordingly and may provide expertise and assistance; medical record should reflect assessments and interventions.
• Prepare for delivery	If interventions are not effective and the bradycardia is of hypoxic etiology, emergent delivery is likely.

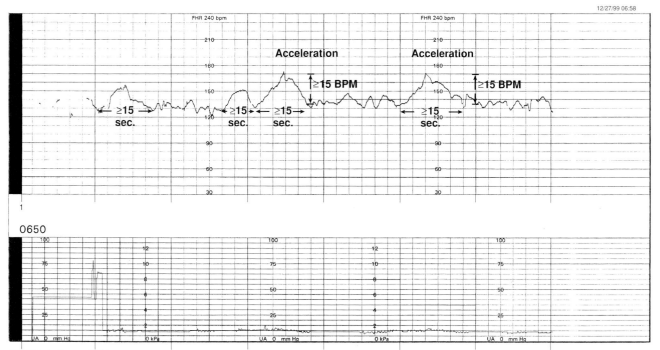

FHR Baseline = 135 bpm

FIGURE 3–10. Spontaneous accelerations (arrows denote 15 beats above FHR baseline, 15 seconds length).

Stork Byte

Functioning at full capacity . . . accelerations of my heart rate tell you that I am getting enough oxygen and my neurologic system is well-oxygenated.

Uniform Accelerations

Some FHR accelerations maintain a very distinctive appearance and have a different etiology than spontaneous or induced accelerations. These are known as *uniform accelerations*. Uniform accelerations are

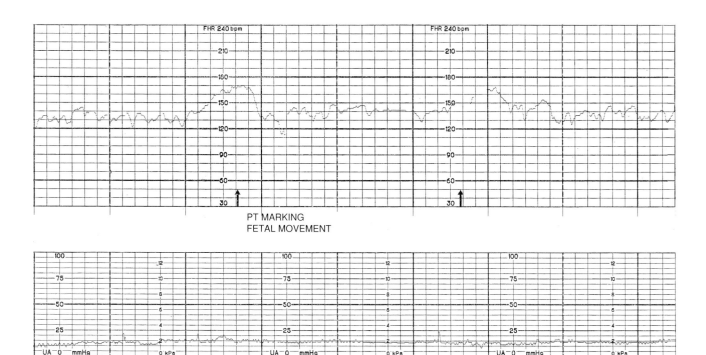

FHR Baseline = 140 bpm

FIGURE 3–11. Accelerations in response to fetal movement.

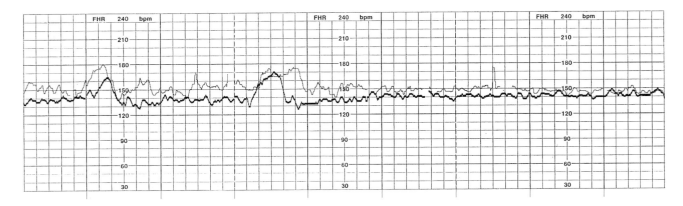

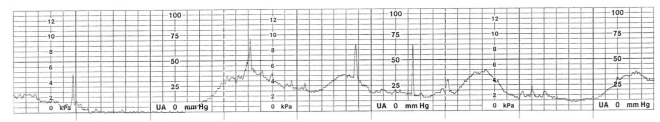

Twin A FHR Baseline = 130 bpm; Twin B FHR Baseline = 150 bpm

FIGURE 3–12. Accelerations of both fetal heart rates in a twin gestation.

a pattern of accelerations that present simultaneously with contractions and maintain a very similar (uniform) shape with each occurrence. The presence of uniform accelerations is usually a benign response to one of two conditions: breech presentation or mild cord compression. Although accelerations are considered a reassuring finding regardless of their etiology, for purposes of appropriate clinical management, it is helpful to understand what is precipitating their appearance.

When the fetus is in a breech position, contractions of the uterus may cause a sympathetic response as the fetal torso is stimulated. Concurrently, there is an absence of parasympathetic stimulation that would normally occur when the fetal head is pressed into the pelvis during contractions. These events result in a pattern of transient increases in the FHR during contractions known as uniform accelerations. If the position of the fetus has not been confirmed and a pattern of uniform accelerations is noted, assessment for presentation is warranted.[6]

Another reason for the appearance of uniform accelerations is that the umbilical cord may be in a position that makes it vulnerable to pressure during a contraction.[19] The force exerted on the umbilical cord may be sufficient to inhibit flow through the umbilical vein, but not of a degree great enough to affect perfusion through the sturdier walls of the

umbilical arteries. The subsequent decrease in blood flow to the fetus caused by compression of the umbilical vein during the contraction elicits a sympathetic response in the fetus. The resulting increases of the FHR noted to occur simultaneously with contractions are uniform accelerations (Figure 3–13).

When uniform accelerations are present, it is important to also consider the possibility that maternal heart rate is being erroneously recorded (discussed in Chapter 2), especially if the baseline heart rate is in the lower ranges of normal or below normal. If this is the case, the increase in a woman's heart rate that occurs as she experiences pain or exerts expulsive efforts during contractions could be mistaken for accelerations of the FHR (Figure 3–14).[20] To eliminate confusion any time there is a question of maternal versus fetal signal, the best method is to palpate the maternal pulse and compare it to the monitor's audible signal. Document these important bedside findings so that they can be clear to any other clinicians who may evaluate the tracing. If the question of maternal signal is an ongoing issue then, additionally (but not to take the place of comparison of the palpated maternal pulse to the audible signal), for documentation purposes, it is useful if the maternal heart rate can also be automatically obtained and printed or trended directly on the fetal strip chart. If there is any uncertainty,

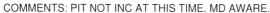

1) 01/17/01 09:34
   BP 112/75 M 90 P 85.
   COMMENTS: PIT NOT INC AT THIS TIME. MD AWARE.

2) 01/17/01 09:38
   COMMENTS: PIT DEC TO 4 MU/MIN PER MD ORDER.

01/17/01 09:39

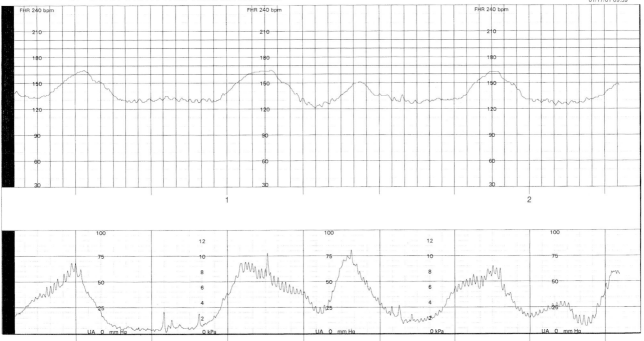

FHR Baseline = 130 bpm

FIGURE 3–13. Uniform accelerations of the FHR.

sonographic evaluation may be useful to visually confirm fetal cardiac activity.

Prolonged Accelerations

When accelerations of the FHR occur for a period at least 2 minutes but continue for less than 10 minutes in duration, they are known as *prolonged accelerations.*[4] As with the accelerations discussed previously, prolonged accelerations peak at amplitude of at least 15 bpm above the FHR baseline. Their distinguishing characteristic, however, is their duration—an interval of between 2 and 10 minutes.

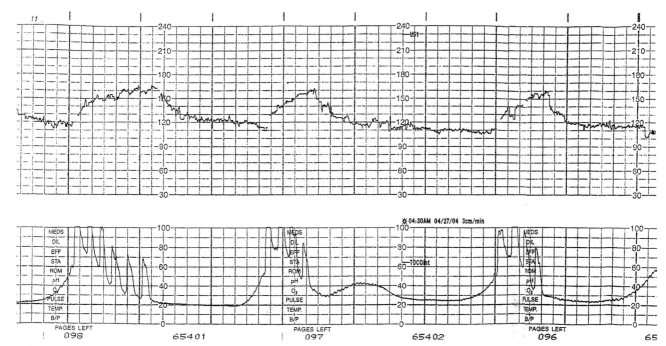

FIGURE 3–14. Maternal heart rate (MHR) showing increases during expulsive efforts.

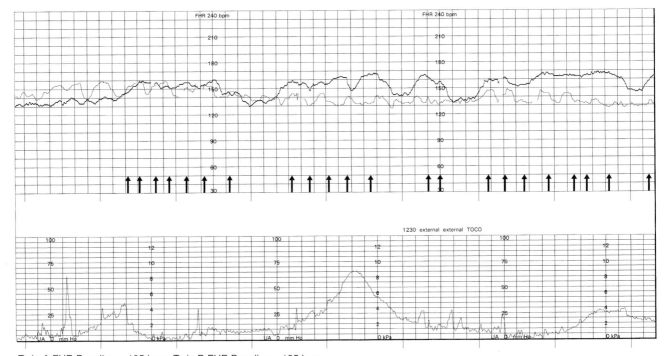

Twin A FHR Baseline = 135 bpm; Twin B FHR Baseline = 135 bpm

FIGURE 3–15. Prolonged accelerations. (Fetus "B," indicated by the heavier density tracing, responds to movement by accelerating its heart rate ≥2 minutes, but ≤10 minutes.)

Prolonged accelerations are a reassuring indication of fetal well-being (Figure 3–15).

Decelerations

Transient decreases in the FHR can occur in relation to the stress of contractions or can be triggered by other physiologic events. There are specific criteria by which such changes of the FHR are evaluated for identification and clinical management purposes. These include:

- Depth (measured in beats per minute)
- Descent (time, in seconds, from the onset of the deceleration to its nadir)
- Duration (length of the deceleration as measured from its onset to recovery)
- Timing (in relation to/in the absence of contractions)
- Other factors that are considered include shape, frequency of occurrence, and the amount of variability present in the FHR baseline.

Early Decelerations

Early decelerations are usually thought to result from compression of the fetal head and are not associated with fetal hypoxia (see Chapter 1). This pattern can occur with cephalopelvic disproportion, fetal descent, cervical examination, forceps application, or as a result of the fetal head being pressed into the pelvis during contractions. Early decelerations are often seen during the later phases of active labor. Pressure exerted on the fetal head during contractions stimulates the parasympathetic nervous system and subsequently slows the FHR. This is a normal physiologic event that does not require treatment (Figure 3–16). See Table 3–5 for the characteristics of early decelerations usually seen on visual assessment of the FHR tracing.

Late Decelerations

Late decelerations indicate a reflex fetal response to hypoxemia resulting from maternal, fetal, or placental conditions that impede the necessary provision of oxygen from the mother to the fetus. Late decelerations maintain many of the same visually apparent attributes as early decelerations; however, they are readily distinguishable by their timing in relation to contractions (Table 3–6; Figure 3–17).

As explained in Chapter 1, only a minimal amount of oxygen at most crosses the placenta during a contraction. The fetus experiencing prolonged periods of hypoxia before the onset of contractions may already be compromised. Therefore, when contractions begin and blood flow diminishes, the FHR slows in response to the level of hypoxemia. The

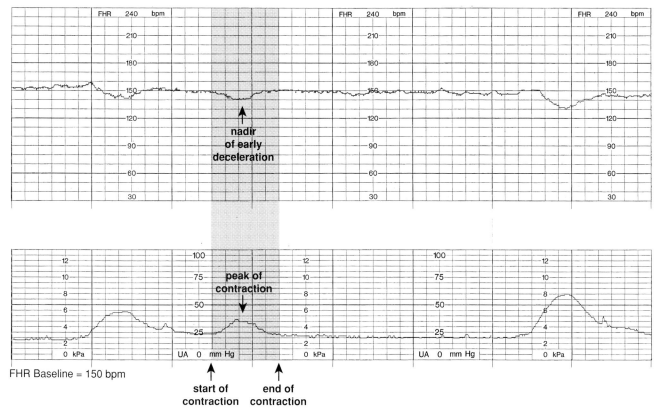

FHR Baseline = 150 bpm

FIGURE 3–16. Early deceleration.

FHR remains lowered until the contraction ends and maternal–fetal exchange resumes. The FHR then slowly returns to the baseline rate.

Stork Byte

How deeply my heart rate drops during late decelerations does not tell you how bad my problem is; I may be in worse condition when my heart rate is falling below the baseline by only a few beats per minute. Be sure to consider my baseline FHR, especially variability!

Previously well-oxygenated fetuses also demonstrate late decelerations when faced with an acute decrease in oxygenation. This often occurs with tachysystole due to oxytocin administration or maternal hypotension secondary to either supine positioning or administration of a regional anesthetic. If the contractions are occurring too close together, uteroplacental blood flow can remain diminished throughout the episode of tachysystole. As well, if maternal blood pressure is low due to her positioning, there may be suboptimal uteroplacental perfusion as blood is diverted to organs more critical

TABLE 3–5 CHARACTERISTICS OF EARLY DECELERATIONS

Descent	Gradual; onset to nadir ≥30 Seconds
Duration	≥15 seconds and <2 minutes; usually about the same length as concurrent contractions
Timing	Simultaneous with contractions; early decelerations usually begin when the contraction starts, reach their nadir as the contraction reaches its peak, and conclude by the time the contraction has ended
Shape	Symmetrical
Frequency of occurrence	Recurrent (appearing with ≥50% of contractions/20 minute window) or intermittent (occurring with <50% of contractions/20 minute window)

Adapted from Macones et al.[1]

TABLE 3–6 CHARACTERISTICS OF LATE DECELERATIONS

Descent	Gradual; onset to nadir ≥30 Seconds
Duration	≥15 seconds and <2 minutes; usually about the same length as concurrent contractions
Timing	Offset from contractions; late decelerations usually begin after the contraction has started and reach their nadir after the contraction has reached its peak; the FHR does not return to baseline rate until after the contraction has ended
Shape	Symmetrical
Frequency of occurrence	Recurrent (appearing with ≥50% of contractions/20 minute window) or intermittent (occurring with <50% of contractions/20 minute window)

Adapted from Macones et al.[1]

to maternal survival (i.e., maternal heart and brain) (Table 3–7).

Variable Decelerations

Variable decelerations are usually considered to occur in relation to compression of the umbilical cord. They have also been identified as resulting from head compression in the second stage of labor secondary to vagal stimulation.[21] Any factor that inhibits the umbilical cord from floating freely (e.g., actions or positioning of the fetus, monoamniotic multiple gestation, nuchal cord, cord entanglement,

short or knotted cord, occult or overt prolapse, oligohydramnios, or thick meconium) may lead to the presence of variable decelerations. If the umbilical cord is compressed, blood flow into or out of the fetal circulation may be impeded. In response, the FHR drops abruptly. Once the cord compression/occlusion is alleviated, the FHR usually returns to its normal baseline rate. If variable decelerations are recurrent, persist over a prolonged period of time, and do not respond to treatment, the fetus may become hypoxic.

Variable decelerations have a very different appearance from other types of decelerations. The

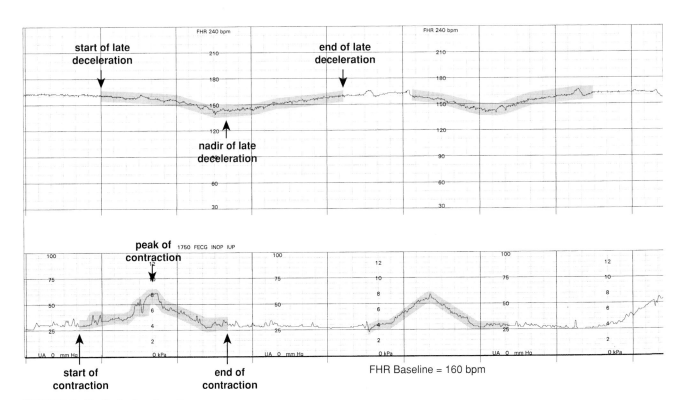

FIGURE 3–17. Late decelerations.

TABLE 3-7 LATE DECELERATIONS

Related to Maternal Conditions	• Hypertension/vascular disease • Cardiac status • Hypotension • Anemia	• Diabetes • Smoking • Tachysystole
Related to Fetal/Placental Conditions	• Postterm • Intrauterine growth restriction • Abruptio placentae	• Chorioamnionitis • Placenta previa/hemorrhage

Goal of Intervention	Rationale
Improve uteroplacental perfusion	Improving the amount and quality of blood flow to the fetus will assist with attempts at recovery

Specific Interventions	Rationale
• Lateral positioning	Improve maternal circulation and perfusion to the placenta.
• Increase IV fluid rate (1,000 mL bolus) unless otherwise contraindicated	Improve maternal circulation and perfusion to placenta.
• Administer oxygen 10 L/min by nonrebreather mask	Hyperoxygenate maternal blood to increase fetal oxygenation.
• Discontinue oxytocin infusion; remove uterotonic agents; consider tocolytics	Eliminate additional stress of decreased blood flow during contractions until further assessment proves the fetus is not acidotic.
• Palpate uterus	Palpation may be the most effective means of determining tachysystole or inadequate uterine resting tone.
• Assess maternal vital signs	Maternal status directly influences FHR patterns.
• Observe for reassuring signs such as accelerations and moderate variability	Accelerations and moderate variability suggest that the fetus is not sufficiently hypoxic to produce acidosis.
• Initiate procedures to assist in determining fetal acid–base status, such as scalp stimulation.	EFM is only a screening device. Adjunct means of assessment may be helpful in affirming suspicions and making a diagnosis.
• Consider internal monitoring	Internal monitoring with a spiral electrode may provide more accurate assessment of the FHR.
• Consider BPP	BPP may be helpful in assessing for signs of hypoxia/asphyxia.
• Observe for other nonreassuring signs such as rising baseline FHR; minimal, absent, or marked variability; variable or prolonged decelerations; bradycardia	These are indicators that the fetal condition is worsening. If interventions are not improving fetal status, operative intervention may be necessary.
• Communicate FHR/UA pattern and interventions to care provider and personnel in charge, and document in medical record	Care provider should assess patient/fetal condition; charge personnel need to plan staffing accordingly and may provide expertise and assistance; medical record should reflect assessments and interventions.
• Prepare for delivery	If interventions are not effective and the late deceleration pattern continues, operative or assisted delivery may be indicated.

TABLE 3–8 CHARACTERISTICS OF VARIABLE DECELERATIONS

Depth	Drop in FHR of ≥15 beats below the FHR baseline
Descent	Abrupt: onset to nadir <30 seconds
Duration	≥15 seconds and <2 minutes
Timing	May occur in relation to contractions (periodic) and may also happen independently of contractions (episodic)
Shape	Inconsistent, irregular: may appear similar to one another or differ; shoulders or overshoots may further differentiate appearance.
Frequency of occurrence	Can appear singularly, or as intermittent (with <50% of contractions in a 20-minute segment), or recurrent (with >50% of contractions in a 20-minute window)

Adapted from Macones et al.[1]

abruptness of their onset and sharp decline of the FHR usually make them readily identifiable. Common characteristics of variable decelerations are shown in Table 3–8 (Figure 3–18).

Stork Byte

Hey, look at me! Sometimes I squeeze my umbilical cord just to get attention!

Variable decelerations can often be eliminated with position changes (Table 3–9). Amnioinfusion is another effective means for remediating the variable deceleration pattern.[22,23] Results are usually seen within half an hour of beginning this procedure. Amnioinfusion is often indicated in cases where cord compression due to decreased amniotic fluid or fluid thickened by meconium is an issue and expedient delivery is not indicated. Amnioinfusion is accomplished by the instillation of sterile normal saline or lactated Ringer's solution into the uterine cavity through a device such as an intra-uterine pressure catheter. This is accomplished by bolus dose or maintenance dose, with or without use of an infusion pump, and with or without use of a blood warmer, depending on hospital protocol. A number of variations of amnioinfusion technique exist and are effective. Amnioinfusion remains a reasonable approach in the treatment of repetitive

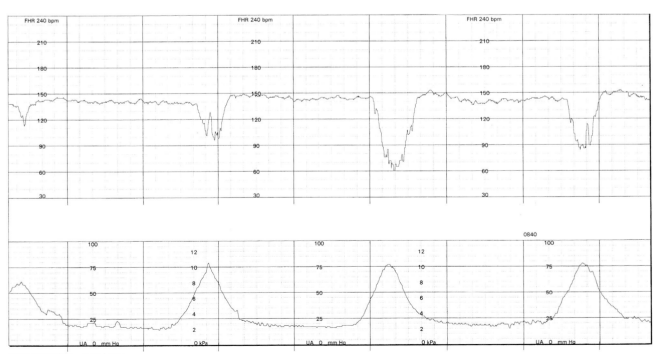

FHR Baseline = 140 bpm

FIGURE 3–18. Variable decelerations.

TABLE 3-9 VARIABLE DECELERATIONS

Related to Maternal/Fetal Conditions	• Positioning • Second-stage labor	• Copious fluid loss with rupture of membranes • Monoamniotic multiple gestation
Related to Intrauterine Conditions	• Oligohydramnios • Meconium • Cord entanglement • Nuchal cord	• Short cord • Knotted cord • Prolapsed cord • Forceps and vacuum

Goal of Intervention	Rationale
Improve blood flow through the umbilical cord	Alleviating compression on the umbilical cord will help it to float freely and not be compressed

Specific Interventions	Rationale
• Vaginal examination	Check for cord prolapse. If prolapse is detected, lift presenting part off cord and continue to do so until delivery of fetus. Continue EFM as best as possible, to determine whether there is improvement with displacement of the presenting part.
• Positioning—left lateral, right lateral, knee–chest	Improve maternal circulation and perfusion to placenta; improve blood flow through the umbilical cord.
• Increase IV fluid rate (1,000 mL bolus) unless otherwise contraindicated	Improve maternal circulation and perfusion to placenta; improve maternal hydration to potentiate greater amniotic fluid volume.
• Administer oxygen 10 L/min by nonrebreather mask	Hyperoxygenate maternal blood to increase fetal oxygenation.
• Amnioinfusion	Create cushioning for the cord and alleviate compression.
• Consider discontinuation of oxytocin infusion, uterotonic agents; consider tocolytics	Additional deoxygenation on the fetus from decreased blood flow during contractions may be too great when recurrent or severe variable decelerations are present. Decrease the stress of contractions on the fetus until further assessment proves the fetus is not acidotic.
• Do not ask patient to "push" with every contraction	Gives fetus a chance to recover/reoxygenate.
• Observe for reassuring signs such as accelerations and moderate variability	Accelerations and moderate variability suggest that the fetus is not sufficiently hypoxic to produce acidosis.
• Initiate procedures to assist in determining fetal acid–base status, such as scalp stimulation.	EFM is only a screening device. Adjunct means of assessment may be helpful in affirming suspicions and making a diagnosis.
• Consider internal monitoring	Internal monitoring with a spiral electrode may provide more accurate assessment of the FHR.
• Consider BPP	BPP may be helpful in assessing for signs of hypoxia/asphyxia.
• Observe for other nonreassuring signs such as rising baseline FHR; minimal, absent, or marked variability; overshoots; late or prolonged decelerations; or bradycardia	These are indicators that the fetal condition is worsening. If interventions are not improving fetal status, operative intervention may be necessary.
• Communicate FHR/UA pattern and interventions to care provider and personnel in charge, and document in medical record	Care provider should assess patient/fetal condition if variable decelerations are recurrent or severe; charge personnel need to plan staffing accordingly and may provide expertise and assistance; medical record should reflect assessments and interventions.
• Prepare for delivery	If interventions are not successful and the variable deceleration pattern continues, operative or assisted delivery may be indicated.

variable decelerations, regardless of amniotic fluid meconium status.[22] When properly performed, this intervention may be helpful in alleviating cord compression before the fetus experiences any further decline in status.

Shoulders

Variable decelerations possess another unique feature—they are the only type of deceleration pattern that, at times, includes an accelerative phase within the context of their occurrence. There are two specific acceleration patterns that can occur as part of the variable deceleration. These are known as *shoulders* and *overshoots*. Shoulders and overshoots are acknowledged in the 2008 NICHD definitions[4] but not described. Shoulders are brief accelerations of the FHR that may immediately precede or follow the decelerative phase of the variable deceleration and denote progressive amounts of pressure being placed on and removed from the umbilical cord, compressing the umbilical vein. When shoulders appear, there is usually a moderate amount of variability present in the FHR baseline as a reassuring sign of fetal status. If there is a shoulder on the concluding end of the variable deceleration, it returns rapidly to FHR baseline (Figure 3–19).[6,10]

Overshoots

Overshoots are another type of acceleration associated with variable decelerations. Overshoots appear only at the end of the variable deceleration, as the FHR is attempting to resolve back to baseline from the variable deceleration. The compromised fetus, in an attempt to recover to baseline rate, raises its heart rate well above (overshoots) the baseline. When overshoots are present, variability in the FHR baseline is usually minimal to absent, and there is no accelerative phase preceding the variable deceleration. The fetus usually maintains the overshoot for a fairly significant period of time before returning to baseline FHR (Figure 3–20).

Prolonged Deceleration

A prolonged deceleration is the most easily recognizable deceleration, characterized simply by its duration. Prolonged decelerations (≥15 bpm below baseline) range in duration from 2–10 minutes (Figure 3–21). The span of the deceleration is measured from the point where the FHR falls from the baseline until its return to baseline FHR. The etiology of the prolonged deceleration is varied. It is related to any acute event that transiently interrupts maternal–fetal perfusion, such as cord compression, tachysystole, or maternal hypotension. Prolonged decelerations usually exhibit the characteristics shown in Table 3–10.

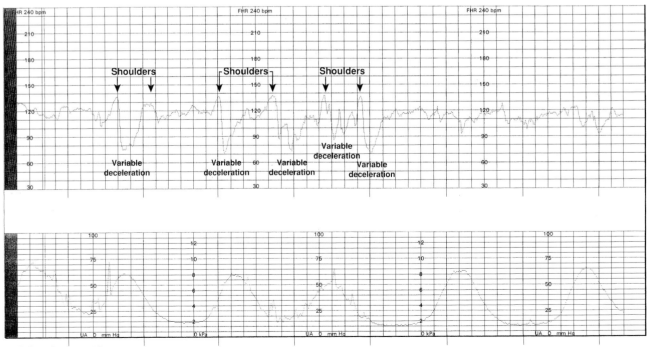

FHR Baseline = 120 bpm

FIGURE 3–19. Variable decelerations with shoulders.

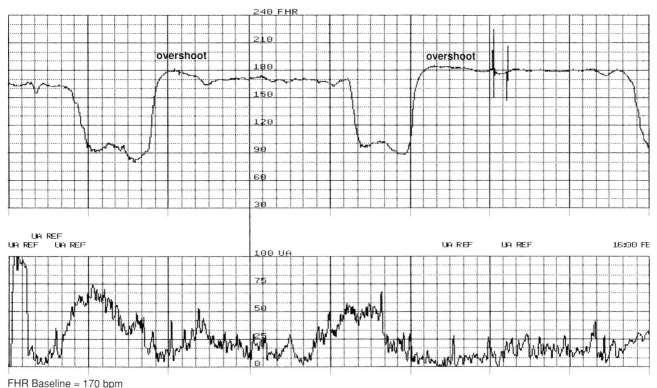

FHR Baseline = 170 bpm

FIGURE 3–20. Variable decelerations with overshoots.

1) 02/13/01 13:30
   UTERUS BEGINNING TO RELAX PER PALPATION AND PT REPORT

2) 02/13/01 13:31
   UTERUS SOFT PER PALPATION

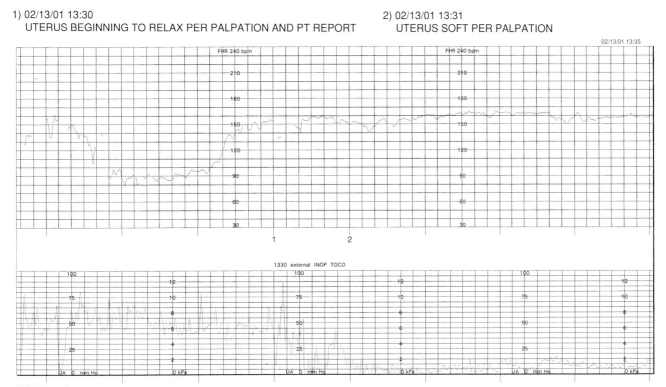

FHR Baseline = 150 bpm

FIGURE 3–21. Prolonged deceleration with tachysystole.

TABLE 3-10 CHARACTERISTICS OF PROLONGED DECELERATIONS

Depth	Drop in FHR of ≥15 beats below the FHR baseline
Duration	≥2 minutes and <10 minutes
Timing	May occur in relation to contractions (periodic) and may also happen independently of contractions (episodic)
Frequency of occurrence	Can appear singularly, or as intermittent (with <50% of contractions in a 20-minute segment), or recurrent (with >50% of contractions in a 20-minute window)

Adapted from Macones et al.[1]

Because the insult initiating the prolonged deceleration is often unknown at the time of its occurrence, interventions are a compilation of those aimed at promoting intrauterine resuscitation. This strategy includes the following actions:

- Increasing uterine blood flow (e.g., discontinuing oxytocin/removing uterotonic agents, administering tocolytics)
- Promoting maternal oxygenation (e.g., hyperoxygenation with O_2)
- Promoting perfusion to and through the uterus, placenta, and umbilical cord (e.g., maternal positioning, hydration, discontinuing oxytocin/removing uterotonic agents, administering tocolytics, vaginal assessment for cord prolapse and fetal descent [Table 3–11])

CLINICAL PERSPECTIVE

The majority of women are admitted to labor and delivery with FHR patterns indicative of normal fetal development and oxygenation (i.e., stable FHR baseline that is within normal limits, has moderate variability and accelerations present, and has no decelerations). It is optimal to observe the FHR and take notice of any changes that begin to appear over time. If late and/or variable decelerations begin to develop, interventions (see Tables 3–7 and 3–9) to resolve these patterns should be employed. If the FHR continues to display components that are concerning, despite appropriate intervention, the tracing should be closely monitored for other elements that may indicate the development or progression of fetal hypoxia. Such changes may include a slowly rising baseline, diminishment and/or the loss of variability, and worsening of deceleration patterns.

During the course of such progression, the FHR may temporarily settle into what can *appear* to be an improved pattern (stable rate that is still within "normal" limits, diminishment and/or disappearance of decelerations, but with variability minimal or absent) if considered only in the present context. When compared against an earlier recording of the FHR, however, it becomes evident that this is not a sign of recovery but rather of compromise. FHR patterns indicative of fetal acidemia usually evolve over a period of time. The literature supports approximately a 1-hour time frame for this progression to acidemia to occur, giving the providers ample time to make decisions and take action.[5]

Preexisting Neurologic Injury

According to the American Academy of Pediatrics (AAP) and ACOG,[24] "Most known conditions associated with either neonatal encephalopathy or cerebral palsy are related to abnormal antepartum conditions rarely amenable to intervention by the health care provider." Two retrospective case studies have demonstrated that when the FHR tracings of neurologically damaged children were reviewed several common features were present.[8,9] Phelan noted that 69% of these children had nonreactive patterns from admission to delivery. Schifrin noted that all 44 children with cerebral palsy in his study showed persistently absent variability and small variable decelerations with overshoots from the onset of intrapartum monitoring. Despite these findings, the care provider cannot rely solely on the FHR tracing as evidence that prior neurologic injury has occurred. Although the negative predictive value of EFM is quite high (~98%) when the FHR tracing is reassuring, it also has a high false-positive rate when the FHR tracing is suggestive of fetal compromise. Further investigation of fetal status is necessary when presented with an FHR tracing

TABLE 3-11 PROLONGED DECELERATIONS

Goal of Intervention	Rationale
Improve uteroplacental blood flow and perfusion through the umbilical cord	Improving the amount and quality of blood flow to the fetus will assist with attempts at recovery

Specific Interventions	Rationale
• Attempt to determine cause	Recognition of causative factors increases efficiency of response.
• Vaginal examination	Check for cord prolapse. If prolapse is detected, lift presenting part off cord and continue to do so and continue monitoring until delivery of the fetus.
• Positioning—left lateral, right lateral, knee–chest	Reposition until successful, giving each position a chance to take effect. Improve maternal circulation and perfusion to the placenta; improve blood flow through the umbilical cord.
• Increase IV fluid rate (1,000 mL bolus) unless otherwise contraindicated	Improve maternal circulation and perfusion to placenta; improve maternal hydration to potentiate greater amniotic fluid volume.
• Administer oxygen 10 L/min by nonrebreather mask	Hyperoxygenate maternal blood to increase fetal oxygenation.
• Discontinue oxytocin infusion; remove uterotonic agents; consider tocolytics	Eliminate additional stress of decreased blood flow during contractions by promoting uterine relaxation until further assessment proves the fetus is not acidotic.
• Palpate uterus	Palpation may be most effective means of determining tachysystole or inadequate uterine resting tone.
• Assess maternal vital signs, particularly BP for hypotension	Maternal status directly affects FHR pattern.
• Observe tracing for reassuring signs such as accelerations and moderate variability	Accelerations and moderate variability suggest that the fetus is not sufficiently hypoxic to produce acidosis.
• Initiate procedures to assist in determining fetal acid–base status, such as scalp stimulation.	EFM is only a screening device. Adjunct means of assessment may be helpful in affirming suspicions and making a diagnosis.
• Consider internal monitoring	Internal monitoring with a spiral electrode may provide more accurate assessment of the FHR.
• Consider BPP	BPP may be helpful in assessing for signs of hypoxia/asphyxia.
• Observe for other nonreassuring signs, such as rising baseline FHR; minimal, absent, or marked variability; presence of variable or late decelerations; progression to bradycardia	These are indicators that the fetal condition is worsening. If interventions are not improving fetal status, operative intervention may be necessary.
• Communicate FHR/UA pattern and interventions to care provider and personnel in charge, and document in medical record	Care provider should assess patient/fetal condition; charge personnel need to plan staffing accordingly and may provide expertise and assistance; medical record should reflect assessment and interventions.
• Prepare for delivery	If interventions are not successful and prolonged decelerations continue to occur, operative or assisted delivery may be indicated.

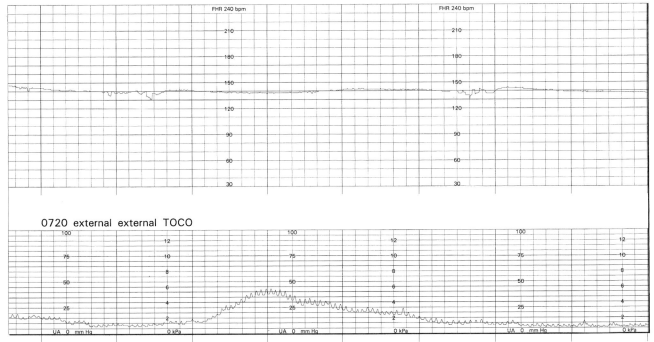

0720 external external TOCO

FHR Baseline = 140 bpm

FIGURE 3–22. Chronic hypoxemia.

that is unusual and/or does not have any reassuring components (Figure 3–22).

UNUSUAL FHR PATTERNS

Although they do not happen frequently, it is necessary to be aware of some of the less common FHR patterns to be able to respond appropriately when one is encountered.

Sinusoidal Pattern

When the rare sinusoidal pattern occurs, the FHR baseline rate remains stable and within normal range, but the tracing has an obviously unusual appearance. The predominant feature of the sinusoidal pattern is that the FHR baseline undulates across the strip chart, repetitively creating a constant, sine-wave-shaped form. These oscillations occur regularly, at a frequency of 2 to 5 times per minute with amplitude of 5 to 15 beats above and below the FHR baseline.[25] The actual FHR baseline is indeterminate when a sinusoidal pattern is present. The FHR baseline variability is absent or minimal,[26] giving the sinusoidal pattern its smooth shape. There are no periods during the FHR tracing with a sinusoidal pattern where the FHR demonstrates normal variability or reactivity (Figure 3–23).[27] This pattern will not resolve

spontaneously. The FHR tracing with a sinusoidal pattern may be complicated by additional nonreassuring elements, such as variable, late, or prolonged decelerations.[11,28]

The possible etiologies of sinusoidal patterns include fetal anemia, fetal hypoxia, or maternal narcotic administration (see Chapter 1). Sinusoidal patterns are most commonly due to fetal anemia secondary to Rh isoimmunization. This was described as the causative factor in the original description of a sinusoidal pattern.[29] Fetal anemia can also result from other maternal–fetal blood incompatibilities, maternal trauma, abruptio placentae, placenta previa, or any fetal–maternal hemorrhage and can present as a sinusoidal pattern. In some cases (such as with blood–antigen incompatibilities), fetal transfusion by way of percutaneous umbilical blood sampling (a.k.a., PUBS or cordocentesis) may temporarily resolve the anemia. Once the anemia is corrected, the FHR tracing will no longer appear sinusoidal. In these instances, it is often necessary to repeat this treatment numerous times during the antepartum. When a sinusoidal pattern is noted, a sonographic examination is performed to observe the fetus for ascites and/or hydrops. Other methods of fetal assessment may also be employed to evaluate fetal oxygenation.

Sinusoidal patterns can result from severe fetal hypoxia. Lack of oxygen affects the fetal ANS,

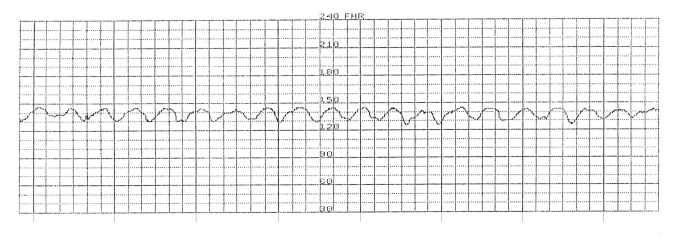

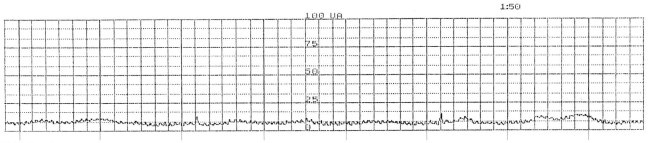

FHR Baseline = Indeterminate

FIGURE 3–23. Sinusoidal pattern.

subsequently altering the fetal heart rhythm. In the majority of these cases, prompt delivery of the fetus is indicated, although it is recognized that some measure of neurologic damage to the fetus may have already occurred.

Most commonly observed is the sinusoidal tracing resulting from narcotic administration. When this occurs, the tracing is referred to as *pseudosinusoidal,* indicating that the causative nature of the sine-wave-shaped undulations is not pathologic. Pseudosinusoidal patterns were originally noted after the administration of alphaprodine and are commonly seen after the administration of butorphanol, morphine sulfate, and meperidine. Various illicit drugs also have this effect on the FHR. It is prudent to obtain a reassuring FHR tracing before dispensing pain medications so that, if a sinusoidal pattern ensues, it can be determined to have resulted from the narcotic rather than the onset of fetal hypoxia or anemia. The benign pseudosinusoidal pattern is usually distinguishable from the ominous sinusoidal pattern through careful history taking and assessment of the FHR tracing. Unlike the sinusoidal pattern, the pseudosinusoidal pattern usually has periods of normal FHR baseline, baseline variability, and other elements such as spontaneous or induced accelerations of the FHR (Figure 3–24) that support an absence of fetal metabolic acidemia.

The pseudosinusoidal pattern is corrected when the drug effects subside.

When a patient presents with a sinusoidal pattern, it is important to ascertain a complete maternal and prenatal history to rule out causes of fetal anemia or fetal hypoxia. Fetal scalp stimulation or vibra-acoustic stimulation can be done to elicit accelerations of the FHR (thus ruling out acidosis). These techniques are discussed in greater detail in Chapters 1 and 4.

Fetal Dysrhythmias

Fetal dysrhythmias are a relatively rare occurrence, affecting about 1% of all pregnancies. Less than 20% pose a serious threat to fetal or neonatal well-being, and most (99%) disappear shortly (hours to weeks) after birth and are of no long-term consequence.[30] Fetal dysrhythmias are recognizable on the strip chart as abrupt changes in rhythm or rate between beats (R–R interval) of the fetal heart. This is demonstrated in the recorded FHR as linear deflections above and/or below the FHR baseline, depending on the type of arrhythmia. These deflections appear in an organized fashion and may be present intermittently or continuously. Fetal dysrhythmias can only be recorded on the strip chart when the signal

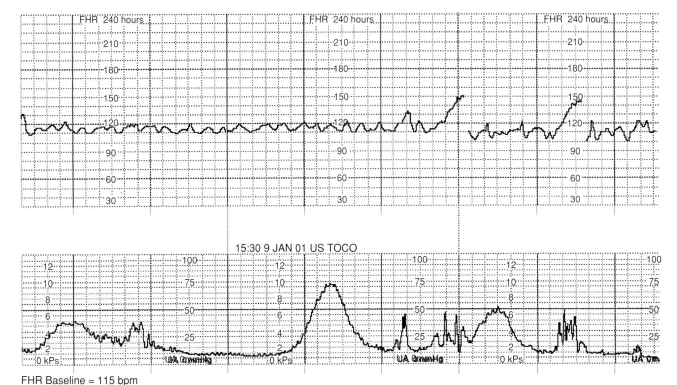

FHR Baseline = 115 bpm

FIGURE 3–24. Pseudosinusoidal pattern. The two accelerations occurring toward the end of this tracing negate the presence of a sinusoidal pattern.

source is the fetal electrocardiogram (FECG) and the FHR is printed without the use of any type of artifact-elimination technology (Figure 3–25). Diagnosis of the specific type of dysrhythmia cannot be accomplished simply by looking at the FHR tracing (equipment issues are discussed in Chapter 2). This is most effectively accomplished either by FECG, fetal echocardiography, or M-mode ultrasound. A printout of the FECG waveform can usually be obtained by connecting the electronic fetal monitor to an adult ECG recorder. M-mode ultrasound (see Chapter 9) can be used to visualize the fetal heart and record the rhythm. Usually, when an irregular FHR is noted, the patient is referred to a perinatologist for evaluation. Once a diagnosis has been made, the risks and benefits of various treatment modalities are weighed. Depending on the type of dysrhythmia and its etiology, expectant management may be the chosen course of action. Other treatment modalities may include administration of antidysrhythmic drugs to the mother (usually orally) or to the fetus (through PUBS), use of steroids or other medications to decrease maternal antibodies, or delivery with planned treatment of the neonate postnatally. During labor, scalp stimulation can be used to assess fetal oxygen status.[31]

Examples of Fetal Dysrhythmias

Premature Ventricular Contractions and Premature Atrial Contractions

Fetal dysrhythmias are most commonly associated with hydrops, hydramnios, intrauterine growth restriction, family history of congenital heart disease, maternal connective tissue disease, and maternal viral disease. Two of the most common types of fetal dysrhythmias are premature ventricular contractions (PVCs) and premature atrial contractions (PACs). PVCs comprise more than half the cases of fetal dysrhythmia. These dysrhythmias are characterized by isolated extrasystoles and may be related to maternal usage of caffeine, tobacco, cocaine, alcohol, adrenergic drugs (pseudoephedrine), or beta-mimetic tocolytics. They are generally considered benign, but do warrant observation because up to 2% of fetuses with PVCs have structural anomalies, and up to 1% may develop a sustained tachydysrhythmia causing risk for fetal hydrops.[32] PVCs may also lead to the dysrhythmic patterns of bigeminy (two PVCs occurring at a time) or trigeminy (three PVCs occurring at a time).

Fetuses with irregular FHRs seldom have significant structural heart defects. If congenital heart disease is diagnosed, however, it is important to

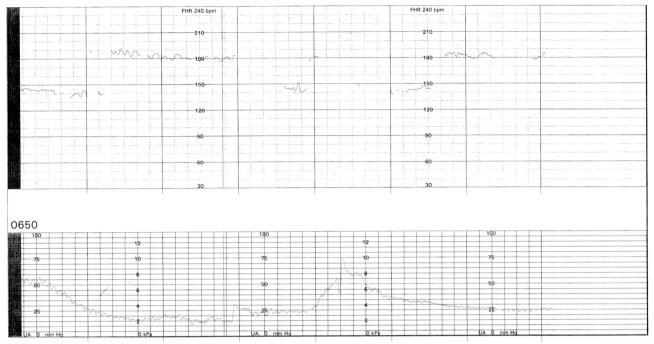

A FHR Baseline = Indeterminate

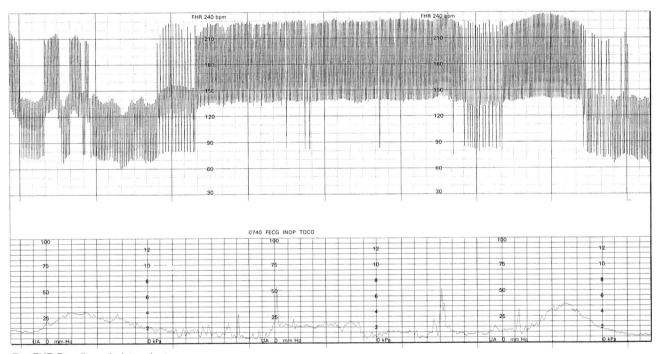

B FHR Baseline = Indeterminate

FIGURE 3–25. Dysrhythmia. **(A)** Signal obtained with ultrasound transducer. **(B)** Same signal obtained with spiral electrode.

rule out chromosomal abnormalities because there is a strong association between these two findings. Although atrial extrasystoles (PACs) (Figure 3–26) appear to be benign, there is a chance that they can precipitate supraventricular tachycardia (SVT), which is a more worrisome dysrhythmia.[33]

Supraventricular Tachycardia

SVT is the most common serious fetal dysrhythmia. It is characterized by an FHR baseline rate of greater than 200 bpm, 1:1 atrial to ventricular activity, and a fixed R–R interval (little or no beat-to-beat variation) (Figure 3–27). Most (~95%) SVTs are caused by

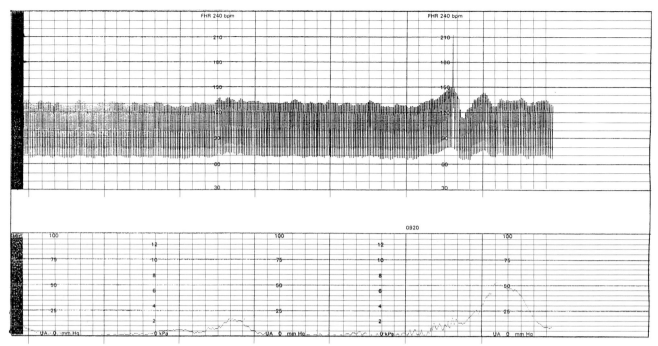

FHR Baseline = Indeterminate

FIGURE 3–26. Fetal extrasystoles.

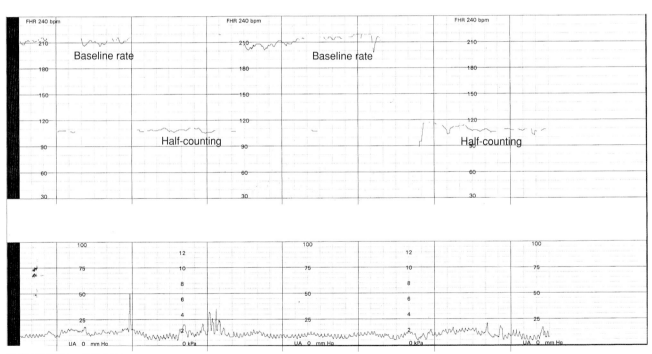

FHR Baseline = 210 bpm

FIGURE 3–27. Supraventricular tachycardia with half-counting. Signal obtained with ultrasound transducer, dysrhythmia later verified.

an electrical impulse that reenters the atrium from the ventricle, an etiology usually responsive to pharmacologic management.[34] Only a small percentage (~5%) of SVTs have an atrial flutter/fibrillation or an ectopic atrial focus, which may require surgical intervention.[34] Sustained SVT can lead to congestive heart failure or hydrops and can put the fetus at risk for demise. Treatment modalities depend on etiology, gestational age, whether the condition is sustained or intermittent in nature, and whether hydrops has occurred. Fetuses with known SVTs or atrial flutter may be followed with antepartum testing, as well as with sonographic evaluation for signs of hydrops or ascites. Even in the presence of hydrops, chances of survival are 73%.[35] Treatment usually includes administration of digoxin or other antiarrhythmic agents (such as procainamide) to the patient (to break the cycle of tachycardia) or delivery of fetus.

Bradydysrhythmia

As described earlier in this chapter, FHR baseline bradycardia is defined as FHR below 110 bpm for ≥10 minutes. The nonhypoxic types of fetal bradycardia that have been described in the literature include response to increased intracranial pressure[10] and fetal bradydysrhythmia.[36]

A fetal bradydysrhythmia (Figure 3–28) can result from cardiac anomalies, incomplete heart block asso-ciated with PAC or SVT, or complete heart block. Diagnosis of the type of dysrhythmia is made by fetal echocardiography or M-mode ultrasound. In most situations, expectant management is recommended in consultation with a perinatologist. In the presence of fetal hydrops or fetal heart failure, delivery may be indicated.[37]

Atrioventricular (AV) block, also known as congenital heart block, is the most concerning bradydysrhythmia. It is characterized by a baseline FHR of 50 to 70 bpm. First-degree AV block is a rare occurrence, marked by a prolonged P–R interval and dropped beats. In second-degree AV block (Figure 3–29), the rapid atrial beats are incompletely conducted to the ventricles, exhibiting as dropped beats. With third-degree AV block, there is complete atrioventricular dissociation, meaning that atrial beats are not conducted to ventricles. About half the fetuses with complete heart block have congenital heart disease, which is associated with poor outcome. If the heart is structurally normal, the outcome is more favorable. Maternal autoimmune disease (systemic lupus erythematosus, anti-SSA/Ro, anti-SSB/La) and viral disease (cytomegalovirus) are common causes of complete heart block when the fetal heart is structurally normal. Steroids or medications to decrease maternal antibodies may be used as treatment in these cases. The

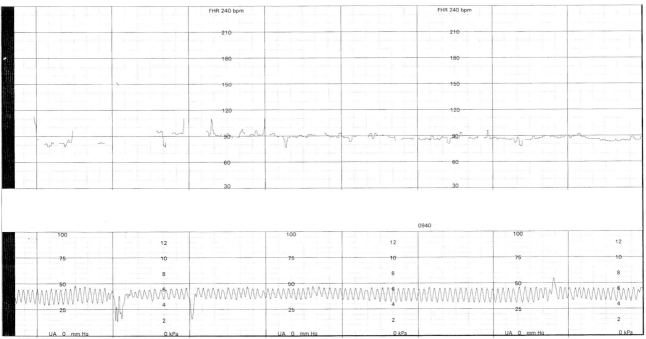

FHR Baseline = 90 bpm

FIGURE 3–28. Fetal bradydysrhythmia.

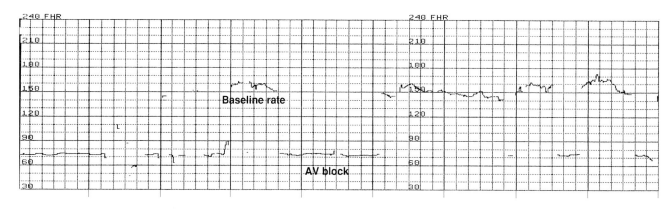

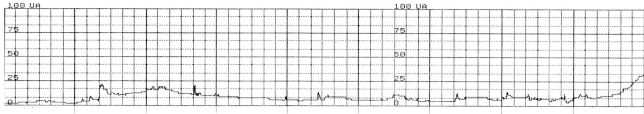

FHR Baseline = 155 bpm

FIGURE 3–29. Atrioventricular block.

fetus must be observed for development of hydrops, an indicator of worsening prognosis.

The primary method of distinguishing between artifact and dysrhythmia is auscultation of the FHR and rhythm. As discussed in Chapter 2, when the spiral electrode is in use, interference with signal acquisition can occur. It is necessary to differentiate this event from the presence of a dysrhythmia.

Auscultation of the FHR with a hand-held Doppler or use of M-mode sonography or fetal echocardiography (see Chapter 9) can assist in this process by providing information about rate and rhythm. Artifact is usually visually discernible from dysrhythmia by its disorganized appearance and presence during events that disrupt the FECG signal, such as maternal movement or vaginal examinations (Figure 3–30).

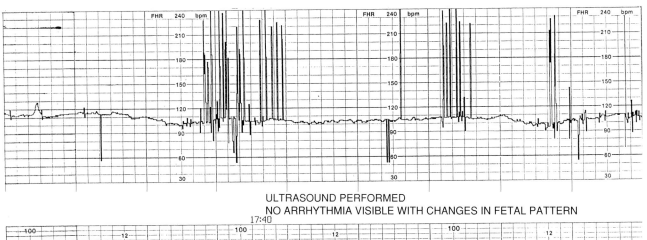

ULTRASOUND PERFORMED
NO ARRHYTHMIA VISIBLE WITH CHANGES IN FETAL PATTERN
17:40

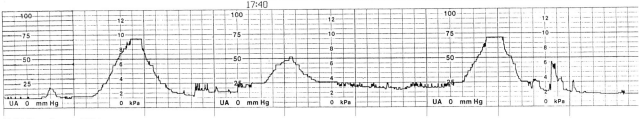

FHR Baseline = 105 bpm

FIGURE 3–30. Artifact.

THREE-TIER FETAL HEART RATE SYSTEM OF INTERPRETATION

In 2008, the NICHD committee introduced a new component to EFM nomenclature: a three-tier system (Table 3–12) for classifying FHR tracings according to FHR patterns and what they did (or did not) demonstrate in regard to reassurance of fetal status. Some rather general guidelines for clinical management were offered for each of the categories introduced; however, the equivocal nature of the largest percentage of FHR tracings (Category II, Indeterminate) persists in clouding the issue of setting firmer management principles. As discussed throughout this book, FHR tracings that demonstrate reassuring elements, such as an FHR within normal limits with accelerations, moderate variability, and no late or variable decelerations (Category I, Normal), very rarely give cause for concern and, if continued,

are highly predictive of a good outcome. Almost as easy to discern are those tracings that are clearly indicative of severe fetal compromise (Category III, Abnormal).

The ongoing dilemma, regardless of the nomenclature or classification assigned, is that most FHR tracings fall into a much less definitive territory (Category II) that is much harder to quantify in regard to management. Clark et al.[38] convened a group of experts to address this topic. Although they note a few caveats to their suggested approach, including not being able to include all identified fetal patterns, a useful algorithm (Figure 3–31) is presented to guide clinicians through a logical, evidence-based approach to Category II tracings.

Many institutions have incorporated the three-tier method into their documentation and/or communication of their systematic assessment of the FHR. It is important for all disciplines working

TABLE 3–12 THREE-TIER FETAL HEART RATE INTERPRETATION SYSTEM

Category	Description

I	FHR tracing shows *all* of the following:
	  Baseline rate: 110–160 bpm
	  Baseline variability: moderate
	  Late or variable decelerations: absent
	  Early decelerations: present or absent
	  Accelerations: present or absent

II	All FHR tracings not categorized as Category I or III; may represent an appreciable fraction of those encountered in clinical care. Examples include the characteristics cited for each of the following:
	Baseline rate
	  Bradycardia without absent baseline variability
	  Tachycardia
	Baseline variability
	  Minimal baseline variability
	  Absent baseline variability with no recurrent decelerations
	  Marked baseline variability
	Accelerations
	  Absence of induced accelerations after fetal stimulation
	Periodic or episodic deceleration
	  Recurrent variable decelerations with minimal or moderate baseline variability
	  Prolonged deceleration ≥2 min, but <10 min
	  Recurrent late decelerations with moderate baseline variability
	  Variable decelerations with other characteristics such as slow return to baseline, "overshoots," or "shoulders"

III	FHR tracing shows either:
	  Absent baseline variability with any of the following:
	    Bradycardia
	    Recurrent variable decelerations
	    Recurrent late decelerations
	  Sinusoidal pattern

Adapted from Macones et al.[1]

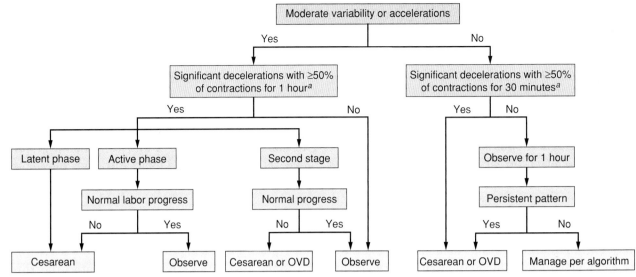

OVD, operative vaginal delivery.

[a]That have not resolved with appropriate conservative corrective measures, which may include supplemental oxygen, maternal position changes, intravenous fluid administration, correction of hypotension, reduction or discontinuation of uterine stimulation, administration of uterine relaxanl, amnioinfusion, and/or changes in second stage breathing and pushing techniques.

> Variability refers to predominant baseline FHR pattern (marked, moderate, minimal, absent) during a 30-minute evaluation period, as defined by NICHD.
> Marked variability is considered same as moderate variability for purposes of this algorithm.
> Significant decelerations are defined as any of the following:
> • Variable decelerations lasting longer than 60 seconds and reaching a nadir more than 60 bpm below baseline.
> • Variable decelerations lasting longer than 60 seconds and reaching a nadir less than 60 bpm regardless of the baseline.
> • Any late decelerations of any depth.
> • Any prolonged deceleration, as defined by the NICHD. Due to the broad heterogeneity inherent in this definition, identification of a prolonged deceleration should prompt discontinuation of the algorithm until the deceleration is resolved.
> Application of algorithm may be initially delayed for up to 30 minutes while attempts are made to alleviate Category II pattern with conservative therapeutic interventions (eg, correction of hypotension, position change, amnioinfusion, tocolysis, reduction or discontinuation of oxytocin).
> Once a Category II FHR pattern is identified, FHR is evaluated and algorithm applied every 30 minutes.
> Any significant change in FHR parameters should result in reapplication of algorithm.
> For Category II FHR patterns in which algorithm suggests delivery is indicated, such delivery should ideally be initiated within 30 minutes of decision for cesarean.
> If at any time tracing reverts to Category I status, or deteriorates for even a short time to Category III status, the algorithm no longer applies. However, algorithm should be reinstituted if Category I pattern again reverts to Category II.
> In fetus with extreme prematurity, neither significance of certain FHR patterns of concern in more mature fetus (eg, minimal variability) or ability of such fetuses to tolerate intrapartum events leading to certain types of Category II patterns are well defined. This algorithm is not intended as guide to management of fetus with extreme prematurity.
> Algorithm may be overridden at any time if, after evaluation of patient, physician believes it is in best interest of the fetus to intervene sooner.

FIGURE 3–31. Algorithm for management of Category II FHR tracings. From Clark SL, Nageotte MP, Garite TJ, et al. Intrapartum management of Category II fetal heart tracings: toward standardization of care. *Am J Obstet Gynecol.* 2013;(209):2:89–97.

together to utilize common terminology. Regardless of the details of how FHR parameters are expressed, it is important to remember that FHR patterns are dynamic, particularly intrapartum. The information about the fetus gleaned from the strip chart is only good for the time that it appears, and ongoing assessment and evaluation is necessary, regardless of the last category or classification to which the fetal tracing may have been assigned. ACOG[39] offers a general but useful algorithm (Figure 3–32) based on the three-tier system to outline management

strategies addressing all three categories. This may be a helpful guide for formulating more institution-specific protocols.

UTERINE ACTIVITY

No discussion of FHR pattern interpretation is complete without inclusion of uterine activity. The physiology and function of the uterus are detailed in Chapter 1. Normal uterine activity is defined as

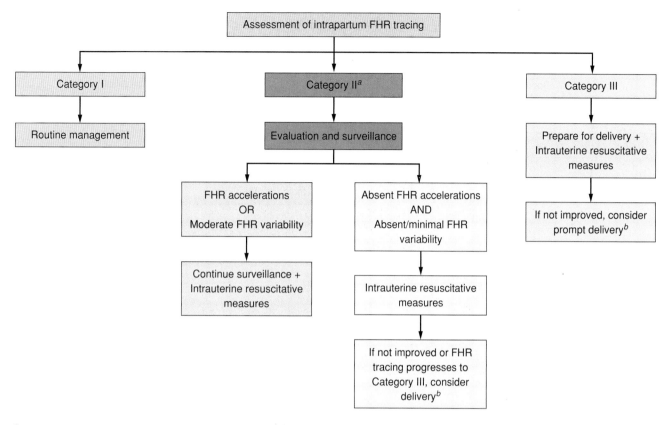

[a]Given the wide variation of FHR tracings in Category II, this algorithm is not meant to represent assessment and management of all potential FHR tracings, but provide an action template for common clinical situations.

[b]Timing and mode of delivery based on feasibility and maternal–fetal status.

FIGURE 3–32. Algorithm for management of intrapartum FHR tracings in accordance with the three-tier category system. From American College of Obstetricians and Gynecologists. *Management of Intrapartum Fetal Heart Rate Tracings*. ACOG Practice Bulletin 116. Washington, DC: Author; 2010.

a frequency of 3 to 5 contractions in 10 minutes and 25 to 75 mm Hg in strength (95–395 Montevideo units).[40] There should be a minimum of 1-minute of uterine relaxation between contractions and contraction length should not exceed ~60 to ~90 seconds in length. Uterine blood flow decreases during contractions, and there is a decrease in the amount of oxygen, carbon dioxide, and nutrients exchanged between fetal and maternal blood during this time. The resulting loss of oxygen to the fetus and buildup of carbon dioxide within the fetal circulation necessitates an adequate period of recovery before the next contraction. It cannot be emphasized enough how important it is to maintain an optimal contraction pattern (i.e., one that is functional for labor progress yet does not compromise blood and oxygen flow to the fetus).

Tachysystole is discussed in detail in Chapter 1 and is presently defined as >5 contractions in 10 minutes, averaged over a 30-minute window and must be qualified by the presence or absence of FHR decelera-tions.[4,39] Despite a growing body of research on patient safety and excessive uterine activity, there has been a good bit of back-and-forth debate regarding whether to treat tachysystole proactively, before the FHR is negatively affected. In a large, retrospective study, Heuser et al.[41] employed the NICHD definitions to investigate tachysystole. They found FHR changes in one-quarter of tachysystole events and that the chances of composite neonatal morbidity are increased with tachysystole, adding to the import of this topic. Factors associated with tachysystole by this study included oxytocin, misoprostol, epidural, hypertension, and labor induction. Oxytocin received attention for the doubling rates of tachysystole and a clear dose–response correlation was reaffirmed. ACOG presents a useful algorithm for managing tachysystole (Figure 3–33) that does include at least some measure of intervention for tachysystole in the presence of a Category I tracing, and this is further expanded on within Practice Bulletin 116.[39] The relatively simple constellation of traditional interventions validated by

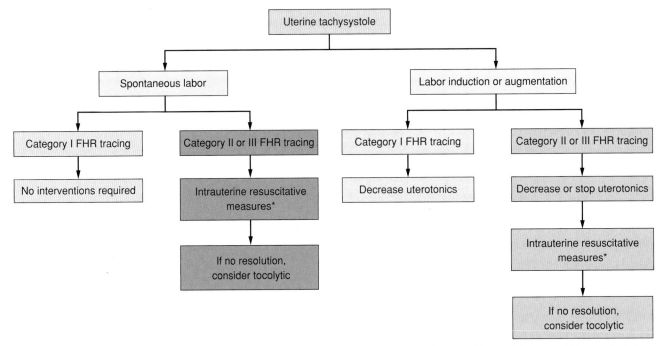

FIGURE 3–33. Algorithm for management of tachysystole. From American College of Obstetricians and Gynecologists. *Management of Intrapartum Fetal Heart Rate Tracings.* ACOG Practice Bulletin 116. Washington, DC: Author; 2010.

Simpson and James[7] that, when performed simultaneously, is commonly known as intrauterine resuscitation is suggested as a method for remediation of Category II and III tracings.

CONCLUSION

This chapter focused mainly on definitions and visual interpretation of the FHR tracing. To integrate this knowledge into practical clinical application, the practitioner must comprehend the underlying physiology of each FHR pattern and subsequently apply this knowledge in the form of appropriate interventions at the bedside. It is important to know that not every FHR pattern can be definitively catalogued or described using existing nomenclature. Some patterns occur so infrequently that they are described in the literature as case reports. Even including such instances, most FHR tracings can usually still be understood at least enough to discern fetal oxygenation status by examining individual recognizable components.

REFERENCES

1. Macones G, Hankin G, Spong CY, et al. The 2008 National Institute of Child Health and Human Development Workshop Report on Electronic Fetal Monitoring Update on Definitions, Interpretation, and Research Guidelines. *Obstet Gynecol.* 2008;112(3):661–666.
2. American College of Obstetricians and Gynecologists. *Intrapartum fetal heart rate monitoring: Nomenclature, Interpretation, and General Management Principles.* ACOG Practice Bulletin 106. Washington, DC: Author; 2009.
3. Association of Women's Health, Obstetric and Neonatal Nurses. *Antepartum and intrapartum fetal heart rate monitoring: clinical competencies and Education Guide.* 5th ed. Washington, DC: Author; 2011.
4. National Institute of Child Health and Human Development Research Planning (NICHD (2008).
5. Parer JT, King T, Flanders S, et al. Fetal acidemia and electronic fetal heart rate patterns: Is there evidence of an association? *J Matern Fetal Neonat Med.* 2006;19(5): 289–294.
6. Schifrin B. *Exercises in Fetal Monitoring.* St. Louis MO: Mosby–Year Book; 1990.
7. Simpson KR, James DC. Efficacy of intrauterine resuscitation techniques in improving fetal oxygen status during labor. *Obstet Gynecol.* 2005;105:1362–1368.
8. Phelan J, Ahn MO. Perinatal observations in forty-eight neurologically impaired term infants. *Am J Obstet Gynecol.* 1994;171(2):424–431.
9. Schifrin B, Hamilton-Rubinstein T, Shields J. Fetal heart rate patterns and the timing of fetal injury. *J Perinatol.* 1994;14(3):174–181.
10. Parer J. *Handbook of Fetal Heart Rate Monitoring.* 2nd ed. Philadelphia, PA: W. B. Saunders; 1997.
11. Schifrin B. *More Exercises in Fetal Monitoring.* St. Louis MO: Mosby–Year Book; 1993.

12. Leung A, Leung E, Paul R. Uterine rupture after previous cesarean delivery: Maternal and fetal consequences. *Am J Obstet Gynecol*. 1993;169(4):945–949.

13. Menihan C. Uterine rupture in women attempting vaginal birth following prior cesarean birth. *J Perinatol*. 1998;18(6):440–443.

14. Miller D, Diaz F, Paul R. Vaginal birth after cesarean: A 10 year experience. *Obstet Gynecol*. 1994;84(2):255–259.

15. Ingemarsson I, Arulkumaran S, Ratnam SS. Single injection of terbutaline in term labor. I. Effect on fetal pH in cases with prolonged bradycardia. *Am J Obstet Gynecol*. 1985;153(8):859–865.

16. Clark SL, Gimovsky ML, Miller FC. The scalp stimulation test: A clinical alternative to fetal scalp blood sampling. *Am J Obstet Gynecol*. 1984;14(3):274–277.

17. Panayotopoulos N, Salamalekis E, Kassanos D, et al. Intrapartum vibratory acoustic stimulation after maternal meperidine administration. *Clin Exp Obstet Gynecol*. 1998;25(4):139–140.

18. Sherer DM, Bentolila E. Blunted fetal response to vibroacoustic stimulation following chronic exposure to propranolol. *Am J Perinatol*. 1998;15(8):495–498.

19. Paul RH, Petrie RH, Rabello YA, Mueller EA. *Fetal Intensive Care*. Wallingford, CT: Corometrics Medical Systems; 1979.

20. Nielson DR, Freeman RK, Mangan S. Signal ambiguity resulting in unexpected outcome with external fetal heart rate monitoring. *Am J Obstet Gynecol*. 2008;198(6):717–724.

21. Ball RH, Parer JT, Caldwell LE, Johnson, J. Regional blood flow and metabolism in ovine fetuses during severe cord occlusion. *Am J Obstet Gynecol*. 1994;117(6):1549–1555.

22. American College of Obstetricians and Gynecologists. *Amnioinfusion Does Not Prevent Meconium Aspiration Syndrome*. ACOG Committee Opinion #346. (2006, reaffirmed 2012.) Washington, DC: Author; 2012.

23. Miyazaki FS, Taylor NA. Saline amnioinfusion for relief of variable or prolonged decelerations. A preliminary report. *Am J Obstet Gynecol*. 1983;146:670–678.

24. American College of Obstetricians and Gynecologists and the American Academy of Pediatrics. *Neonatal encephalopathy and cerebral palsy: Defining the pathogenesis and pathophysiology*. Washington, DC: Author; 2003.

25. Mondanlou HD, Freeman RK. Sinusoidal fetal heart rate pattern: Its definition and clinical significance. *Am J Obstet Gynecol*. 1982;142(8):1033–1038.

26. Garite T. Sinusoidal pattern from anemia. *Contemporary OB/GYN*. 1988, May:42–46.

27. Modanlou HD, Murata Y. Sinusoidal heart rate pattern: Reappraisal of its definition and clinical significance. *J Obstet Gynaecol Res*. 2004;Jun;30(3):169–180.

28. Mondanlou HD. Guide to sinusoidal patterns. *Contemp OB/GYN*. 1983;August:94–98.

29. Rochard F, Schifrin B, Goupil F, et al. Nonstressed fetal heart monitoring in the antepartum period. *Am J Obstet Gynecol*. 1976;126(6):699–706.

30. Clement D, Schifrin B. Diagnosis and management of fetal arrhythmias. *Perinatal/Neonatal*. 1987;11:9–20.

31. Wax J, Emmerich M, Eggleston M. Intrapartum fetal atrial bigeminy—Diagnostic and therapeutic role of the fetal scalp stimulation test. *Am J Obstet Gynecol*. 1996;174:1649–1650.

32. Simpson LL, Marx GR. Diagnosis and treatment of structural fetal cardiac abnormality and dysrhythmia. *Semin Perinatol*. 1994;18(3):215–227.

33. Copel J, Liang R, Demasio K, et al. The clinical significance of the irregular fetal heart rhythm. *Am J Obstet Gynecol*. 2000;182:813–819.

34. Kleinman CS, Copel JA. Electrophysiological principles and fetal antiarrhythmic therapy. *Ultrasound Obstet Gynecol*. 1991;1:286–297.

35. Simpson J, Sharland G. Fetal tachycardias: Management and outcome of 127 consecutive cases. *Heart*. 1998;79:576–581.

36. Copel JA, Friedman AH, Kleinman CS. Management of fetal cardiac arrhythmias. *Obstet Gynecol Clin N Am*. 1997;24(1):201–211.

37. Bayer-Zuoirello LA, Kanaan CM, Benner R, et al. Fetal heart rate monitoring casebook: Persistent bradycardia. *J Perinatol*. 1995;15(6):514–516.

38. Clark SL, Nageotte MP, Garite TJ, et al. Intrapartum management of category II fetal heart tracings: toward standardization of care. *Am J Obstet Gynecol*. 2013;(209):2:89–97.

39. American College of Obstetricians and Gynecologists. *Management of Intrapartum Fetal Heart Rate Tracings*. ACOG Practice Bulletin 116. Washington, DC: Author; 2010.

40. American College of Obstetricians and Gynecologists. Dystocia and Augmentation of Labor. ACOG Practice Bulletin 49. Washington, DC: Author; 2003, reaffirmed 2013.

41. Heuser CC, Knight S, Esplin MS, et al. Tachysystole in term labor: incidence, risk factors, outcomes, and effect on fetal heart tracings. *Am J Obstet Gynecol*. 2013;209:32.e1–6.

SUGGESTED READINGS

Association of Women's Health, Obstetric and Neonatal Nurses. *Fetal Heart Monitoring*. Washington, DC: Author; 2008.

National Institute of Child Health and Human Development Research Planning Workshop. Electronic fetal heart monitoring: Research guidelines for interpretation. *J Obstet, Gynecol Neonat Nurs*. 1997;26(6):635–640.

CHAPTER 4

Antepartum Fetal Assessment

The methods and means for assessing the fetus during the antepartum are selected based on gestational age, patient history and presentation, patient and practitioner preferences, and available technology. The purpose of antepartum testing is to screen for adequacy of uteroplacental function and to determine whether the fetus can safely remain in utero. It is important to consider that antepartum tests currently available are very effective for predicting fetal well-being but are not capable of making definitive diagnosis of fetal hypoxia/acidosis. Antepartum surveillance is also indicated for other conditions affecting or suspected to affect the maternal–fetal unit (see Table 4–1). The American Academy of Pediatrics (AAP) and American College of Obstetricians and Gynecologists (ACOG) have issued research-based guidelines that delineate testing criteria and procedures.[1,2]

Understanding maternal–fetal physiology is essential to selecting, performing, and managing antepartum testing. The fetal central nervous system matures as gestation advances, and the resulting behaviors that the fetus demonstrates develop in a specific order. Antepartum testing methods assess the fetus for its ability to perform behaviors appropriate to its gestational age in an effort to identify or rule out developing fetal asphyxia. An insidious, chronic loss of oxygenation causes the term or near-term fetus to lose the ability to perform expected functions. This decline in fetal status occurs on a continuum, in an opposite order from which abilities develop (Figure 4–1). Fetal tone begins to be evident by sonographic evaluation at approximately 7.5 to 8 weeks' gestation followed by fetal movement, which starts to occur at approximately 9 weeks. Fetal breathing becomes regular at 20 to 21 weeks. Heart rate control (the ability to accelerate and decelerate) is last to develop, presenting at the end of the second or beginning of the third trimester.

NONSTRESS TEST

The nonstress test (NST) involves the application of an electronic fetal monitor (EFM) to the maternal abdomen for the purpose of evaluating the fetus's

TABLE 4–1 INDICATIONS FOR ANTEPARTUM FETAL SURVEILLANCE

Preexisting Indications	Obstetric Indications
Type 1 diabetes mellitus	Post-term gestation
Chronic hypertension	Polyhydramnios or
Previous unexplained fetal	oligohydramnios
demise	Decreased fetal movement
Autoimmune disease	Intrauterine growth
Chronic renal disease	restriction
Endocrine disease	Multiple gestation
Cyanotic heart disease	Isoimmunization
Hemoglobinopathies	Chronic abruptio placentae
Antiphospholipid syndrome	Pregnancy-induced
Systemic lupus	hypertension
erythematosus	Gestational diabetes
Hyperthyroidism	Any factor ↑ risk for
	antepartum fetal demise

Data from AAP & ACOG, 2012; ACOG 2012; Signore et al., 2009.

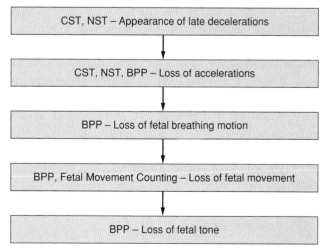

FIGURE 4–1. Utility of antenatal testing methods with respect to the progression of fetal hypoxia. Loss of oxygenation leads to a loss of fetal heart rate reactivity. Prior to loss of reactivity, decelerations may appear (Freeman, 1985). Next on the continuum is a decrease or loss of fetal breathing movements and then a decrease in amniotic fluid. Finally, there is a loss of fetal movement and, ultimately, the loss of fetal tone (Manning). BPP, biophysical profile; CST, contraction stress test; NST, nonstress test.

ability to perform a specified number of fetal heart rate (FHR) accelerations within a specified period of time. If the fetus is able to accomplish this task, the test is deemed *reactive*. If the fetus is not able to produce the desired amount of FHR accelerations within the allotted time frame, the test is considered to be *nonreactive*. The fetus is typically given at least 40 minutes of testing time to produce a reactive NST. This is to allow for the possibility that the time of testing might coincide with a period of fetal sleep. The NST is noninvasive and relatively easy to perform. Activities that affect fetal movement patterns and uteroplacental perfusion (e.g., maternal nutrition, hydration, smoking habits, medication effects, positioning, and time of day) should be considered when scheduling and performing the NST.

The occurrence of two or more accelerations, each rising to ≥15 beats above the FHR baseline and lasting for a period of ≥15 seconds, accomplished within a 20-minute time frame constitutes a reactive NST.[1,3,4] A detailed explanation of accelerations is provided in Chapter 3. It is expected that the fetus should be able to meet these criteria by 32 weeks' gestation. Although not included in the standard definition of a reactive NST, it is reasonable to expect that a fetus meeting these criteria will also demonstrate moderate baseline FHR variability. The FHR baseline would also be expected to fall within normal limits (110–160 bpm).

Some fetuses are able to produce a reactive NST as early as 24 to 28 weeks' gestation; however, there is a high false-positive rate (as much as 50%) in this population.[4] Between 28 and 32 weeks' gestation, there is a 15% chance that the NST will be nonreactive because the fetal autonomic nervous system may not have reached the maturity necessary to accelerate the fetal heart per NST criteria.[5,6] However, when such development is exhibited at an early gestational age, it is expected that the fetus will continue to achieve a reactive result of the same or better standard during all subsequent monitoring sessions.

Stork Byte

I am growing up so quickly!
Now that I am mature enough to give you a reactive NST, I should do this well or even better every time you test me! If not, beware!

There are variations in the parameters used to define the NST and its results. Both the period of time in which the NST is performed and the number of accelerations required during the defined period to deem the test reactive differ among institutions. Another variation of the NST includes the definition of a qualifying acceleration. Although the standard definition is that the accelerations rise above the baseline by ≥15 bpm and last ≥15 seconds, this definition may vary based on gestational age. For a fetus of less than 32 weeks' gestation, accelerations of ≥10 bpm that last ≥10 seconds in length are acceptable,[7] providing that the fetus has not previously demonstrated ≥15 bpm × ≥15 second accelerations. Implicit understanding of NST performance requirements and results in various institutions may differ to some degree. For example, some institutions may require documentation and/or correlation of instances of perceived fetal movement with accelerations during the NST (Figure 4–2). For clarity and accuracy, it is necessary to be aware of and follow institutional policy.

When the result of the NST is reactive, the patient will most likely be scheduled for testing on a weekly or twice-weekly basis, depending on gestational age and the indication for antepartum surveillance. Women who have maternal or obstetric indications that require twice-weekly testing include, but are not limited to, those with a post-term gestation, intrauterine growth restriction, type 1 diabetes mellitus, and pregnancy-induced hypertension.[1,2] Some high-risk conditions may warrant testing on a more frequent basis. Isolated episodes that occur during a normal-risk pregnancy that warrant performance of an NST (such as complaint of decreased fetal movement) and are subsequently ruled out might not be followed with any regular schedule of testing. A reactive NST has a negative predictive value of 99.8%, meaning that the possibility of stillbirth occurring within 1 week after a reactive NST is extremely low.[8]

If the NST is reactive, but the FHR demonstrates additional components such as variable, late, or prolonged decelerations (Category II tracing), continued monitoring and further evaluation are indicated. If variable decelerations are brief (<30 seconds in length) and occur infrequently, they do not require intervention.[9] If repetitive variable decelerations are present, measurement of the amniotic fluid volume by sonographic examination will determine if oligohydramnios is the underlying cause of this pattern (Figure 4–3). It is well established that oligohydramnios is associated with increased perinatal morbidity and mortality[10] and requires immediate attention and possible intervention. Further sonographic

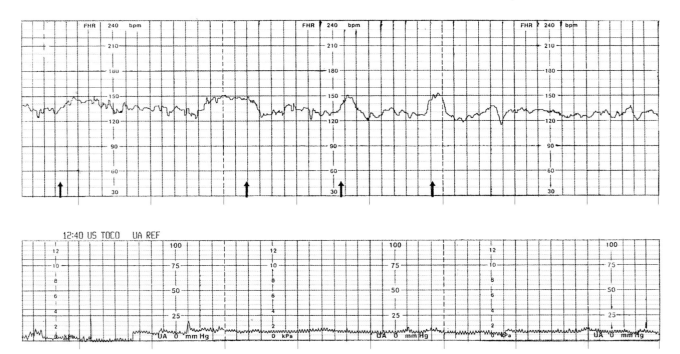

FIGURE 4-2. Reactive nonstress test with marks indicating perceived fetal movement.

examination may reveal structural anomalies of the maternal–fetal unit that may be causing decelerations of the FHR to occur.

If the NST is judged to be nonreactive, meaning that there are no accelerations or an insufficient number of accelerations produced during a 40-minute time period (extended length of time to account for fetal sleep cycles), additional testing of the fetus is indicated. Intervention is not based solely on a nonreactive NST because 80% to 90% of the nonreactive tracings are due to fetal sleep and are not the result of hypoxia (Figure 4–4).[11,12]

A nonreactive NST that also demonstrates nonreassuring signs, particularly in combination (e.g., variable, late, or prolonged decelerations; marked or minimal/absent variability; a baseline rate that is not within normal limits; or a sinusoidal pattern), is of great concern. Such findings warrant immediate investigation and possible consideration of the need for delivery.

In summary, whether the tracing is considered reactive or nonreactive, if any part of the tracing is indicative of a FHR pattern not predictive of normal fetal acid–base status, further evaluation is needed.

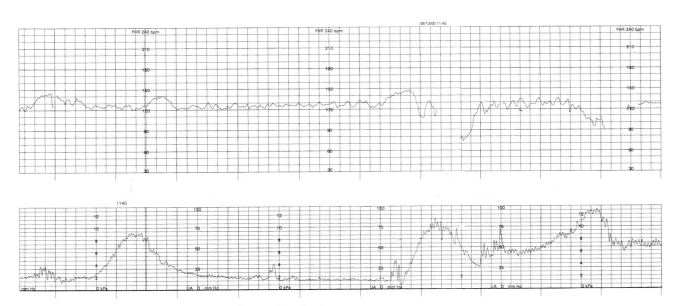

FIGURE 4-3. Reactive nonstress test with variable decelerations.

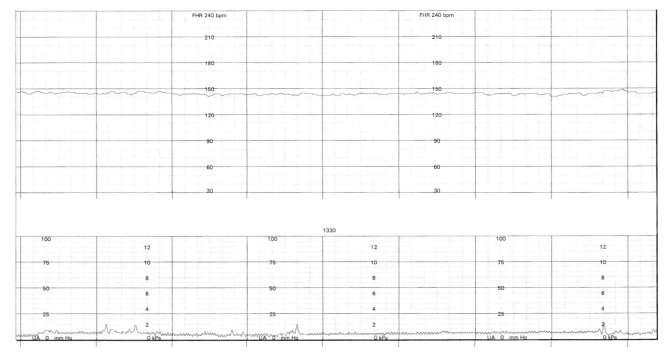

FIGURE 4–4. Nonreactive nonstress test.

This may consist of any one or a combination of the tests mentioned in this chapter. It is important to understand that, although the NST is an effective screening tool for the evaluation of fetal well-being and is often used as the primary method of testing, it has poor positive predictive value for determining fetal hypoxia/acidosis.[13] Adjunct methods of assessment should be employed any time fetal status is in question.

FETAL ACOUSTIC STIMULATION TEST/ VIBRA-ACOUSTIC STIMULATION

A combination of vibratory and acoustic stimulation can be used to elicit acceleration(s) of the FHR valid in the prediction of fetal well-being (Figure 4–5),[2] thus decreasing false nonreactive NSTs and safely reducing the testing time of the NST.[1,14] The FHR tracing is then judged to be either reactive or nonreactive based on the same criteria explained previously in regard to the NST. A prolonged acceleration(s) is frequently observed in response to the fetal acoustic stimulation test (FAST)[15] and is interpreted as a reactive test. For this reason, it is important to have established the baseline FHR before applying vibra-acoustic stimulation (VAS). Fetal movement elicited through VAS is almost always associated with a reactive NST.[16] The positive correlation between fetal movement, FHR, and fetal well-being is the basis for

the well-established screening method of fetal movement counting and continues to factor into the study of potential new methods of fetal assessment.[17] A fetus that shows no response to the applied stimulus will require further evaluation. The concern in this instance is that a fetus without the ability to produce accelerations may be neurologically compromised or acidotic.

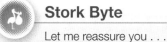

Stork Byte

Let me reassure you . . .
If I can raise my heart rate at least 15 beats above my FHR baseline for at least 15 seconds, then you don't need to worry that I have metabolic acidemia!

The fetal acoustic stimulator is an artificial larynx, adapted for this particular use and attached by a connector to the EFM. It annotates directly on the fetal strip chart when stimulation is given, so that the mark it leaves may be correlated with the fetal response. The patient end of the fetal acoustic stimulator is placed on the maternal abdomen in the area of the fetal head and up to a 3-second stimulus is applied. If no reaction occurs, stimulation may be repeated after 1 minute. A total of three attempts at fetal acoustic stimulation may be made, each at a minimum of 1-minute intervals. Some advantages to using fetal acoustic stimulation are not only that it may decrease both testing time and the incidence of

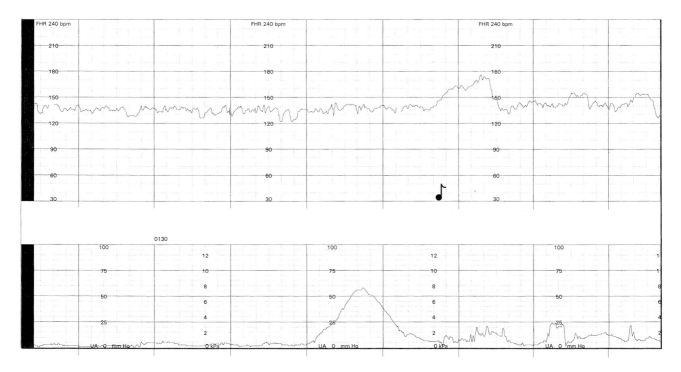

FIGURE 4–5. Acceleration in response to fetal acoustic stimulation (musical note).

nonreactive NSTs,[16,18] but also that the procedure is noninvasive and easy to perform. If fetal hypoxia/acidosis is suspected, an alternative method to assess fetal status should be used.

Some limitations to the use of fetal acoustic stimulation include the possibility of variable decelerations or tachycardia in response to the stimulus. The occurrence of either result prompts further monitoring and investigation. If the fetus fails to respond to acoustic stimulation by producing a reactive NST, further testing is indicated, such as with a contraction stress test or biophysical profile. It is also important to note that when magnesium sulfate is being administered to the patient, FHR accelerations may be blunted and fetal movements reduced in response to VAS.[19] In this clinical circumstance, if fetal hypoxia/acidosis is suspected, an alternative method to assess fetal status should be used. Accordingly, fetal acoustic stimulation is not presently supported by research for use in labor; therefore, it is important to categorize it as an antepartum screening technique only.[20]

CONTRACTION STRESS TEST

The contraction stress test (CST) is another screening test that involves observing the FHR response to three palpable contractions (≥40 seconds' duration) that occur within a 10-minute period. The FHR pattern is assessed for the presence of late decelerations, which represent possible evidence of uteroplacental insufficiency. The advantage of using the CST is that, in progressive fetal compromise, late decelerations may appear before the disappearance of accelerations. As such, the CST may be an earlier predictor of declining fetal status than the NST.[21] Additionally, if performed as an adjunct assessment after a nonreactive NST, the CST can assist in determining whether the nonreactive result is indicative of hypoxia/acidosis.

There are variations in how the contraction pattern for the performance of the CST is initiated. These include assessing the patient who is experiencing spontaneous contractions, having the patient perform nipple stimulation to elicit contractions, or by administering oxytocin intravenously (also referred to as an *oxytocin challenge test*). Nipple stimulation is the most efficient means of eliciting a contraction pattern for the purposes of the CST. This can be accomplished by having the patient rub one nipple through her clothing until contractions occur. If this activity does not prompt an adequate contraction pattern within 2 minutes, the patient is instructed to stop performing stimulation. She may attempt this technique again after 5 minutes.[2,22]

If nipple stimulation is not successful in generating an adequate contraction pattern, administration of oxytocin may produce the desired results. Oxytocin is administered intravenously with the aid of an infusion pump, starting at a rate of 0.5 mU/min. The dosage may be doubled at a frequency of 20-minute intervals until an adequate contraction pattern is initiated.[2]

Some limitations to performing the CST include that it is not always possible to elicit enough contractions or, of greater concern, it is possible to cause too many contractions (tachysystole). It is not currently a popular choice for testing for a variety of reasons, including that it is not especially convenient to perform and there are other combinations of options available in most settings (Appendix B). Performing an NST first and obtaining a reactive tracing can rule out the need for this test. Administration of oxytocin requires the placement of an intravenous catheter, an invasive procedure that carries risk and may cause maternal discomfort, and the CST is often time-consuming and carries a high false-positive rate (late decelerations are present during testing, but the fetus is tolerant of subsequent labor induction) of 35% to 50%.[23,24] Finally, care must be taken not to perform this test in cases where the presence of contractions would present risk to the patient or fetus, such as when preterm labor, uterine rupture, or bleeding might ensue. Interpretation of the results of the CST is as follows:

- *Negative:* Absence of late decelerations observed during testing (Figure 4–6)

- *Positive:* Late decelerations occurring in response to 50% or more of the contractions (Figure 4–7)
- *Equivocal (suspicious):* Intermittent late decelerations or significant variable decelerations; (hyperstimulatory) decelerations related to tachysystole (Figure 4–8)
- *Unsatisfactory:* Inability to achieve the three required contractions within the 10-minute time frame or the tracing is of poor quality (Figure 4–9)

In most instances, a negative CST will be followed with weekly repeat testing. This may be prescribed in addition to more frequent performance of NSTs or biophysical profiles (discussed later in this chapter and in more detail in Chapter 13). Any result other than a negative CST requires immediate follow-up investigation. If the fetus is mature, the patient with a nonreactive NST and a positive CST should be immediately followed with a sonographic examination to rule out anomalies and, barring their existence, considered for delivery. These test results indicate that the fetus may not be adequately oxygenated by way of the placenta, and there is no reassurance that the fetus is in a supportive intrauterine environment. A preterm fetus may be either further evaluated by adjunct methods and repeat testing in a timely manner, or it

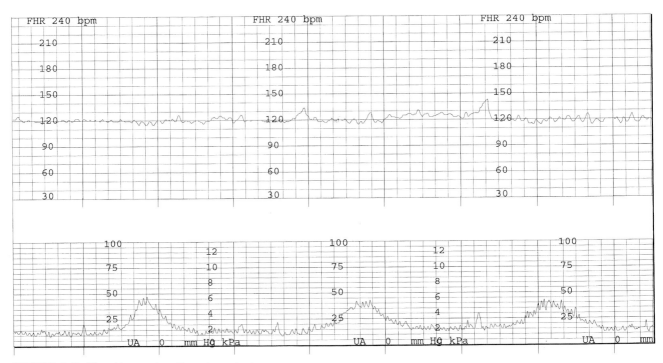

FIGURE 4–6. Negative contraction stress test.

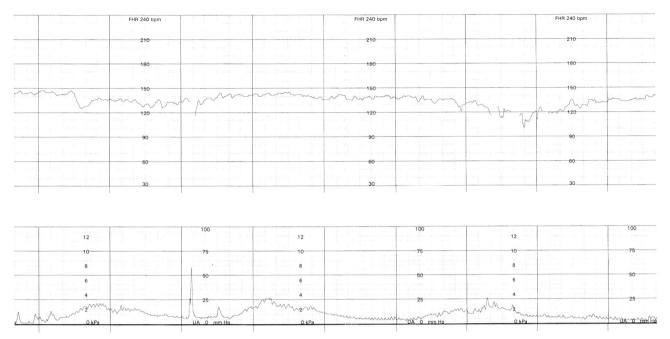

FIGURE 4–7. Positive contraction stress test.

may be decided that extrauterine life would be more beneficial. This decision requires the evaluation of test results within the context of the entire clinical situation.

An equivocal or unsatisfactory test result presents a more challenging situation. Repeating the CST within 24 hours[2,23] or performing immediate evaluation with a biophysical profile is warranted.

BIOPHYSICAL PROFILE

The biophysical profile (BPP) involves evaluating the fetus with a combination of EFM and real-time sonography. The fetus is assessed on five separate criteria: the presence or absence of a reactive NST, the presence or absence of fetal breathing movements, the presence or absence of fetal movement and visualization of fetal

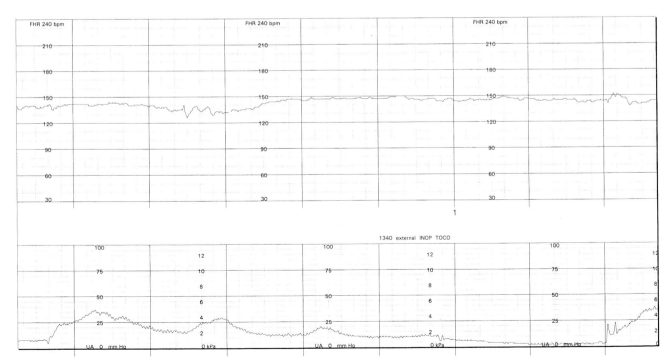

FIGURE 4–8. Equivocal (suspicious) contraction stress test.

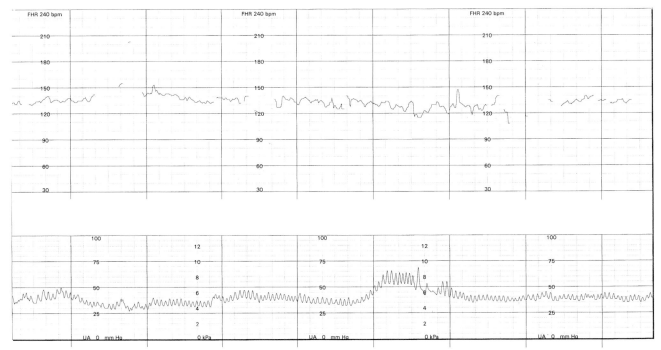

FHR Baseline = Indeterminate

FIGURE 4–9. Unsatisfactory contraction stress test.

tone as evidenced by flexion and extension, and the measurement of amniotic fluid volume.[25,26] A number of variations in biophysical testing have evolved since its inception. With the Manning criteria,[2] a possible score of 2 points is assigned for the satisfaction of each parameter and a score of 0 is assigned to each criterion that is not met. No partial credit is given. The highest and most reassuring BPP test result, therefore, is a score of 10 (Table 4–2).[25]

Interpretation of the BPP is as follows:

- 10/10, 8/10: Reassuring
- 6/10: Equivocal
- 4/10, 2/10, 0/10: Nonreassuring

The Vintzileos[26] scoring system is on a 12-point scale and is seldom used. This variation of the BPP

includes the addition of a sixth component, placental grading. If the placenta is observed to be appropriate for gestational age, 2 points are assigned. This raises the total possible score for the BPP to 12.[26] Additionally, if the fetus moves, breathes, or demonstrates tone yet in an amount insufficient to satisfy the criteria for a full score, a partial score of 1 is given for that behavior.

The third variation is the "modified BPP." This involves first performing the NST and then measuring the amniotic fluid index by sonography. If both parameters are reassuring, it can be assumed that the result is equivalent to a BPP of 8/10. This conclusion is derived from the assumption that, if the NST is reactive, fetal movement and fetal tone are likely to be present.[27] More recently, it has been shown

TABLE 4–2 MANNING BIOPHYSICAL PROFILE (BPP)

Criteria for Evaluation	Nonreassuring Results	Reassuring Results
NST	Nonreactive = 0	Reactive = 2
Fetal breathing movements	Absent or ↓ = 0	Present (≥1 episodes sustained for ≥30 seconds occurring within 30 minutes of observation) = 2
Fetal movement	Absent or ↓ = 0	Present (≥3 episodes of body or limb movements occurring within 30 minutes of observation) = 2
Fetal tone	–Flexion/–episode(s) of extension/flexion = 0	Present (≥1 episode of extension of an extremity with return to flexion or opening and closing of a hand) = 2
Amniotic fluid volume	↓ Fluid = 0	Adequate fluid (>2 cm vertical pocket) = 2

Adapted from Manning et al.[25]

that using fetal acoustic stimulation early in the BPP testing can shorten the testing time and reduce the number of nonreassuring test results.[28]

Any fetus with a score of less than 8/10 (per Manning criteria) on the BPP requires further observation and possible intervention. The equivocal score is managed the same as that of an equivocal CST; the test is to be repeated within 24 hours, preferably sooner. Gestational age is also taken into consideration when determining management strategies. Manning and associates found that there was a significantly lower incidence of cerebral palsy in fetuses at risk who were tested with BPP than in untested patients.[29,30] Any fetus found to have oligohydramnios, regardless of the result of the BPP, requires further evaluation. Please see Chapter 13 for more detailed information about BPP.

The specific antepartum screening test selected may vary depending on resources, location, or practitioner preference (see Appendix B). Regardless of the type of test(s) chosen or the order of their performance, antepartum testing is a highly predictive indicator of fetal well-being.

REFERENCES

1. American Academy of Pediatrics and American College of Obstetricians and Gynecologists. *Guidelines for Perinatal Care.* 7th ed. Washington, DC: ACOG; 2012.
2. American College of Obstetrics and Gynecology (ACOG). *Antepartum Fetal Surveillance.* Practice Bulletin No. 9 (Replaces Technical Bulletin No. 188; 1999, reaffirmed 2012). Washington, DC: Author; 2012.
3. American College of Obstetricians and Gynecologists. *Intrapartum fetal Heart Rate Monitoring: Nomenclature Interpretation and General Management Principles.* ACOG Practice Bulletin #106. Washington, DC: Author; 2009.
4. Bishop EH. Fetal acceleration test. *Am J Obstet Gynecol.* 1981;141:905–909.
5. Druzin ML, Fox A, Kogut E, Carlson C. The relationship of the nonstress test to gestational age. *Am J Obstet Gynecol.* 1985;153:386–389.
6. Lavin JP, Miodovnik M, Barden TP. Relationship of nonstress test reactivity and gestational age. *Obstet Gynecol.* 1984;63:338–344.
7. Macones G, Hankin G, Spong CY, et al. The 2008 National Institute of Child Health and Human Development Workshop Report on Electronic Fetal Monitoring Update on Definitions, Interpretation, and Research Guidelines. *Obstet Gynecol.* 2008;112(3):661–666.
8. Freeman RK, Anderson G, Dorchester W. A prospective multi-institutional study of antepartum fetal heart rate monitoring. I. Risk of perinatal mortality and morbidity according to antepartum fetal heart rate test results. *Am J Obstet Gynecol.* 1982;143:771–777.
9. Meis PJ, Ureda JR, Swaim M, et al. Variable decelerations during testing are not a sign of fetal compromise. *Am J Obstet Gynecol.* 1986;154:586–590.
10. Casey BM, McIntire DD, Bloom SL, et al. Pregnancy outcomes after antepartum diagnosis of oligohydramnios at or beyond 34 weeks' gestation. *Am J Obstet Gynecol.* 2000;182:909–912.
11. Evertson LR, Gauthier RJ, Schifrin BS, Paul RH. Antepartum fetal heart rate testing. I. Evolution of the nonstress test. *Am J Obstet Gynecol.* 1979;133:29–33.
12. Evertson L, Paul R. Antepartum fetal heart rate testing: The nonstress test. *Am J Obstet Gynecol.* 1978;132:895–900.
13. Salamalekis E, Loghis C, Panayotopoulos N, et al. Nonstress test: A fifteen-year clinical appraisal. *Clin Exp Obstet Gynecol.* 1997;24(2):79–81.
14. Smith CV, Phelan JP, Platt LD, et al.; FAST II. A randomized clinical comparison with the nonstress test. *Am J Obstet Gynecol.* 1986;155:131–134.
15. Miller-Slade D, Gloeb DJ, Bailey S, et al. Acoustic stimulation induced fetal response compared to traditional nonstress testing. *J Obstet Gynecol Neonat Nurs.* 1991; 20(2):160–167.
16. Marden D, McDuffie RS, Allen R, Abitz D. A randomized controlled trial of a new fetal acoustic stimulation test for fetal well-being. *Am J Obstet Gynecol.* 1997;176(6): 1386–1388.
17. Signore C, Freeman RK, Spong CY. Antenatal testing: A reevaluation. Executive summary of a Eunice Kennedy Shriver National Institute of Child Health and Human Development Workshop. *Obstet Gynecol.* 2009;113(3):687–701.
18. Saracoglu F, Gol K, Sahin I, et al. The predictive value of fetal acoustic stimulation. *J Perinatol.* 1999;19(2): 103105.
19. Sherer DM. Blunted response to vibroacoustic stimulation associated with maternal IV magnesium sulfate therapy. *Am J Perinatol.* 1994;11(6):401–403.
20. East C. Vibroacoustic stimulation for fetal assessment in labour in the presence of a nonreassuring fetal heart rate trace. *Cochrane Database Syst Rev.* 2012;(1):doi:10.1002/14651858.CD004664.pub3
21. Freeman RK. Early indications of placental insufficiency. *Contemp OB/GYN.* 1985;28(47):145–161.
22. Huddleston JF, Sutliff G, Robinson D. Contraction stress test by intermittent nipple stimulation. *Obstet Gynecol.* 1984;63:669–673.
23. Schifrin B, Lapidus M, Doctor GS. Contraction stress test for antepartum evaluation. *Obstet Gynecol.* 1975;45: 433–438.
24. Staisch KJ, Westlake JR, Bashore RA. Blind oxytocin challenge test and perinatal outcome. *Am J Obstet Gynecol.* 1980;138(4):399–403.
25. Manning FA, Baskett TF, Morrison I, Lange I. Fetal biophysical scoring: A prospective study in 1,184 high risk patients. *Am J Obstet Gynecol.* 1981;140(3):289–294.
26. Vintzileos AM, Campbell WA, Ingardia CJ, Nochimson D. The biophysical profile and its predictive value. *Obstet Gynecol.* 1983;62(2):271–278.
27. Miller DA, Rabello YA, Paul RH. The modified biophysical profile: Antepartum testing in the 1990s. *Am J Obstet Gynecol.* 1996;174:812–817.

28. Pinette MG, Blackstone J, Wax JR, Cartin A. Using fetal acoustic stimulation to shorten the biophysical profile. *J Clin Ultrasound.* 2005; 33(5):223–225.
29. Manning FA, Bondagji N, Harman CR, et al. Fetal assessment based on the fetal biophysical profile score: Relationship of last BPS result to subsequent cerebral palsy. *Journal de Gynecologie Obstetrique et Biologie de la Reproduction.* 1997;26(7):720–729.
30. Manning FA, Bondagji N, Harman CR, et al. Fetal assessment based on biophysical profile scoring. VIII. The incidence of cerebral palsy in tested and untested perinates. *Am J Obstet Gynecol.* 1998;178(4):696–706.

SUGGESTED READINGS

Association of Women's Health, Obstetric, and Neonatal Nurses. *Antepartum and Intrapartum Fetal Heart Rate Monitoring: Clinical Competencies and Education Guide.* 5th ed. Washington, DC: Author; 2011.
Clark SL, Gimovsky ML, Miller FC. The scalp stimulation test: A clinical alternative to fetal scalp blood sampling. *Am J Obstet Gynecol.* 1984;148(3):274–277.
Smith CV, Davis SR, Rayburn WF, Nelson R M. Fetal habituation to vibroacoustic stimulation in uncomplicated term pregnancies. *Am J Perinatol.* 1991;8(6):380–382.

CHAPTER 5

Exercises in Electronic Fetal Monitoring

The exercises presented in this chapter are meant to facilitate the integration of the didactic information contained within the text of this book into the processes of critical thinking necessary for practicing the skill of electronic fetal monitoring (EFM). In each of the following case studies, select portions of the fetal strip chart are presented along with the contemporaneous nurse's notes. When gaps in the data occur, the passage of time is denoted at the start of the subsequent portion of the fetal strip chart.

Proper completion of the exercises includes comparison of one's interpretation of the fetal strip with the Guide to Interpretation that is located at the end of this chapter. It is necessary to recognize that the information presented within the case studies has been preserved for the purpose of being as accurately reflective of actual circumstances as is possible without breaching confidentiality. Therefore, the interpretations and interventions presented within each case study are not necessarily reflective of the best practices or current standard of care. Comparison with the Guide to Interpretation (located in the second half of this chapter) and with current, evidence-based practice is essential in promoting appropriate clinical decision making. The Guide to Interpretation is based upon the reasoning and parameters for evaluating EFM data as have been explained throughout the preceding chapters. Minor variations in interpretation are expected to occur as a result of multiple factors (as discussed in Chapters 3 and 7); that is, there may be some insignificant differences between readers' interpretations or between the reader and authors' interpretations.

For purposes of confidentiality, all proper pronouns have been removed from the case studies. All other identifying data have been altered to protect the privacy of the patient. Only the clinical designation of the person mentioned (e.g., RN, CNM, MD, etc.) is presented.

The commentary appearing above the strip chart corresponds with the numerical annotations located in the center margin of the paper strip chart. Abbre-

viations and nomenclature may vary from case to case, based on regional or individual differences in expression (e.g., use of the terms *UC* or *CTX* to express *uterine contraction*).

For the purposes of clarity and consistency, the Guide to Interpretation at the end of this chapter utilizes the terminology suggested by the 2008 National Institute of Child Health and Human Development Workshop Report on Electronic Fetal Monitoring (see Chapter 3).[1] When the case studies present monitoring of uterine activity (UA) through use of an intrauterine pressure catheter (IUPC), the strength of contractions is expressed in a peak-minus-baseline format. It is necessary to recognize that the selected methods for expressing interpretation of the strip chart employed in the Guide to Interpretation may not be reflective of individual institutional standards or culture. Additionally, minor interobserver variations in interpretation are likely to occur. Such differences should be viewed objectively and utilized as a catalyst for discussion and continued learning.

The case studies are presented on strip charts that are printed with 30–240 bpm paper scaling. Because the examples are presented at 3 cm/min paper speed, each regularly occurring vertical marker represents the passage of 10 seconds of time. Every sixth vertical line is emphasized to represent the passage of 1 minute of time (six 10-second segments).

It is necessary assess both the mother and fetus at regular intervals as dictated by institutional policy. These assessments should be documented, and any necessary interventions performed should be communicated to the care provider and to any other personnel who may need to know, such as the charge nurse. Regular assessment of the fetus includes systematic evaluation of the fetal heart rate (FHR) as described in Chapter 3. Common, standardized, and descriptive terminology should be used by care providers and registered nurses to communicate information about the FHR.[2] Such assessments are ordinarily performed at least every 30 minutes during the active phase of the first stage of labor and at least every 15 minutes during the second stage. In the presence of risk factors, or with use of oxytocin, the FHR is usually evaluated at least every 15 minutes during the active phase of the first stage of labor and at least every 5 minutes during the second stage.[2–4]

It is important to be aware of institutional policies on evaluation and documentation and also utilize clinical judgment to respond appropriately to individual clinical circumstances. The exercises in this chapter (Box 5–1) provide the opportunity to practice systematic assessment of the FHR. These FHR strips are available on http://solution.lww.com and additional exercises will be added to this website periodically.

REFERENCES

1. Macones G, Hankin G, Spong CY, et al. The 2008 National Institute of Child Health and Human Development Workshop Report on Electronic Fetal Monitoring Update on Definitions, Interpretation, and Research Guidelines. *Obstet Gynecol.* 2008;112(3).
2. Association of Women's Health, Obstetric and Neonatal Nurses. *Fetal heart Monitoring.* Washington, DC: Author; 2008.
3. American Academy of Pediatrics and American College of Obstetricians and Gynecologists. *Guidelines for Perinatal Care.* 7th ed. Washington, DC: ACOG; 2012.
4. American College of Obstetricians and Gynecologists. *Intrapartum Fetal Heart Rate Monitoring: Nomenclature, Interpretation, and General Management Principles.* ACOG Practice Bulletin 106. Washington, DC: Author; 2009.

BOX 5-1 | **Case Review Worksheet for Chapter 5 Exercises**

Photocopy the blank worksheet for convenience in practicing charting on segments of the example tracings.

STRIP CHART

Fetal Heart Rate	*Uterine Activity*		
Baseline:	Frequency:		
Variability:	Duration:		
Periodic/Episodic Changes:	Strength:		
	Resting Tone:		
Category (circle one):	I	II	III

STRIP CHART

Fetal Heart Rate	*Uterine Activity*		
Baseline:	Frequency:		
Variability:	Duration:		
Periodic/Episodic Changes:	Strength:		
	Resting Tone:		
Category (circle one):	I	II	III

STRIP CHART

Fetal Heart Rate	*Uterine Activity*		
Baseline:	Frequency:		
Variability:	Duration:		
Periodic/Episodic Changes:	Strength:		
	Resting Tone:		
Category (circle one):	I	II	III

STRIP CHART

Fetal Heart Rate	*Uterine Activity*		
Baseline:	Frequency:		
Variability:	Duration:		
Periodic/Episodic Changes:	Strength:		
	Resting Tone:		
Category (circle one):	I	II	III

Case Examples

HX OF PATIENT A: 19 Y.O., G1P0, 40 1/7 WEEKS', PRESENTS WITH SROM x 1 HOUR, CLEAR FLUID NOTED. T98². UNREMARKABLE PRENATAL HX.

1) FHR1: TACHYCARDIA

2) ALERT ACKNOWLEDGEMENT

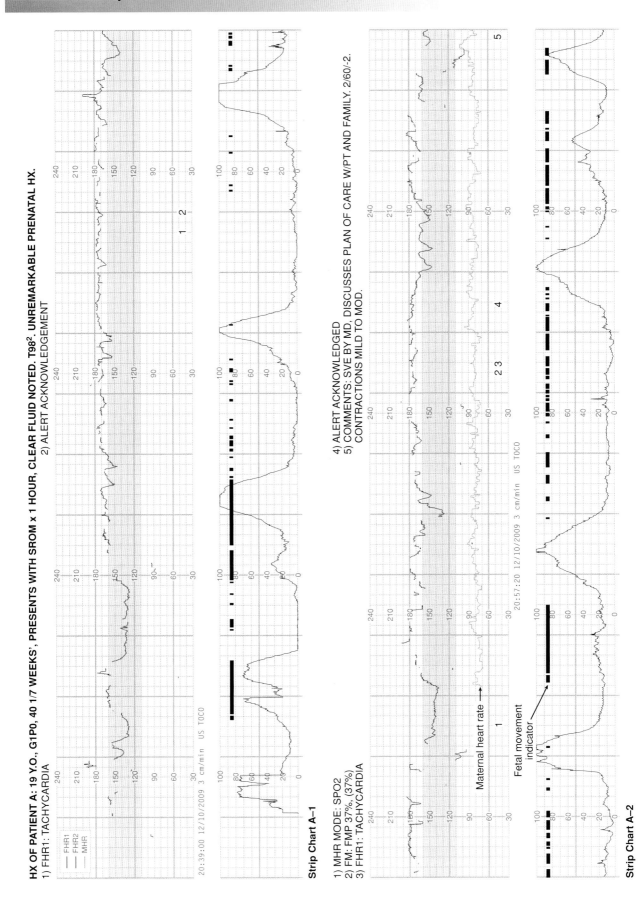

Strip Chart A-1

1) MHR MODE: SPO2
2) FM: FMP 37%, (37%)
3) FHR1: TACHYCARDIA

4) ALERT ACKNOWLEDGED
5) COMMENTS: SVE BY MD, DISCUSSES PLAN OF CARE W/PT AND FAMILY. 2/60/-2. CONTRACTIONS MILD TO MOD.

Maternal heart rate →

Fetal movement indicator

Strip Chart A-2

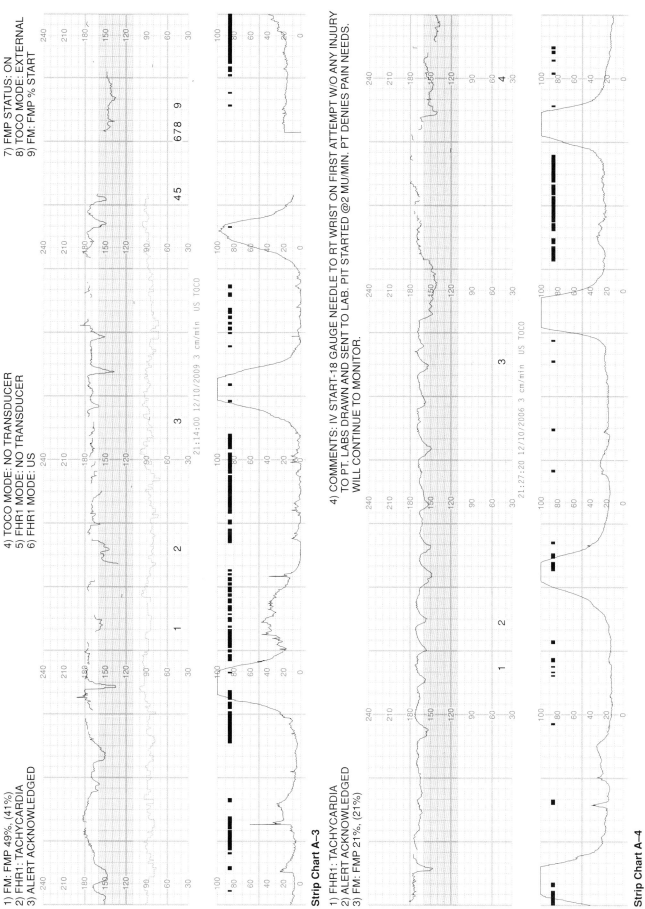

7) FMP STATUS: ON
8) TOCO MODE: EXTERNAL
9) FM: FMP % START

4) TOCO MODE: NO TRANSDUCER
5) FHR1 MODE: NO TRANSDUCER
6) FHR1 MODE: US

1) FM: FMP 49%, (41%)
2) FHR1: TACHYCARDIA
3) ALERT ACKNOWLEDGED

21:14:00 12/10/2009 3 cm/min US TOCO

Strip Chart A–3

1) FHR1: TACHYCARDIA
2) ALERT ACKNOWLEDGED
3) FM: FMP 21%, (21%)

4) COMMENTS: IV START-18 GAUGE NEEDLE TO RT WRIST ON FIRST ATTEMPT W/O ANY INJURY
TO PT. LABS DRAWN AND SENT TO LAB. PIT STARTED @2 MU/MIN. PT DENIES PAIN NEEDS.
WILL CONTINUE TO MONITOR.

21:27:20 12/10/2006 3 cm/min US TOCO

Strip Chart A–4

~ **1 HOUR LATER.**
1) FM: FMP 30%, (33%)

2) OXYTOCIN TO 4 MU/MIN

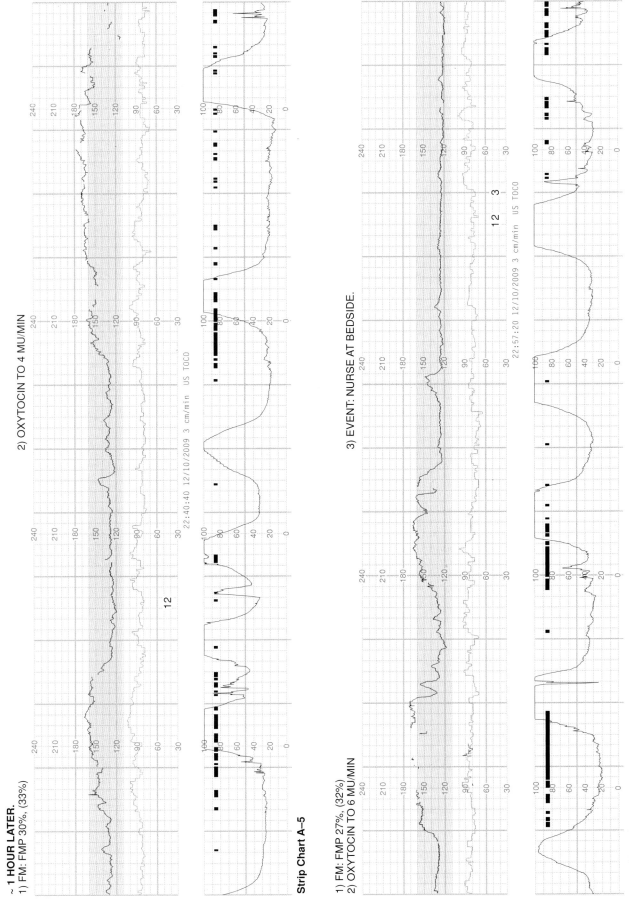

22:40:40 12/10/2009 3 cm/min   US TOCO

Strip Chart A–5

1) FM: FMP 27%, (32%)
2) OXYTOCIN TO 6 MU/MIN

3) EVENT: NURSE AT BEDSIDE.

22:57:20 12/10/2009 3 cm/min   US TOCO

Strip Chart A–6

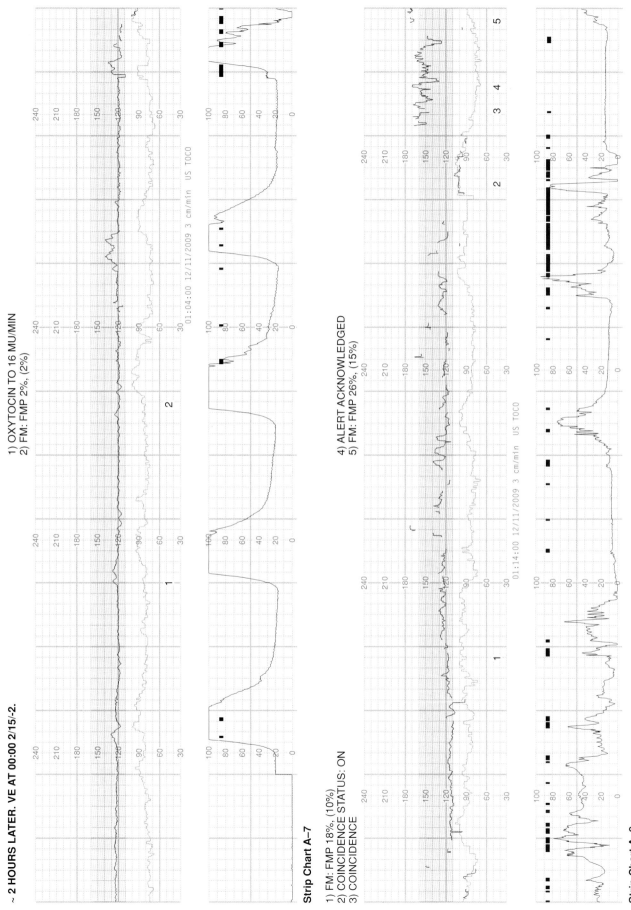

~ 2 HOURS LATER. VE AT 00:00 2/15/-2.

1) OXYTOCIN TO 16 MU/MIN
2) FM: FMP 2%, (2%)

01:04:00 12/11/2009 3 cm/min US TOCO

Strip Chart A–7

1) FM: FMP 18%, (10%)
2) COINCIDENCE STATUS: ON
3) COINCIDENCE

4) ALERT ACKNOWLEDGED
5) FM: FMP 26%, (15%)

01:14:00 12/11/2009 3 cm/min US TOCO

Strip Chart A–8

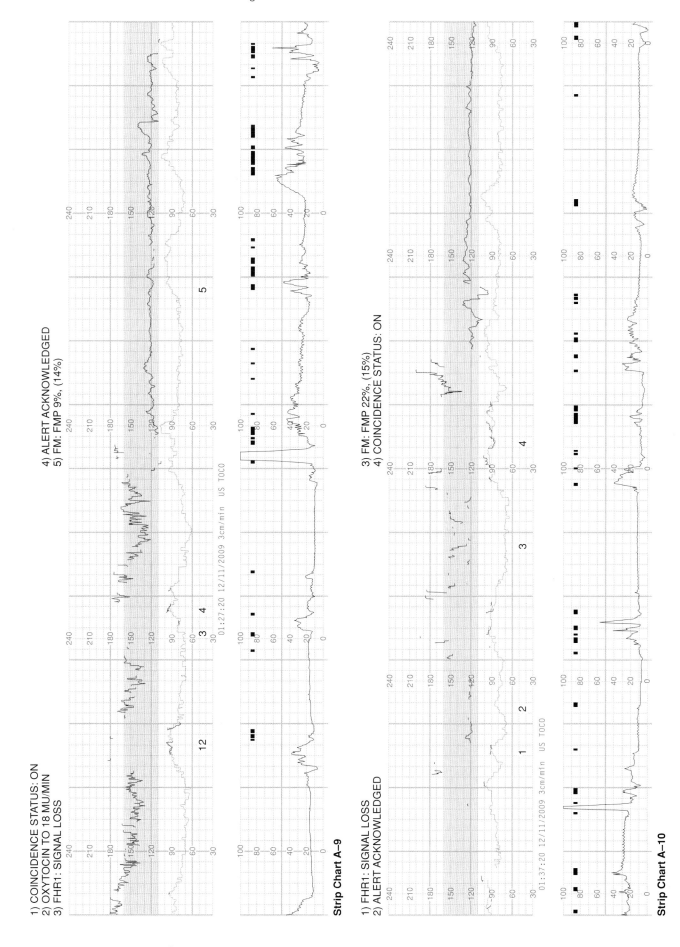

1) COINCIDENCE STATUS: ON
2) OXYTOCIN TO 18 MU/MIN
3) FHR1: SIGNAL LOSS

4) ALERT ACKNOWLEDGED
5) FM: FMP 9%, (14%)

Strip Chart A–9

01:27:20 12/11/2009 3cm/min   US TOCO

1) FHR1: SIGNAL LOSS
2) ALERT ACKNOWLEDGED

3) FM: FMP 22%, (15%)
4) COINCIDENCE STATUS: ON

Strip Chart A–10

01:37:20 12/11/2009 3cm/min   US TOCO

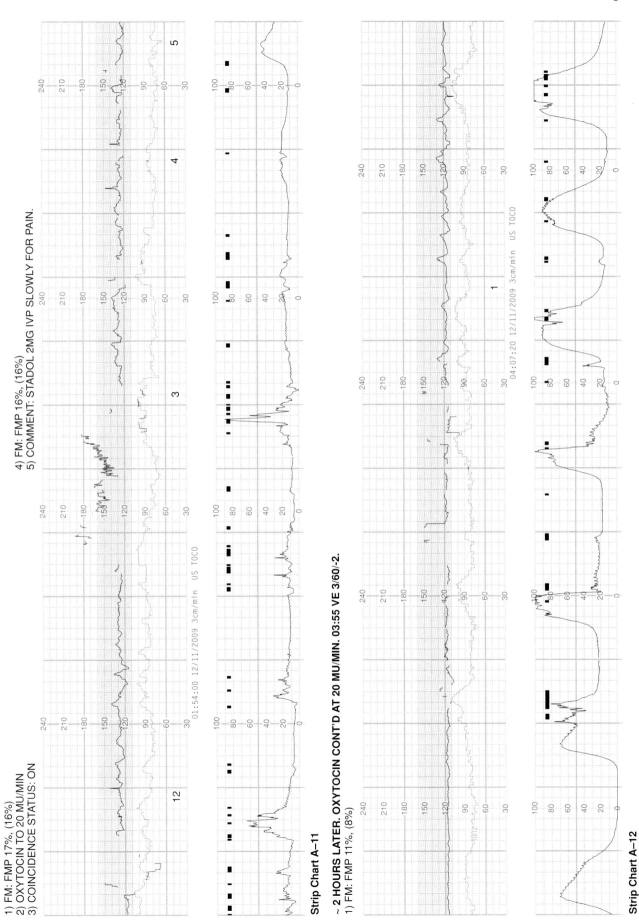

1) FM: FMP 17%, (16%)
2) OXYTOCIN TO 20 MU/MIN
3) COINCIDENCE STATUS: ON

4) FM: FMP 16%, (16%)
5) COMMENT: STADOL 2MG IVP SLOWLY FOR PAIN.

01:54:00 12/11/2009 3cm/min US TOCO

Strip Chart A-11

~ 2 HOURS LATER. OXYTOCIN CONT'D AT 20 MU/MIN. 03:55 VE 3/60/-2.
1) FM: FMP 11%, (8%)

04:07:20 12/11/2009 3cm/min US TOCO

Strip Chart A-12

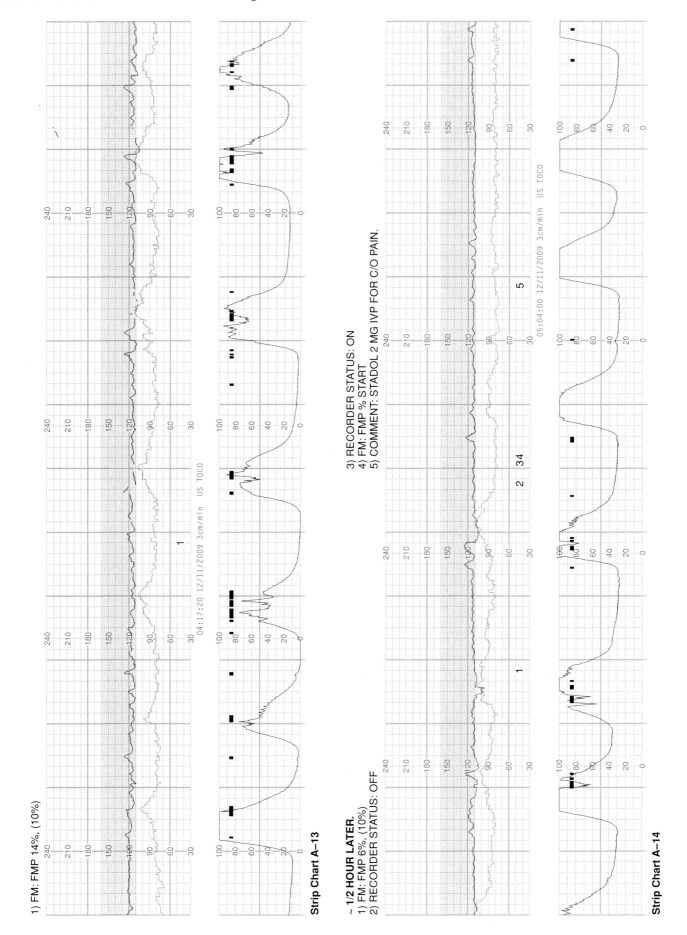

1) FM: FMP 14%, (10%)

04:17:20 12/11/2009 3cm/min US TOCO

Strip Chart A–13

~ 1/2 **HOUR LATER.**
1) FM: FMP 6%, (10%)
2) RECORDER STATUS: OFF

3) RECORDER STATUS: ON
4) FM: FMP % START
5) COMMENT: STADOL 2 MG IVP FOR C/O PAIN.

05:04:00 12/11/2009 3cm/min US TOCO

Strip Chart A–14

1) FM: FMP 2%, (2%)
2) FM: FMP 0%, (1%)

1) FM: FMP 1%, (1%)

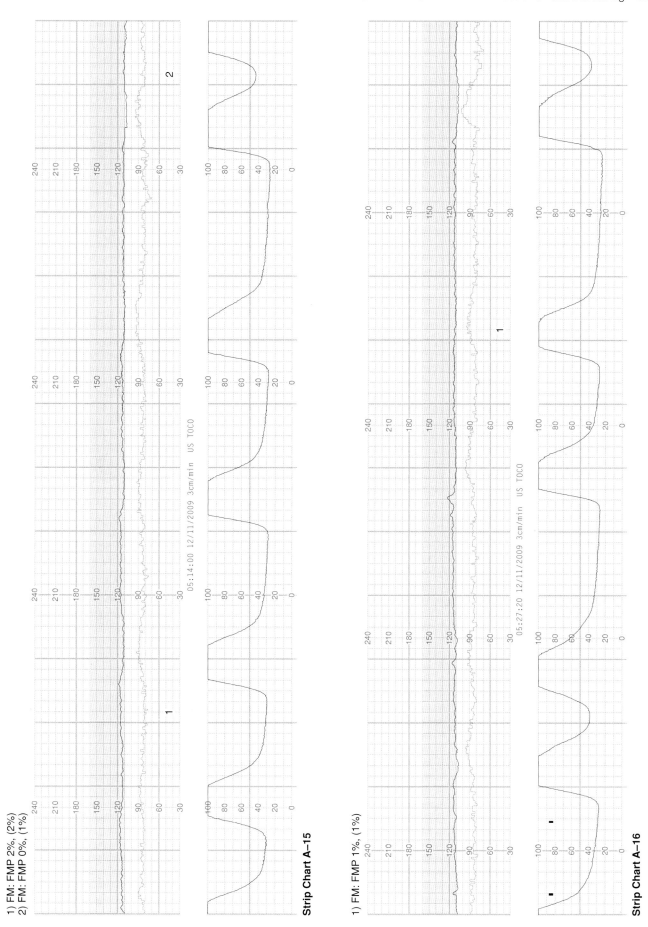

05:14:00 12/11/2009 3cm/min   US TOCO

05:27:20 12/11/2009 3cm/min   US TOCO

Strip Chart A–15

Strip Chart A–16

~ 2 HOURS AND 20 MIN LATER. PT WAS 4/50% AT 06:45. L LATERAL WITH O2 AT 8L/MIN. OXYTOCIN CONTINUES AT 20 MU/MIN. PT BREATHING THROUGH CONTRACTIONS WITH FAMILY SUPPORT, DOES NOT WANT EPIDURAL YET.

1) COINCIDENCE STATUS: ON
2) FM: FMP 27%,(9%)

3) FHR1: BRADYCARDIA
4) ALERT ACKNOWLEDGED

5) COINCIDENCE STATUS: ON
6) SVE 5-6/100/0

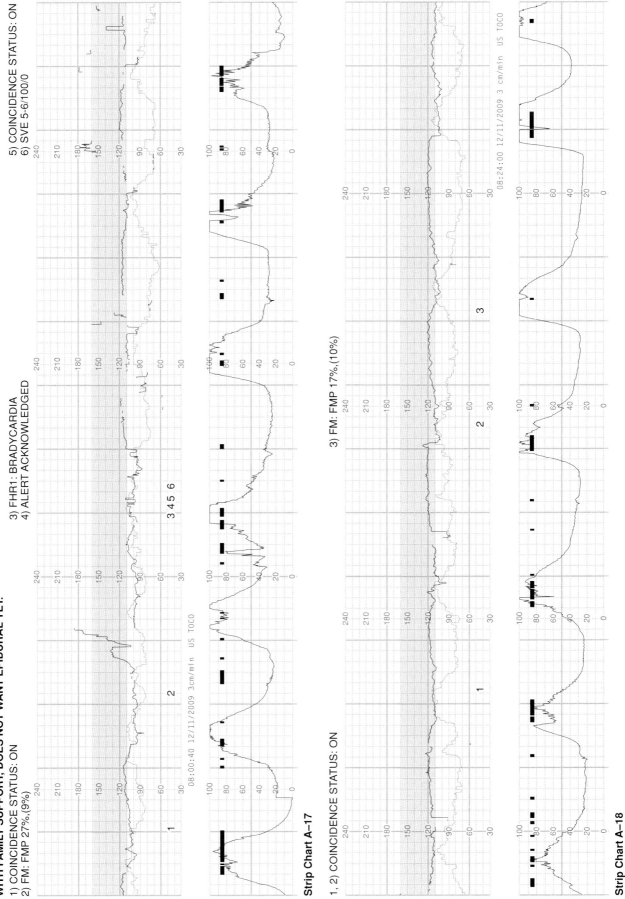

Strip Chart A–17

1, 2) COINCIDENCE STATUS: ON

3) FM: FMP 17%,(10%)

Strip Chart A–18

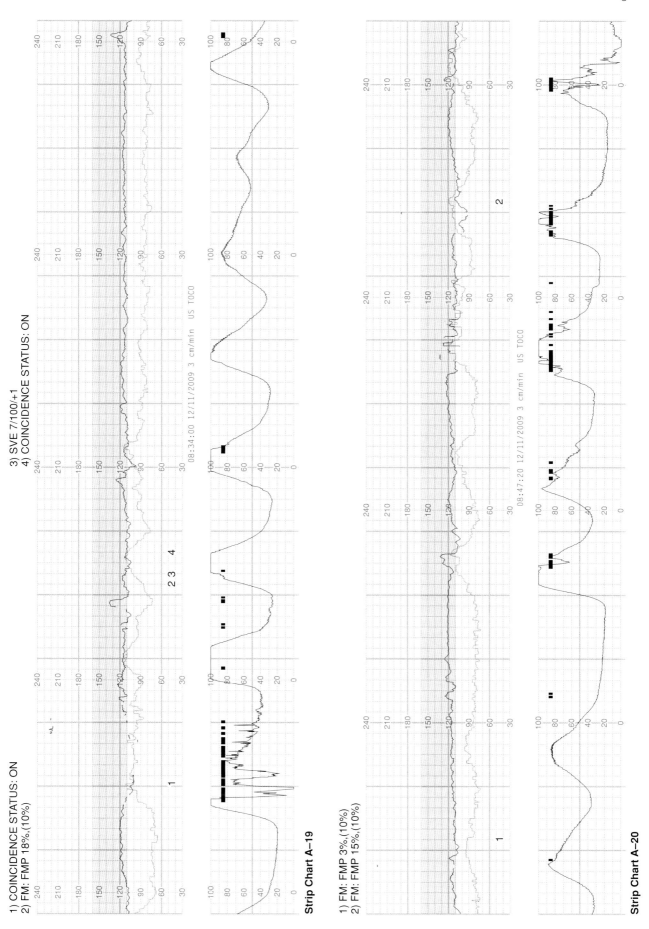

1) COINCIDENCE STATUS: ON
2) FM: FMP 18%,(10%)

3) SVE 7/100/+1
4) COINCIDENCE STATUS: ON

08:34:00 12/11/2009 3 cm/min US TOCO

Strip Chart A–19

1) FM: FMP 3%,(10%)
2) FM: FMP 15%,(10%)

08:47:20 12/11/2009 3 cm/min US TOCO

Strip Chart A–20

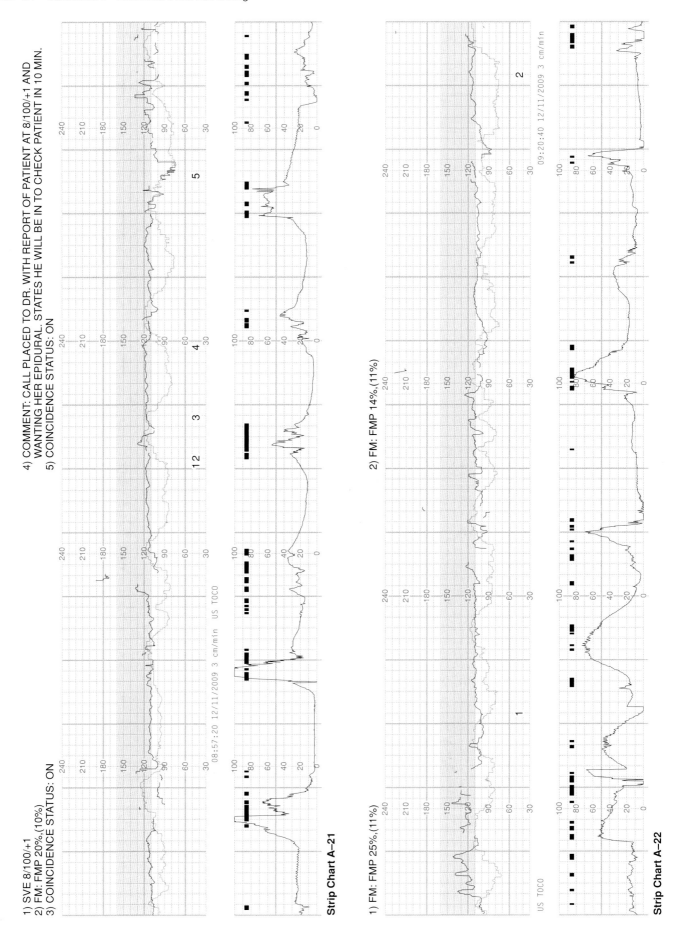

1) SVE 8/100/+1
2) FM: FMP 20%,(10%)
3) COINCIDENCE STATUS: ON

4) COMMENT: CALL PLACED TO DR. WITH REPORT OF PATIENT AT 8/100/+1 AND
   WANTING HER EPIDURAL. STATES HE WILL BE IN TO CHECK PATIENT IN 10 MIN.
5) COINCIDENCE STATUS: ON

1) FM: FMP 25%,(11%)

2) FM: FMP 14%,(11%)

08:57:20 12/11/2009 3 cm/min US TOCO

09:20:40 12/11/2009 3 cm/min

Strip Chart A–21

Strip Chart A–22

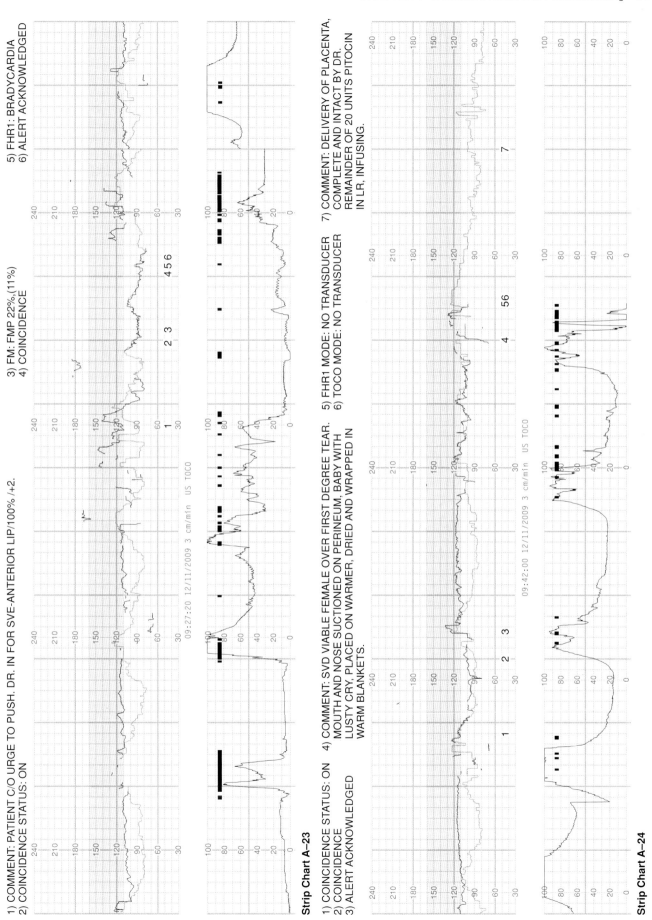

1) COMMENT: PATIENT C/O URGE TO PUSH. DR. IN FOR SVE-ANTERIOR LIP/100% /+2.
2) COINCIDENCE STATUS: ON
3) FM: FMP 22%,(11%)
4) COINCIDENCE
5) FHR1: BRADYCARDIA
6) ALERT ACKNOWLEDGED

09:27:20 12/11/2009 3 cm/min US TOCO

Strip Chart A–23

1) COINCIDENCE STATUS: ON
2) COINCIDENCE
3) ALERT ACKNOWLEDGED
4) COMMENT: SVD VIABLE FEMALE OVER FIRST DEGREE TEAR. MOUTH AND NOSE SUCTIONED ON PERINEUM, BABY WITH LUSTY CRY, PLACED ON WARMER, DRIED AND WRAPPED IN WARM BLANKETS.
5) FHR1 MODE: NO TRANSDUCER
6) TOCO MODE: NO TRANSDUCER
7) COMMENT: DELIVERY OF PLACENTA, COMPLETE AND INTACT BY DR. REMAINDER OF 20 UNITS PITOCIN IN LR, INFUSING.

09:42:00 12/11/2009 3 cm/min US TOCO

Strip Chart A–24

HX OF PATIENT B: PT BEING ADMITTED, APPEARS IN ACTIVE LABOR. LABORING SINCE MIDNIGHT, SROM 05:00. G3P2L2, ONE PRIOR C/S, DESIRING VBAC. BREATHING THROUGH CONTRACTIONS.

1) 12/14/10 15:37 BP 125/87 P 136

2) 12/14/10 15:42 COMMENT: MD IN TO CHECK PATIENT. 8/80%/-3. SPIRAL ELECTRODE APPLIED AS FHR NOT RECORDING WELL. PT IN PAIN WITH AND BETWEEN CTX BUT DECLINES EPIDURAL. BREATHING THROUGH CTX WITH HUSBAND'S SUPPORT.

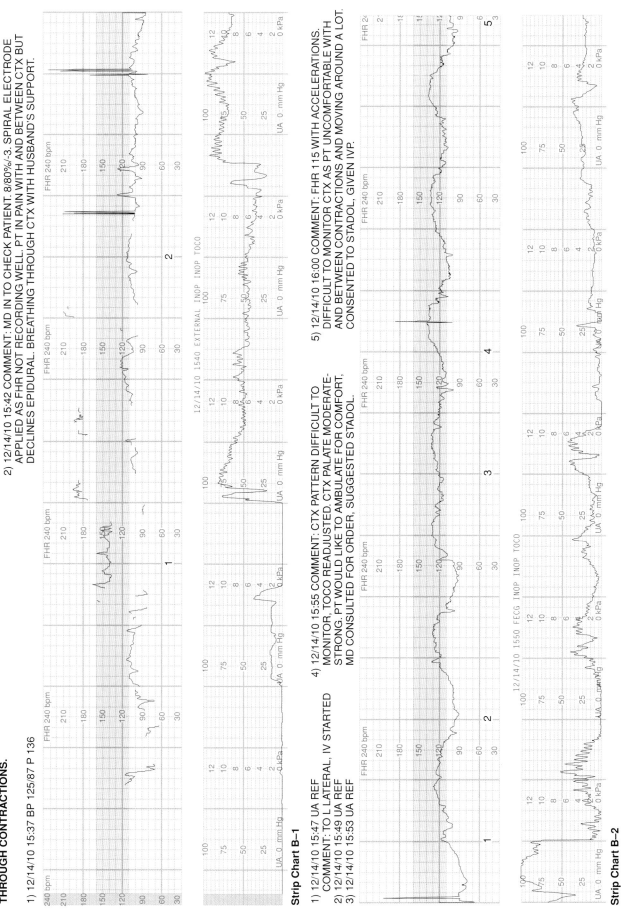

Strip Chart B–1

1) 12/14/10 15:47 UA REF
   COMMENT: TO L LATERAL, IV STARTED
2) 12/14/10 15:49 UA REF
3) 12/14/10 15:53 UA REF

4) 12/14/10 15:55 COMMENT: CTX PATTERN DIFFICULT TO MONITOR, TOCO READJUSTED. CTX PALATE MODERATE-STRONG. PT WOULD LIKE TO AMBULATE FOR COMFORT, MD CONSULTED FOR ORDER, SUGGESTED STADOL.

5) 12/14/10 16:00 COMMENT: FHR 115 WITH ACCELERATIONS. DIFFICULT TO MONITOR CTX AS PT UNCOMFORTABLE WITH AND BETWEEN CONTRACTIONS AND MOVING AROUND A LOT. CONSENTED TO STADOL, GIVEN IVP.

Strip Chart B–2

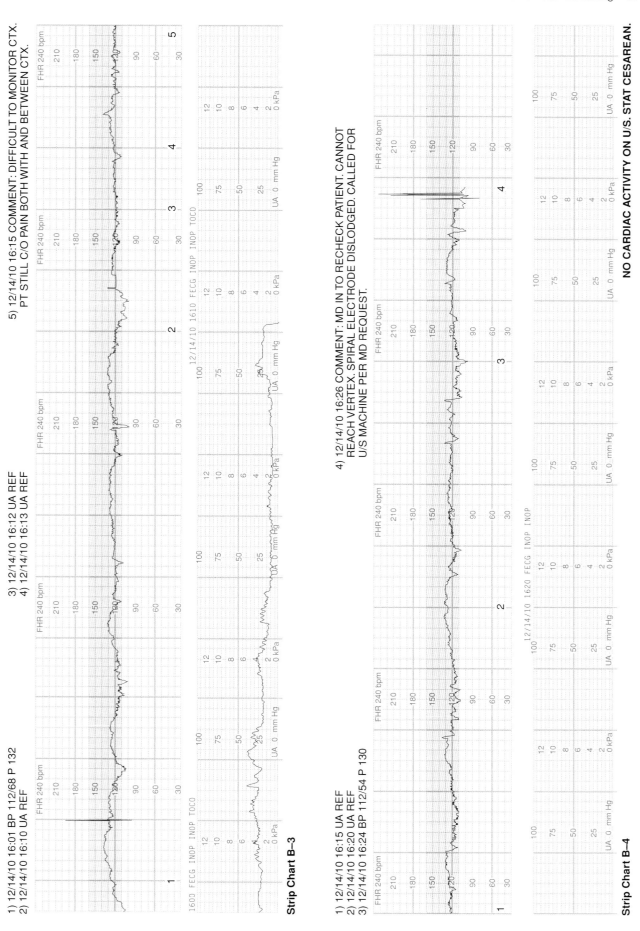

1) 12/14/10 16:01 BP 112/68 P 132
2) 12/14/10 16:10 UA REF

3) 12/14/10 16:12 UA REF
4) 12/14/10 16:13 UA REF

5) 12/14/10 16:15 COMMENT: DIFFICULT TO MONITOR CTX. PT STILL C/O PAIN BOTH WITH AND BETWEEN CTX.

Strip Chart B–3

1) 12/14/10 16:15 UA REF
2) 12/14/10 16:20 UA REF
3) 12/14/10 16:24 BP 112/54 P 130

4) 12/14/10 16:26 COMMENT: MD IN TO RECHECK PATIENT. CANNOT REACH VERTEX. SPIRAL ELECTRODE DISLODGED. CALLED FOR U/S MACHINE PER MD REQUEST.

NO CARDIAC ACTIVITY ON U/S. STAT CESAREAN.

Strip Chart B–4

HX OF PATIENT C: 41 Y.O., G4P3L2A1, 41 2/7 WEEKS', PRIOR CESAREAN (FAILURE TO PROGRESS) AND VBAC (PRECIPITOUS DELIVERY), BOTH PREVIOUS INFANTS >4,000G. ABNORMAL 1 HOUR GTT, DECLINED 3 HOUR GTT. ADMISSION FOR SROM AT 15:00, MECONIUM STAINING NOTED.

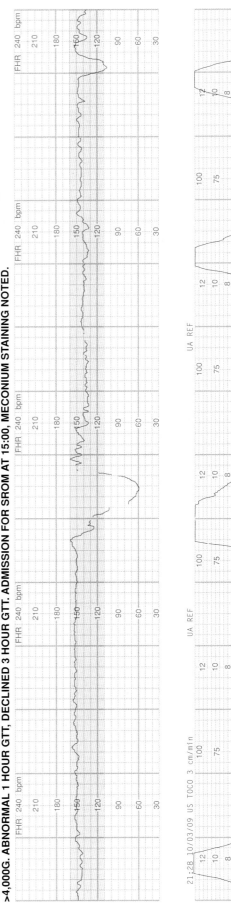

Strip Chart C-1

1) 21:48 COMMENT: IV STARTED AND PATIENT TURNED TO LEFT LATERAL.

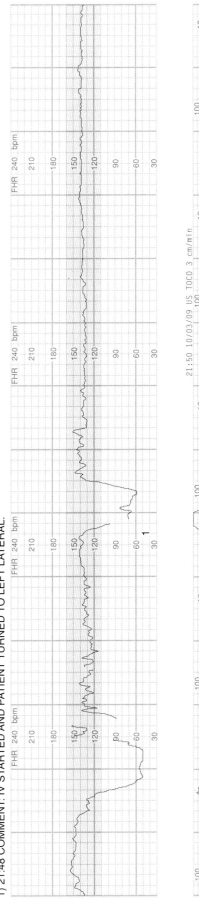

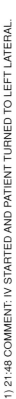

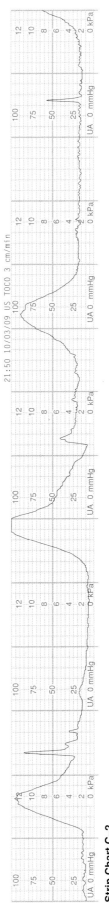

Strip Chart C-2

1) 22:00 COMMENT: VE PERFORMED BY DR, 5-6/90%/0. INTERNAL MONITORS PLACED, CONTRACTIONS PALPATE MILD TO MOD, PT DOES NOT WANT EPIDURAL OR PAIN MEDS AT THIS TIME.

2) 22:02 COMMENT: TO L LATERAL, SUPPORT PERSON PRESENT.

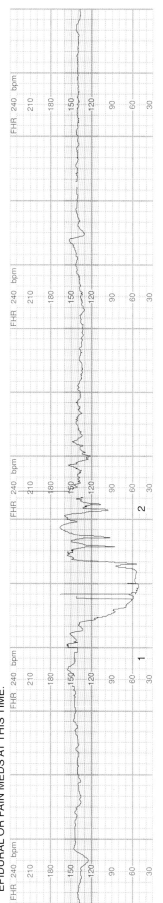
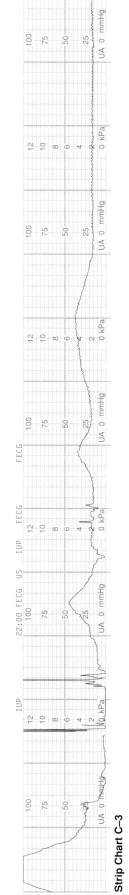

Strip Chart C–3

~ 1 HOUR 20 MIN LATER. OXYTOCIN WAS STARTED AT 2 MU/MIN AT 23:15 AFTER REPEAT VE SHOWED THE CERVIX UNCHANGED. FETUS IN ROP POSITION.

1) 23:34 COMMENT: TO R LATERAL FOR COMFORT.

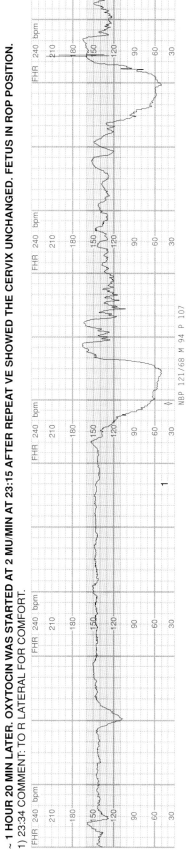
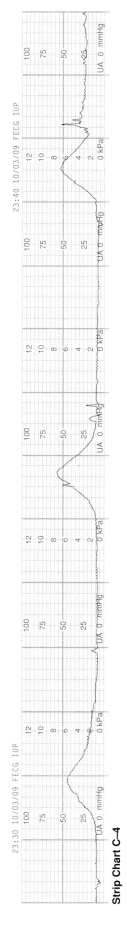

Strip Chart C–4

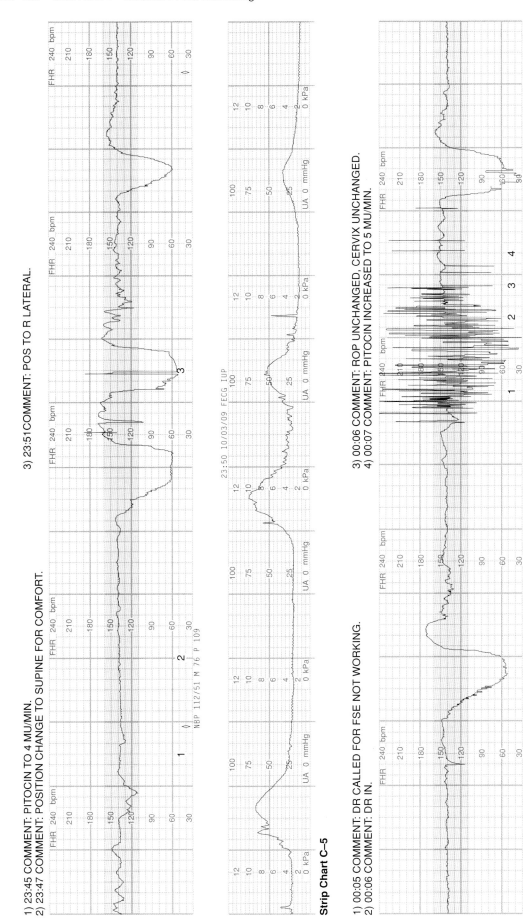

1) 23:45 COMMENT: PITOCIN TO 4 MU/MIN.
2) 23:47 COMMENT: POSITION CHANGE TO SUPINE FOR COMFORT.

3) 23:51 COMMENT: POS TO R LATERAL.

Strip Chart C–5

1) 00:05 COMMENT: DR CALLED FOR FSE NOT WORKING.
2) 00:06 COMMENT: DR IN.

3) 00:06 COMMENT: ROP UNCHANGED, CERVIX UNCHANGED.
4) 00:07 COMMENT: PITOCIN INCREASED TO 5 MU/MIN.

Strip Chart C–6

1) 00:13 COMMENT: POS TO L LATERAL

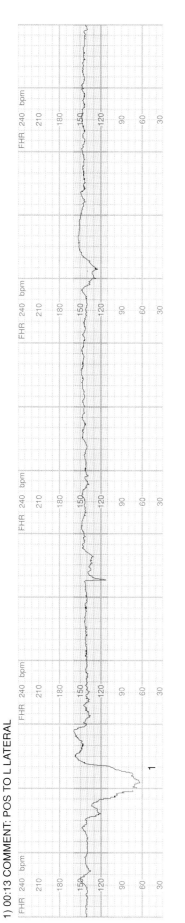

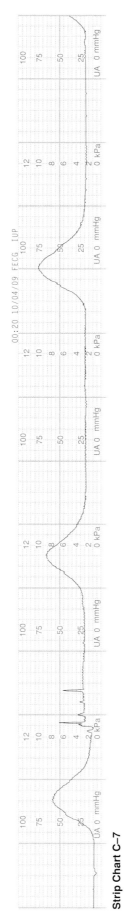

Strip Chart C–7

1) 00:30 COMMENT: PITOCIN INCREASED TO 6 MU/MIN. PT ON R SIDE FOR COMFORT.
2) 00:36 COMMENT: DR IN TO VIEW TRACING.

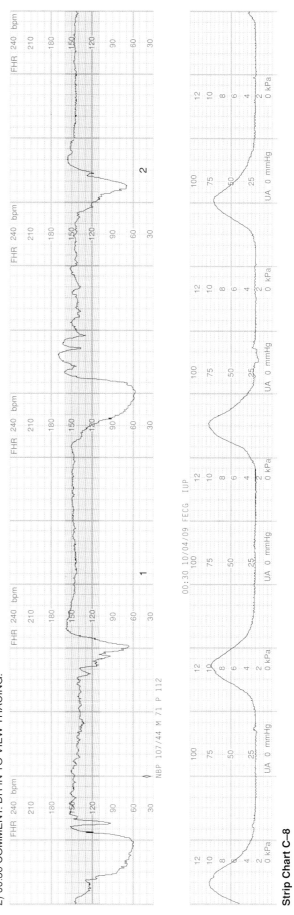

Strip Chart C–8

1) 00:41 COMMENT: TO L LATERAL
2) 00:48 COMMENT: DR IN TO VIEW TRACING. PITOCIN TO 8 MU/MIN.

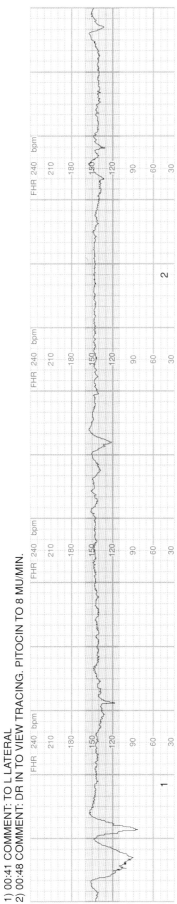

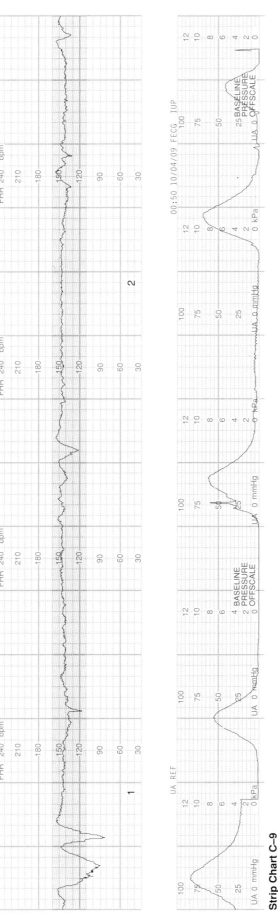

Strip Chart C–9

~ 1 HOUR LATER. MD IN AT 01:30 FOR VE, 7-8CM. OXYTOCIN AT 10 MU/MIN.

1) 01:49 COMMENT: ANESTHESIA IN
2) 01:50 COMMENT: BOLUS IV FLUID.

3) 01:50 COMMENT: TO R LATERAL

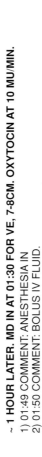

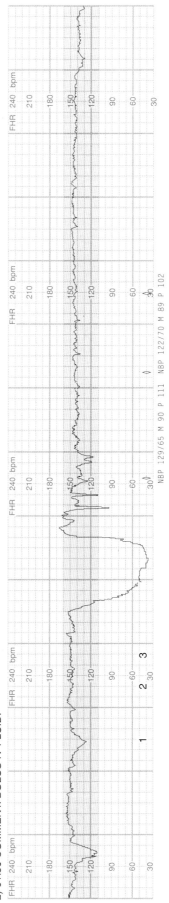

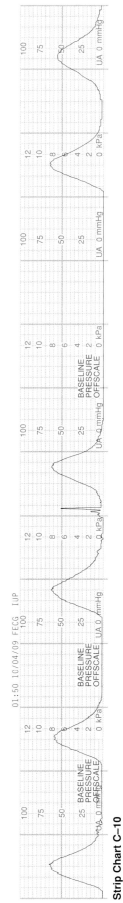

Strip Chart C–10

~ **1 HOUR AND 10 MINUTES LATER. OXYTOCIN AT 14 MU/MIN.**
1) 03:20 COMMENT: PT TO L LATERAL, COMFORTABLE WITH EPIDURAL.

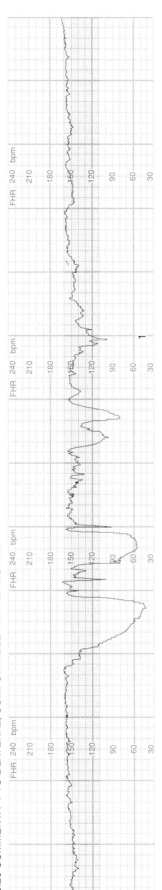

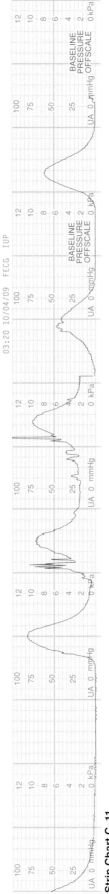

Strip Chart C–11

1) 03:35 COMMENT: PITOCIN INCREASED TO 16 MU/MIN.
2) 03:38 COMMENT: ADJUSTED POSITION

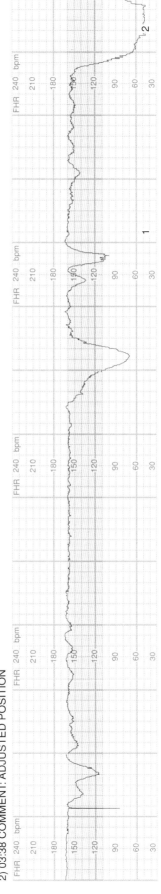

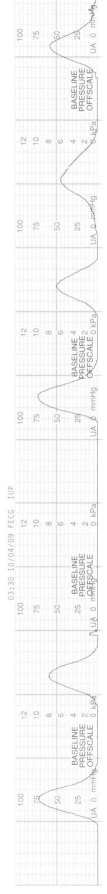

Strip Chart C–12

~ 1/2 HOUR LATER.

1) 04:13 COMMENT: VE - FULLY/+1. BEGIN PUSHING. DR NOTIFIED.

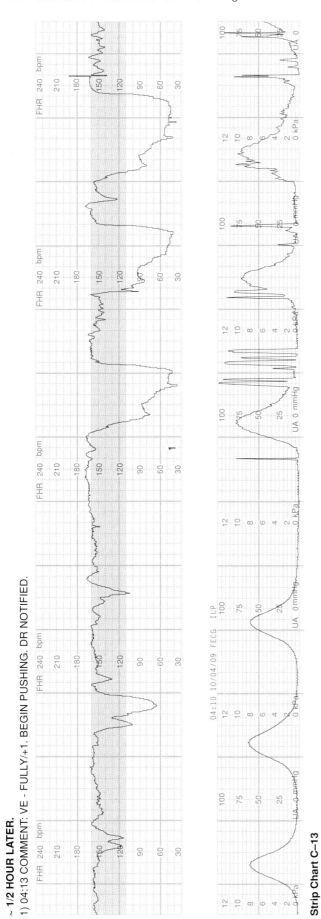

04:10 10/04/09 FECG IUP

Strip Chart C-13

2) 04:34 COMMENT: DR IN, REVIEWS STRIP.

1) 04:25 COMMENT: PUSHING.

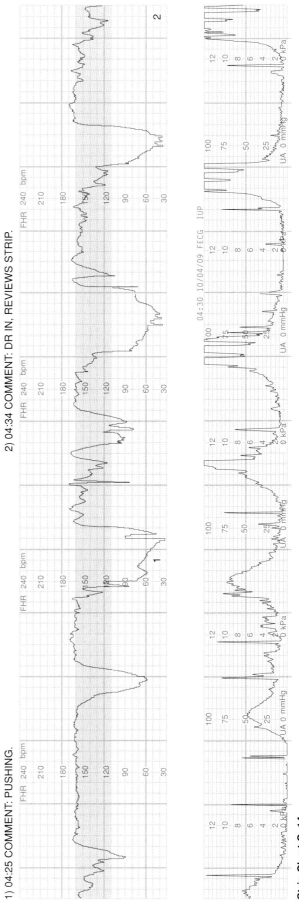

04:30 10/04/09 FECG IUP

Strip Chart C-14

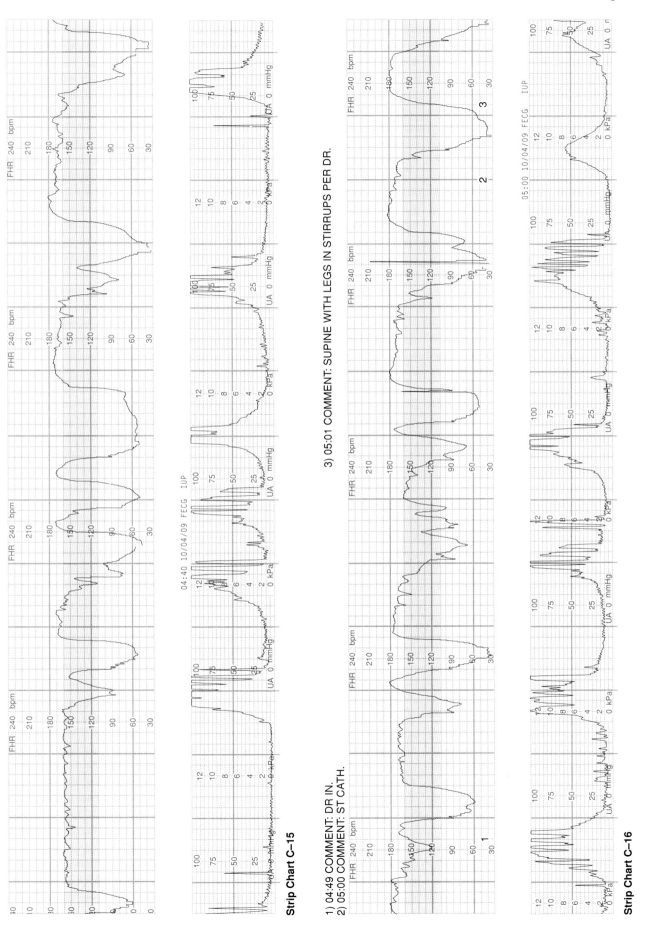

Strip Chart C–15

1) 04:49 COMMENT: DR IN.
2) 05:00 COMMENT: ST CATH.

3) 05:01 COMMENT: SUPINE WITH LEGS IN STIRRUPS PER DR.

Strip Chart C–16

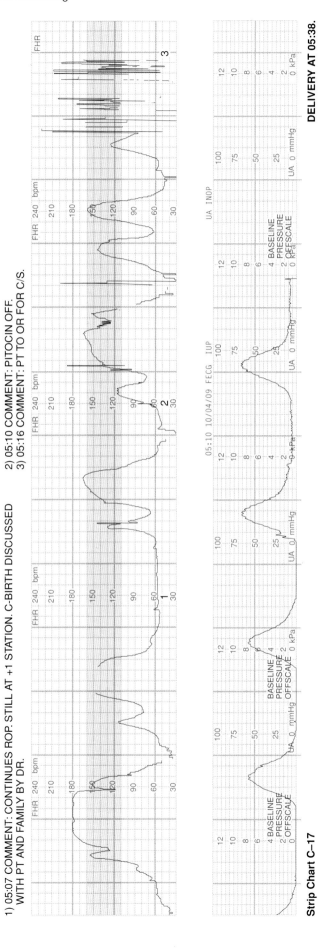

1) 05:07 COMMENT: CONTINUES ROP. STILL AT +1 STATION. C-BIRTH DISCUSSED
WITH PT AND FAMILY BY DR.

2) 05:10 COMMENT: PITOCIN OFF.
3) 05:16 COMMENT: PT TO OR FOR C/S.

Strip Chart C–17

DELIVERY AT 05:38.

HX OF PATIENT D: G1P0, ADMITTED FOR OXYTOCIN INDUCTION FOR POSTDATES AT 40 6/7 WEEKS'. UNREMARKABLE PRENATAL HISTORY. CONTRACTIONS PRESENT ON ADMIT PALPATE MILD-MODERATE; PATIENT SPEAKING EASILY THROUGH THEM AND IS WITHOUT COMPLAINT. CERVICAL EXAM 2-3/50%/-2, MEMBRANES INTACT.

1) COMMENT: IV STARTED IN L WRIST. PLAN OF CARE, INDUCTION PROCESS REVIEWED WITH PATIENT. PT COMFORTABLE AND W/O COMPLAINT.

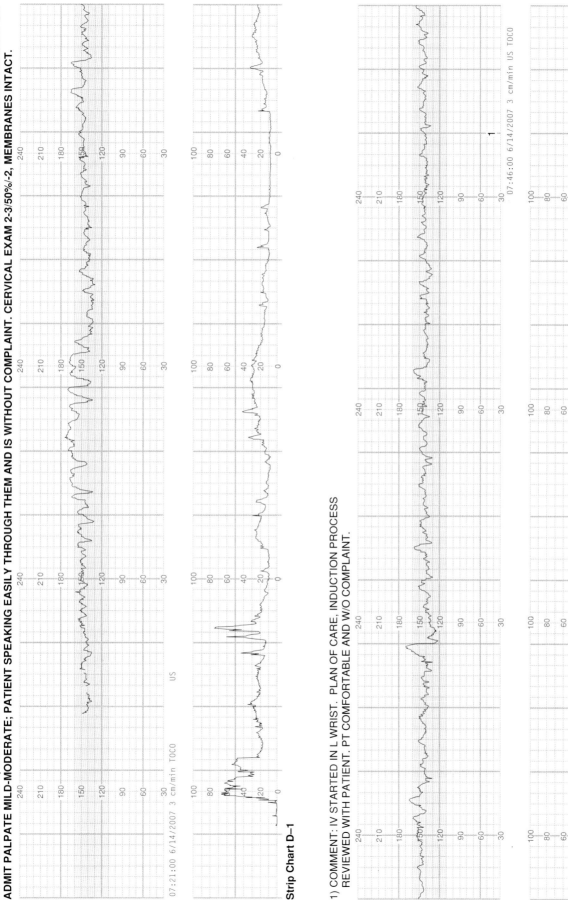

07:21:00 6/14/2007 3 cm/min TOCO

US

Strip Chart D–1

07:46:00 6/14/2007 3 cm/min US TOCO

Strip Chart D–2

~ 15 MINUTES LATER.

1) 08:12 COMMENT: OXYTOCIN BEGUN AT 2 MU/MIN.

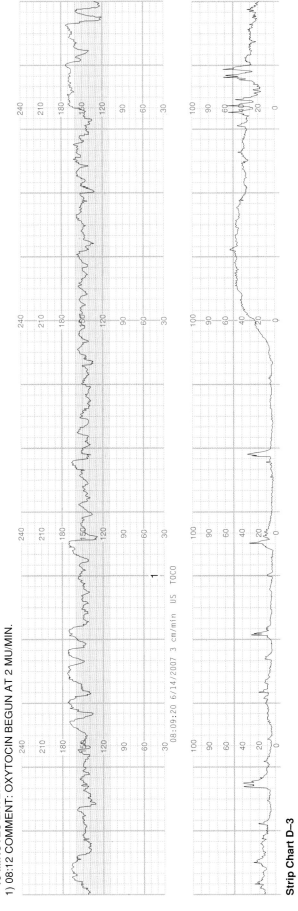

08:09:20 6/14/2007 3 cm/min US TOCO

Strip Chart D–3

~ 25 MINUTES LATER.

1) 08:47 COMMENT: OXYTOCIN TO 3 MU/MIN. CONTRACTIONS PALPATE MILD-MOD.
PT FEELS THEM BUT CAN STILL TALK THROUGH THEM EASILY.

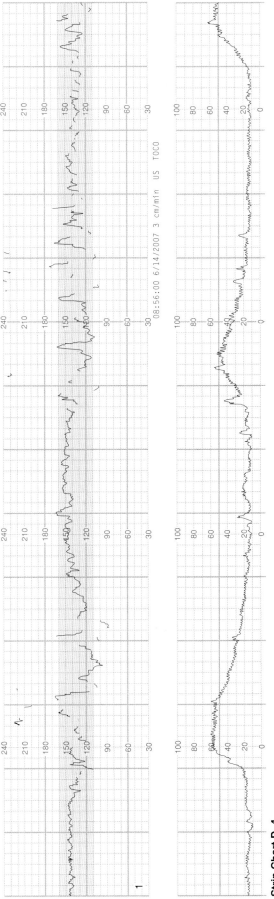

08:56:00 6/14/2007 3 cm/min US TOCO

Strip Chart D–4

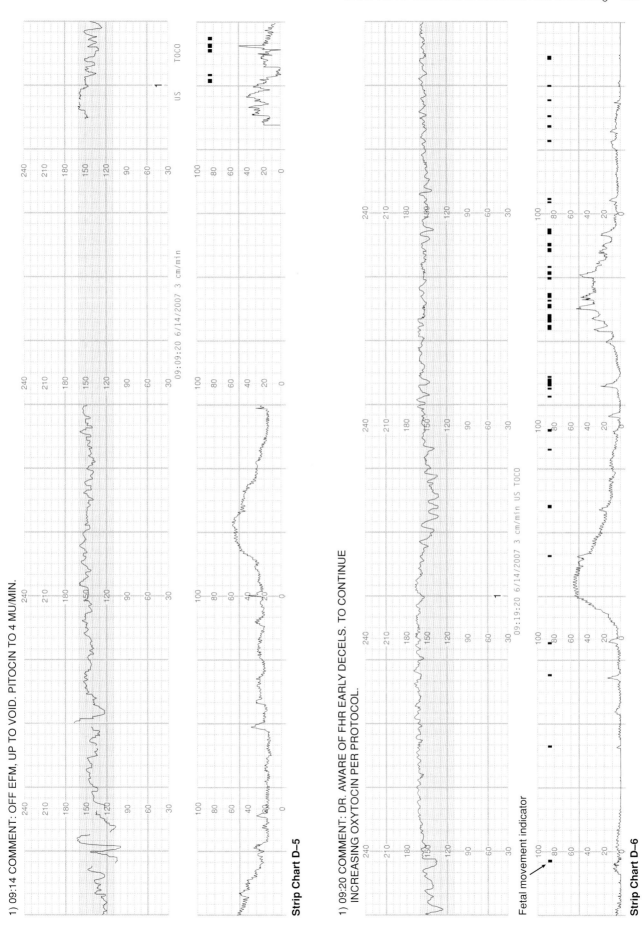

1) 09:14 COMMENT: OFF EFM, UP TO VOID. PITOCIN TO 4 MU/MIN.

09:09:20 6/14/2007 3 cm/min

US   TOCO

Strip Chart D–5

1) 09:20 COMMENT: DR. AWARE OF FHR EARLY DECELS. TO CONTINUE
INCREASING OXYTOCIN PER PROTOCOL.

09:19:20 6/14/2007 3 cm/min US TOCO

Fetal movement indicator

Strip Chart D–6

~ 1 HOUR LATER. PITOCIN AT 8 MU/MIN SINCE 10:15. CONTRACTIONS NOTED TO PALPATE MODERATE.

1) 10:42 COMMENT: PITOCIN DOSE CUT IN HALF DUE TO DECELERATION. NURSE SUPERVISOR IN.

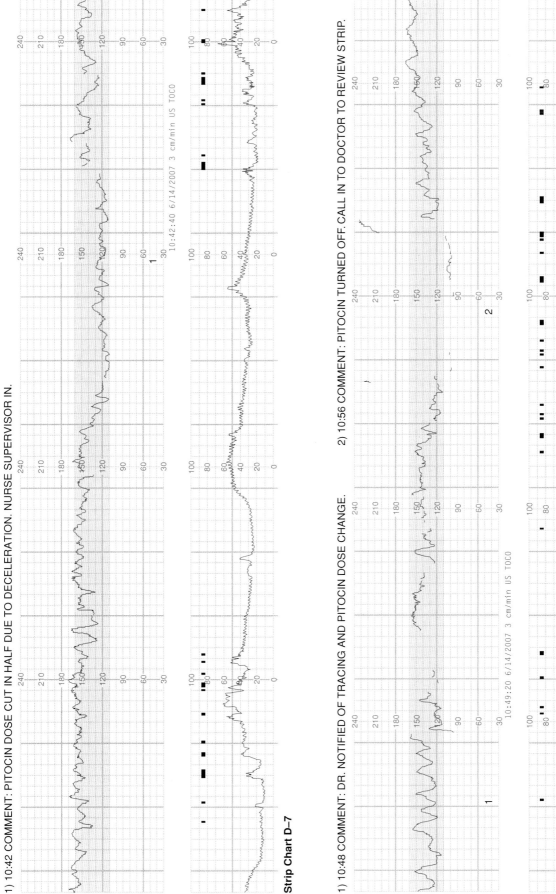

10:42:40 6/14/2007 3 cm/min US TOCO

Strip Chart D–7

1) 10:48 COMMENT: DR. NOTIFIED OF TRACING AND PITOCIN DOSE CHANGE.

2) 10:56 COMMENT: PITOCIN TURNED OFF. CALL IN TO DOCTOR TO REVIEW STRIP.

10:49:20 6/14/2007 3 cm/min US TOCO

Strip Chart D–8

1) 11:04 COMMENT: SUPERVISOR SPOKE WITH DR, WHO WISHES TO KEEP
PITOCIN ON.

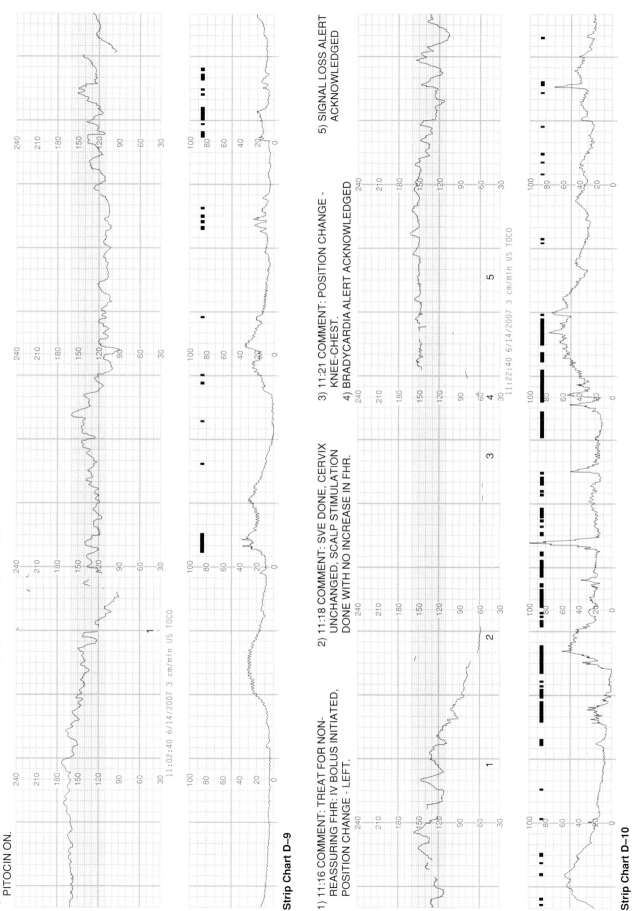

11:02:40 6/14/2007 3 cm/min US TOCO

Strip Chart D–9

1) 11:16 COMMENT: TREAT FOR NON-
REASSURING FHR: IV BOLUS INITIATED,
POSITION CHANGE - LEFT.

2) 11:18 COMMENT: SVE DONE, CERVIX
UNCHANGED, SCALP STIMULATION
DONE WITH NO INCREASE IN FHR.

3) 11:21 COMMENT: POSITION CHANGE -
KNEE-CHEST.
4) BRADYCARDIA ALERT ACKNOWLEDGED

5) SIGNAL LOSS ALERT
ACKNOWLEDGED

11:22:40 6/14/2007 3 cm/min US TOCO

Strip Chart D–10

1) 11:27 COMMENT: DR IN TO REVIEW TRACING. PITOCIN REMAINS OFF. 2-3/50%.

2) 11:40 COMMENT: DR GOING INTO ANOTHER DELIVERY. HAS RESUMED OXYTOCIN AT 6 MU/MIN. ORDER FOR C/S PAPERWORK SIGNED IN CASE NO PROGRESS BY NEXT CHECK.

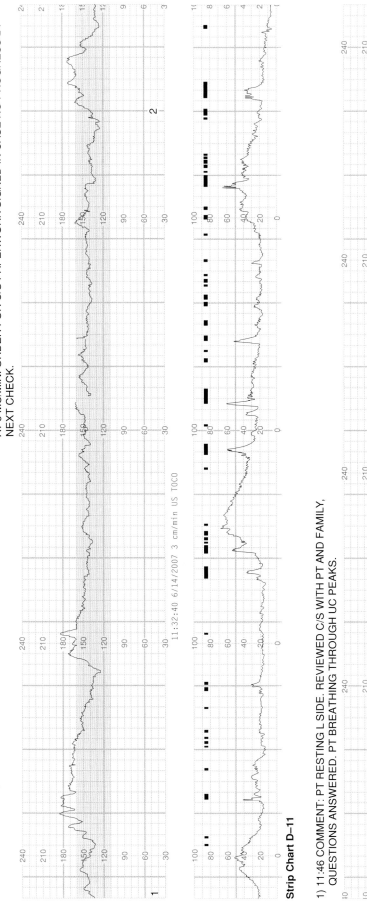

Strip Chart D–11

1) 11:46 COMMENT: PT RESTING L SIDE. REVIEWED C/S WITH PT AND FAMILY, QUESTIONS ANSWERED. PT BREATHING THROUGH UC PEAKS.

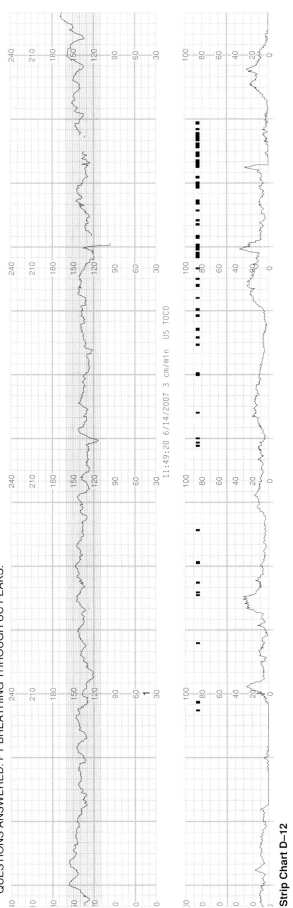

Strip Chart D–12

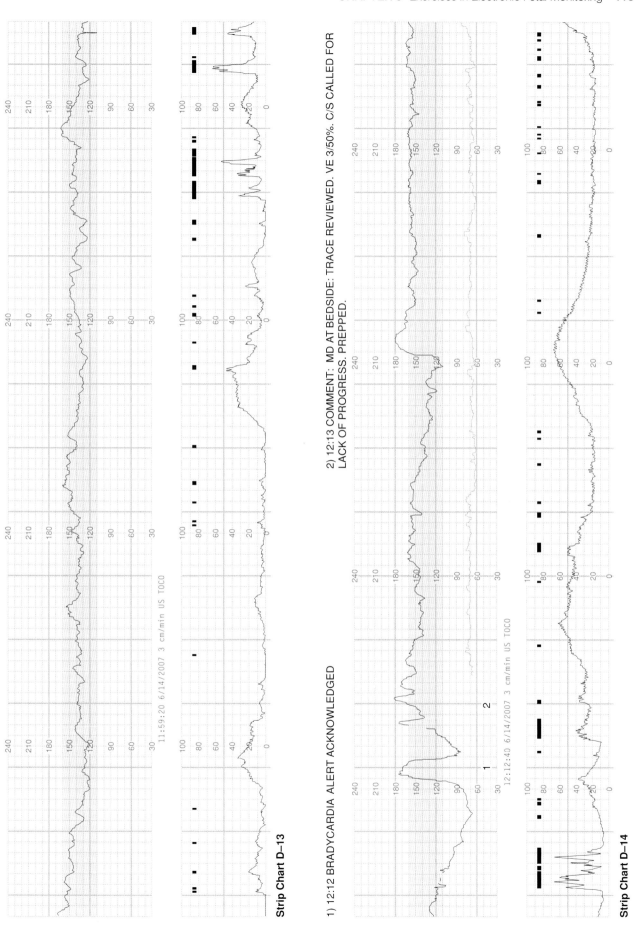

11:59:20 6/14/2007 3 cm/min US TOCO

Strip Chart D–13

1) 12:12 BRADYCARDIA ALERT ACKNOWLEDGED

2) 12:13 COMMENT: MD AT BEDSIDE: TRACE REVIEWED. VE 3/50%. C/S CALLED FOR LACK OF PROGRESS. PREPPED.

12:12:40 6/14/2007 3 cm/min US TOCO

Strip Chart D–14

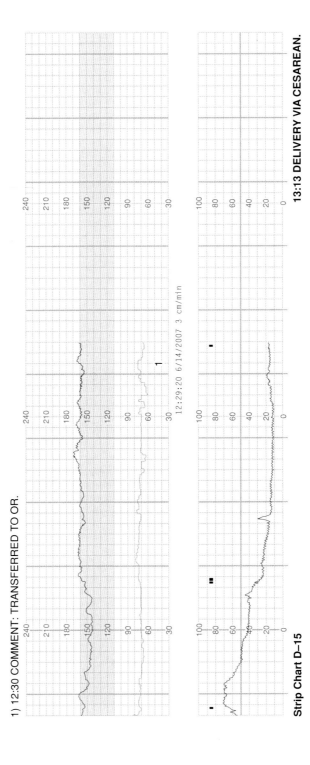

1) 12:30 COMMENT: TRANSFERRED TO OR.

12:29:20 6/14/2007 3 cm/min

1

Strip Chart D–15

13:13 DELIVERY VIA CESAREAN.

HX OF PATIENT E: 30 Y.O., G3P0. C/O LABOR SINCE 02:00. CONTRACTIONS MODERATE. WAS 2 CM IN MD OFFICE YESTERDAY. MEMBRANES INTACT.

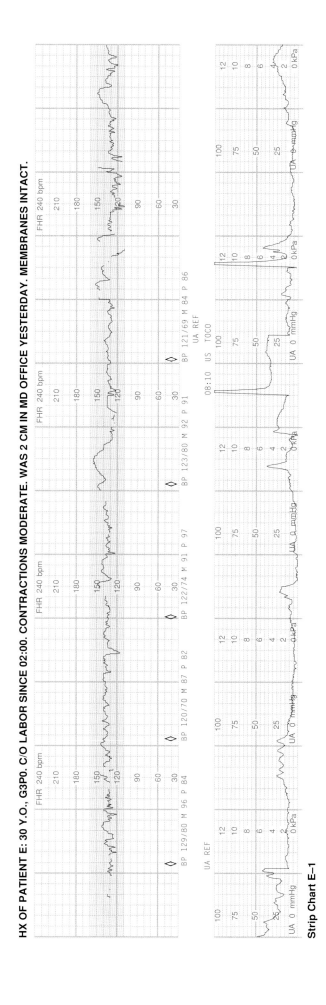

Strip Chart E-1

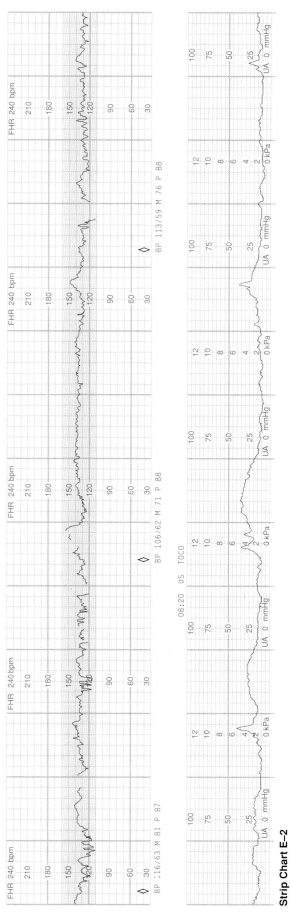

Strip Chart E-2

1) COMMENT: 08:41 VE 4-5/80%/-2. ANESTHESIA EXPLAINING EPIDURAL TO PT.
TO START PITOCIN WHEN PT COMFORTABLE.

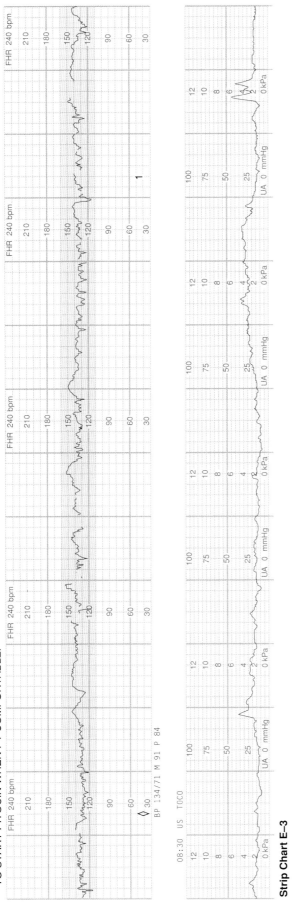

Strip Chart E–3

~ 1 HOUR LATER. EPIDURAL IN PLACE. OXYTOCIN BEGUN AT 2 MU/MIN AND INCREASED BY 2 MU/MIN EVERY 15-30 MIN., NOW AT 8 MU/MIN.

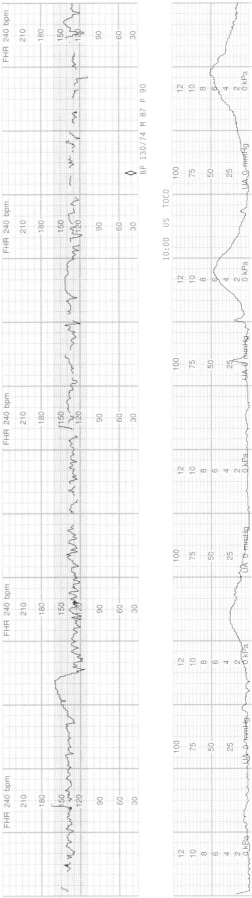

Strip Chart E–4

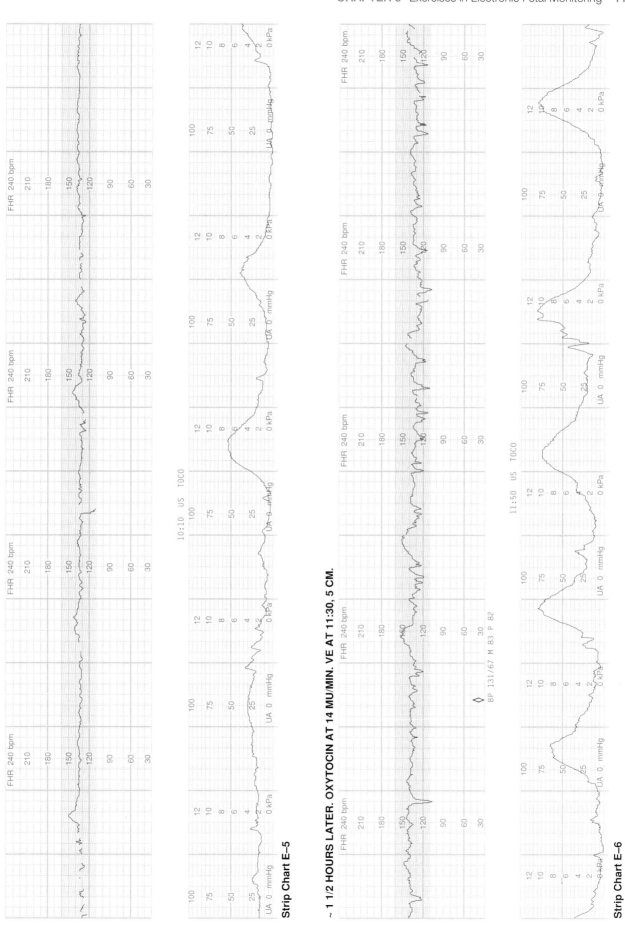

10:10 US TOCO

Strip Chart E–5

~ 1 1/2 HOURS LATER. OXYTOCIN AT 14 MU/MIN. VE AT 11:30, 5 CM.

BP 131/67 M 83 P 82

11:50 US TOCO

Strip Chart E–6

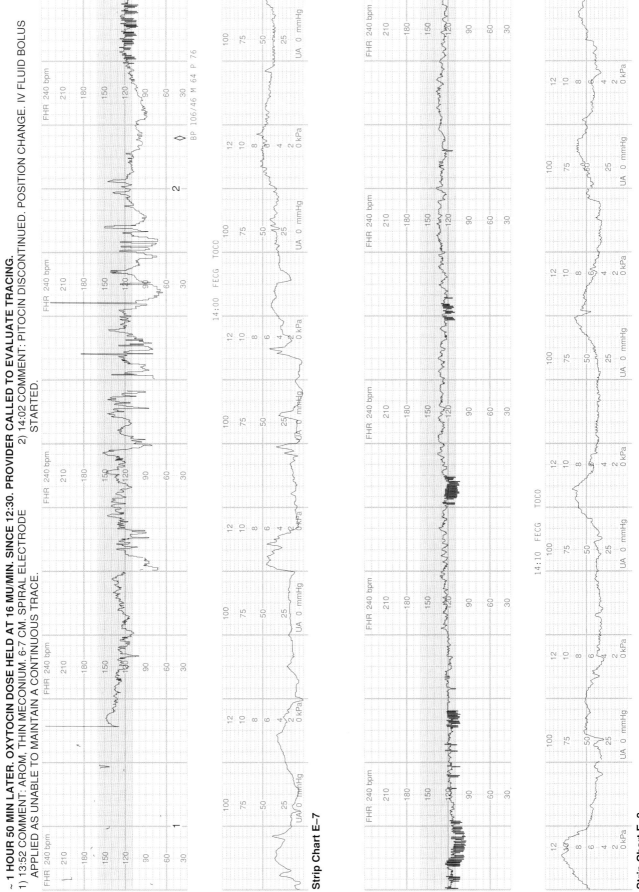

~ 1 HOUR 50 MIN LATER. OXYTOCIN DOSE HELD AT 16 MU/MIN. SINCE 12:30. PROVIDER CALLED TO EVALUATE TRACING.

1) 13:52 COMMENT: AROM, THIN MECONIUM. 6-7 CM. SPIRAL ELECTRODE APPLIED AS UNABLE TO MAINTAIN A CONTINUOUS TRACE.

2) 14:02 COMMENT: PITOCIN DISCONTINUED. POSITION CHANGE. IV FLUID BOLUS STARTED.

Strip Chart E–7

Strip Chart E–8

~ 1 HOUR LATER. OXYTOCIN RESTARTED AT 8 MU/MIN AT 14:45, AFTER VE BY PROVIDER. 8/80%/-2, IUPC PLACED.

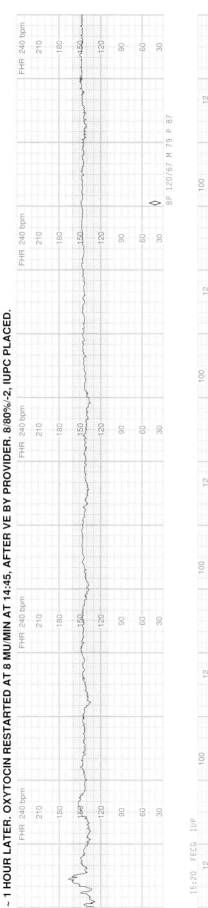

Strip Chart E–9

~ 1 1/2 HOURS LATER. OXYTOCIN CONTINUES RUNNING AT 8 MU/MIN. WAS 8-9 CM AT LAST EXAM.

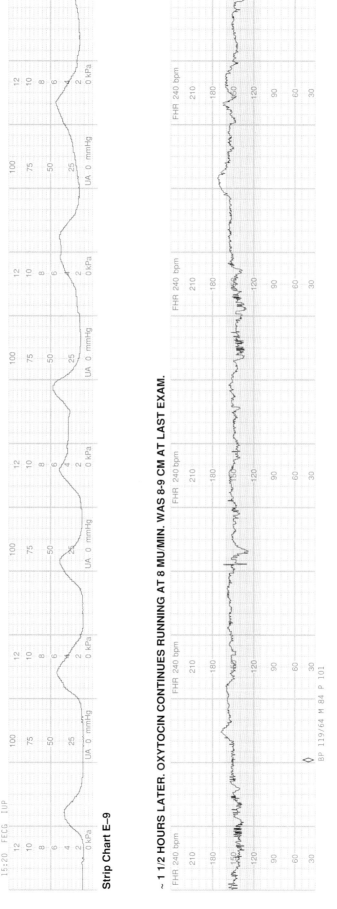

Strip Chart E-10

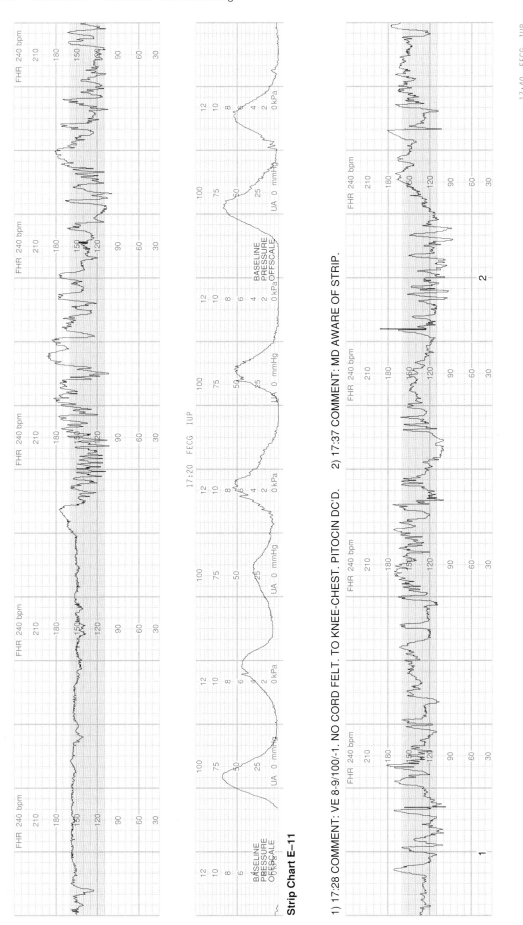

Strip Chart E–11

1) 17:28 COMMENT: VE 8-9/100/-1. NO CORD FELT. TO KNEE-CHEST. PITOCIN DC'D.   2) 17:37 COMMENT: MD AWARE OF STRIP.

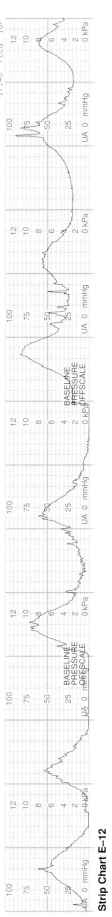

Strip Chart E–12

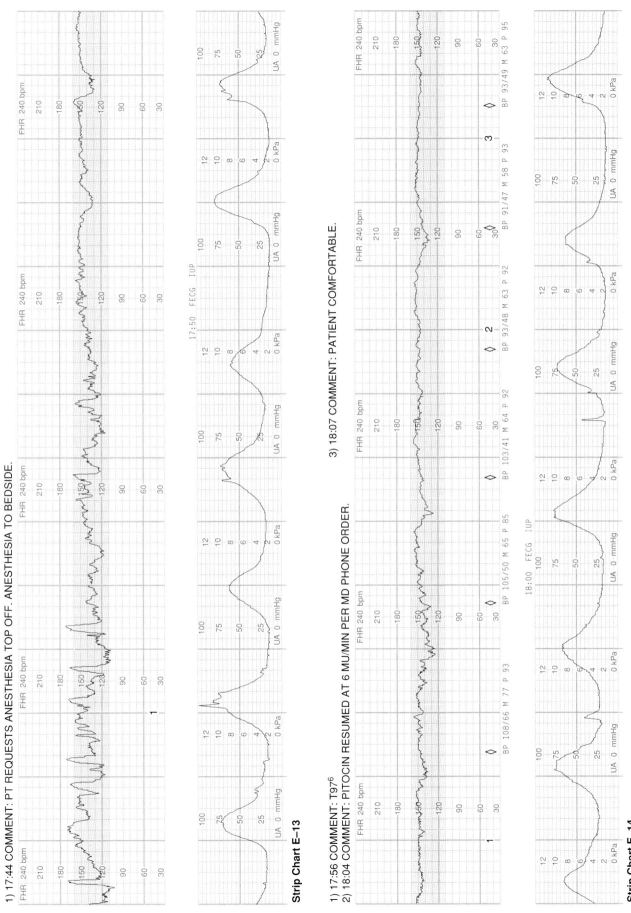

1) 17:44 COMMENT: PT REQUESTS ANESTHESIA TOP OFF. ANESTHESIA TO BEDSIDE.

Strip Chart E–13

1) 17:56 COMMENT: T97⁶

2) 18:04 COMMENT: PITOCIN RESUMED AT 6 MU/MIN PER MD PHONE ORDER.

3) 18:07 COMMENT: PATIENT COMFORTABLE.

Strip Chart E–14

~ 1 HOUR LATER. OXYTOCIN REMAINS AT 6 MU/MIN. CHANGE OF SHIFT. ONCOMING RN CONTACTS PROVIDER, ORDER TO CONTINUE OXYTOCIN.

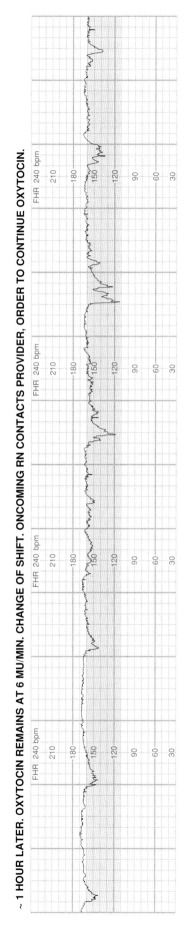

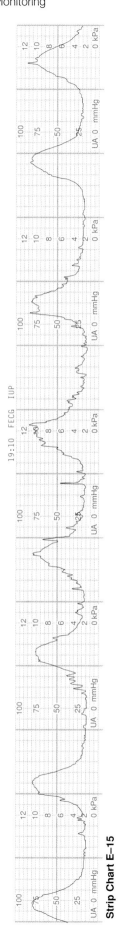

Strip Chart E–15

1) 19:23 COMMENT: T98[4]

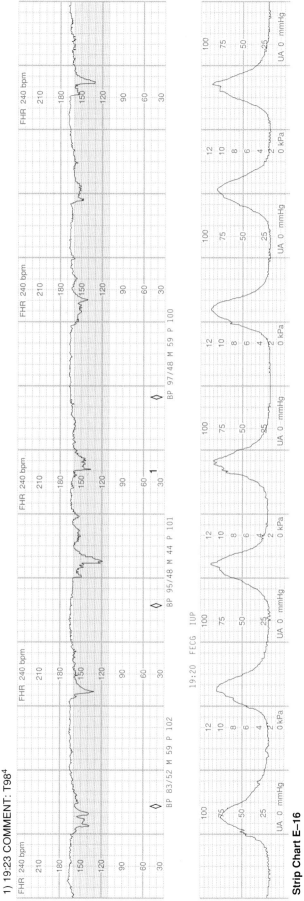

Strip Chart E–16

~ 40 MIN LATER. PITOCIN CONTINUES AT 6 MU/MIN.

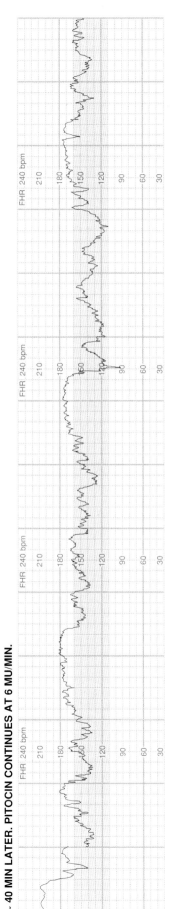

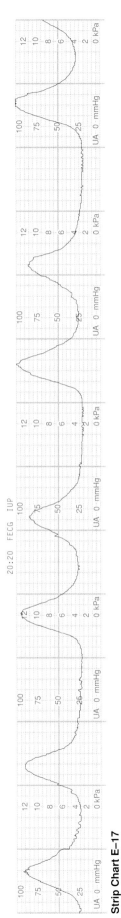

Strip Chart E-17

1) 20:34 COMMENT: VE FULLY. PT DOES NOT FEEL URGE TO PUSH.

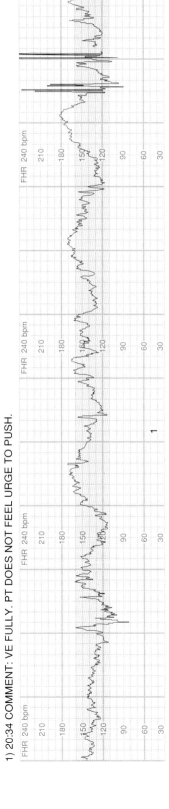

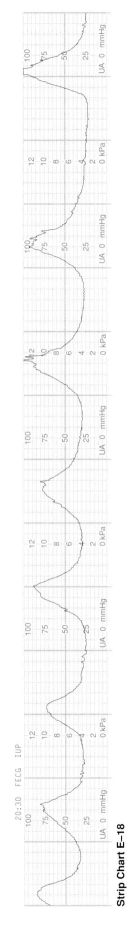

Strip Chart E-18

~ 20 MIN LATER. PT FEELS THE URGE AND BEGINS PUSHING. IUPC REMOVED.

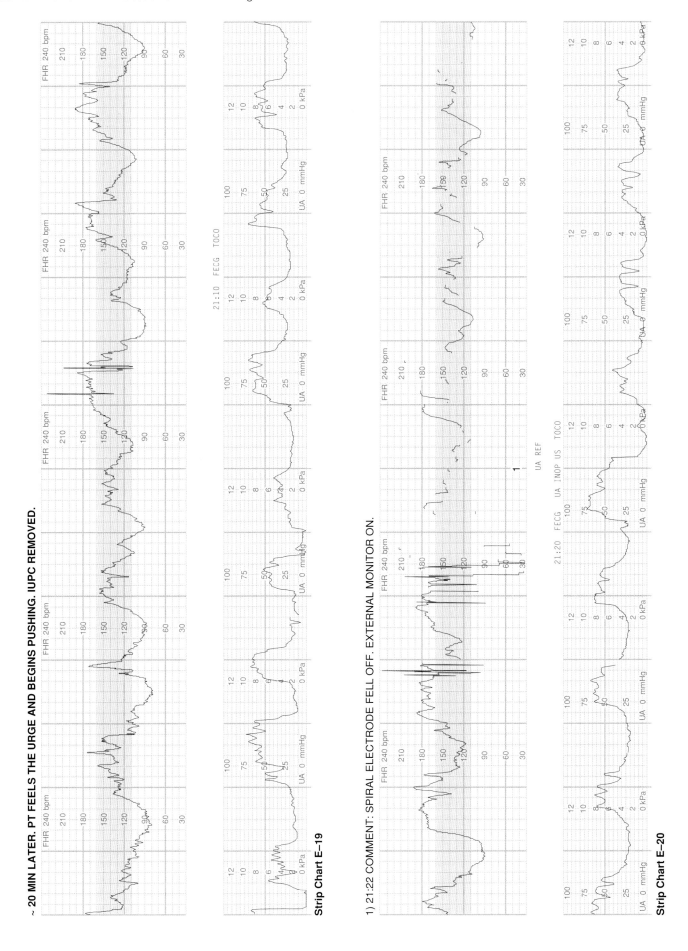

Strip Chart E-19

1) 21:22 COMMENT: SPIRAL ELECTRODE FELL OFF. EXTERNAL MONITOR ON.

Strip Chart E-20

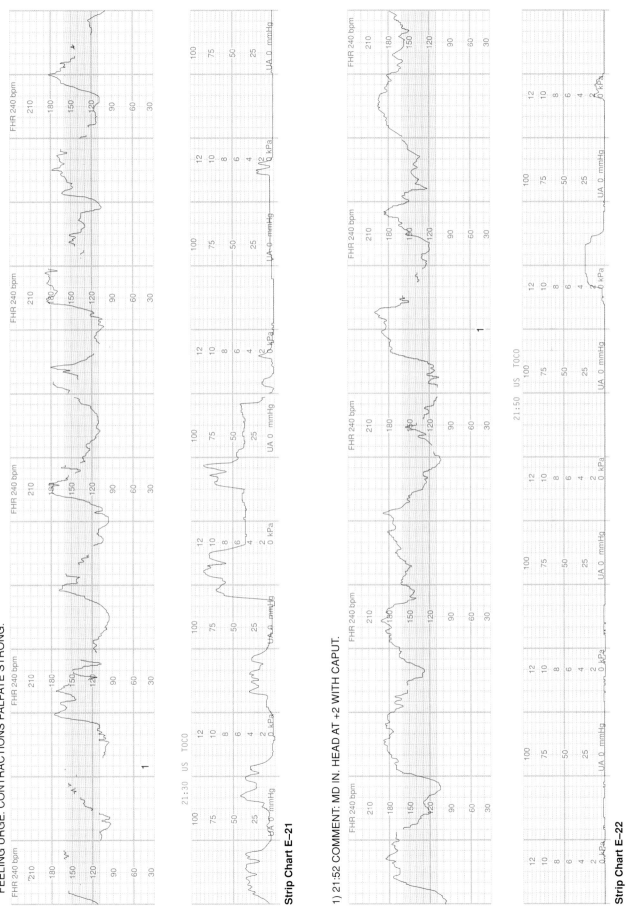

1) 21:31 COMMENT: PATIENT ENCOURAGED WITH PUSHING EFFORTS. STILL NOT FEELING URGE. CONTRACTIONS PALPATE STRONG.

Strip Chart E–21

1) 21:52 COMMENT: MD IN. HEAD AT +2 WITH CAPUT.

Strip Chart E–22

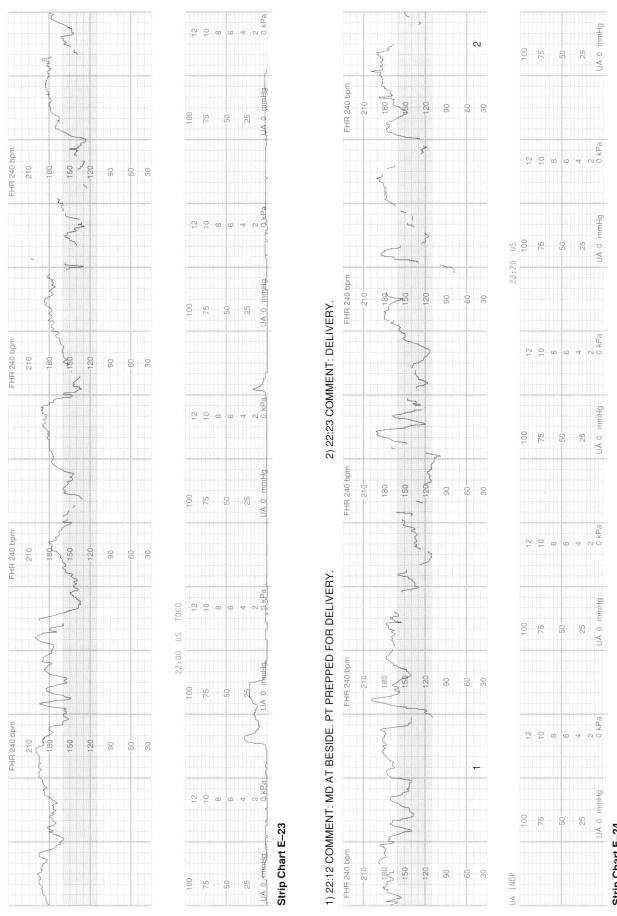

Strip Chart E–23

1) 22:12 COMMENT: MD AT BESIDE. PT PREPPED FOR DELIVERY.

2) 22:23 COMMENT: DELIVERY.

Strip Chart E–24

HX OF PATIENT F: 32 Y.O., G3P1, 40 2/7 WEEKS'. SEEN IN ANTEPARTUM CLINIC FOR SCHEDULED NST AND AFI YESTERDAY. AFI 4.2, TRACING NONREACTIVE WITH VARIABLE DECELERATIONS. INDUCTION SCHEDULED FOR SAME DAY. PATIENT LEFT AMA TO PICK UP HER CHILD FROM SCHOOL AND DID NOT RETURN UNTIL 09:15 THIS AM.

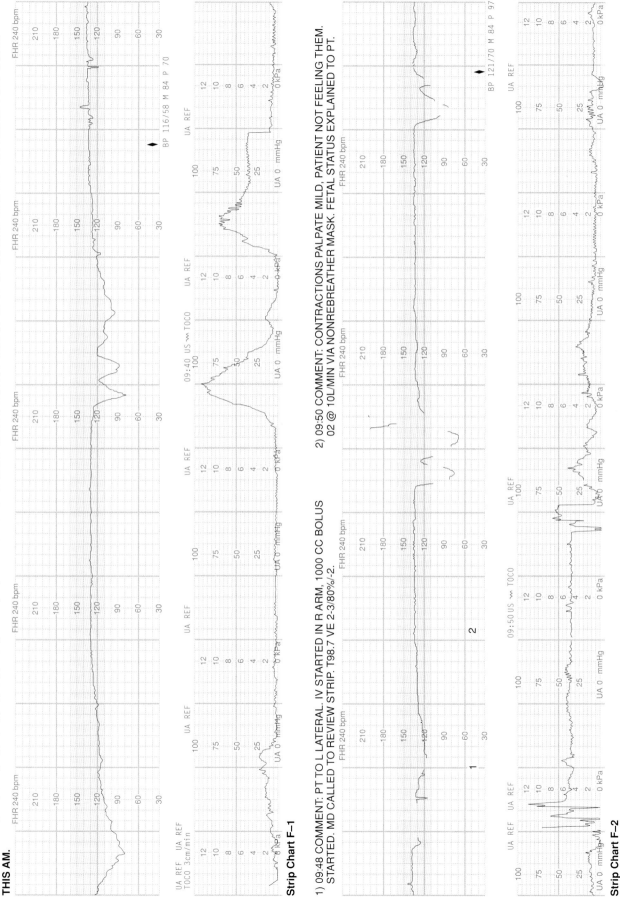

Strip Chart F–1

1) 09:48 COMMENT: PT TO L LATERAL. IV STARTED IN R ARM, 1000 CC BOLUS STARTED. MD CALLED TO REVIEW STRIP. T98.7 VE 2-3/80%/-2.

2) 09:50 COMMENT: CONTRACTIONS PALPATE MILD, PATIENT NOT FEELING THEM. O2 @ 10L/MIN VIA NONREBREATHER MASK. FETAL STATUS EXPLAINED TO PT.

Strip Chart F–2

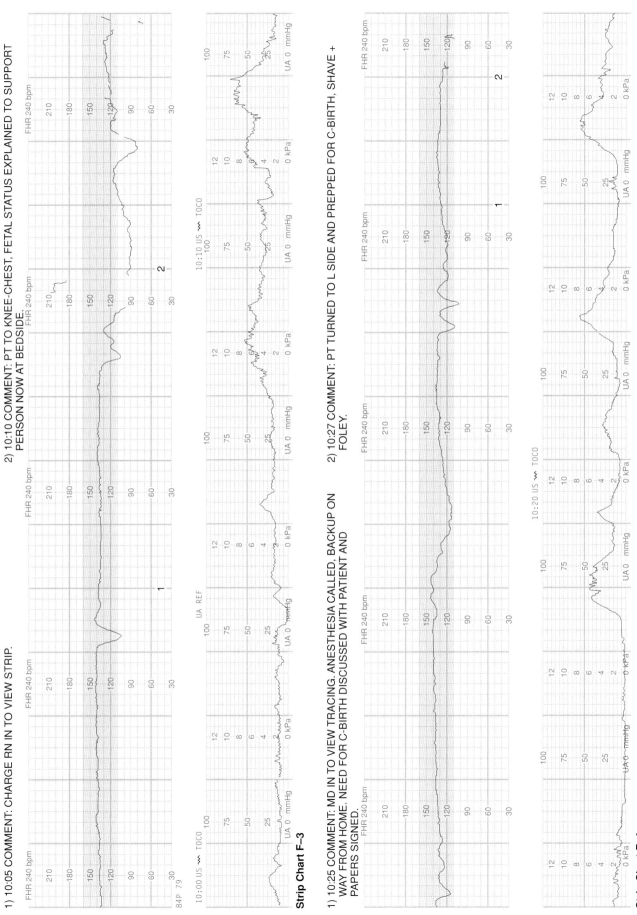

1) 10:05 COMMENT: CHARGE RN IN TO VIEW STRIP.

2) 10:10 COMMENT: PT TO KNEE-CHEST, FETAL STATUS EXPLAINED TO SUPPORT PERSON NOW AT BEDSIDE.

Strip Chart F–3

1) 10:25 COMMENT: MD IN TO VIEW TRACING. ANESTHESIA CALLED, BACKUP ON WAY FROM HOME. NEED FOR C-BIRTH DISCUSSED WITH PATIENT AND PAPERS SIGNED.

2) 10:27 COMMENT: PT TURNED TO L SIDE AND PREPPED FOR C-BIRTH, SHAVE + FOLEY.

Strip Chart F–4

1) 10:42 COMMENT: PT TO OR #1 FOR DELIVERY. ANESTHESIA TO ARRIVE SHORTLY, IN THE BUILDING.

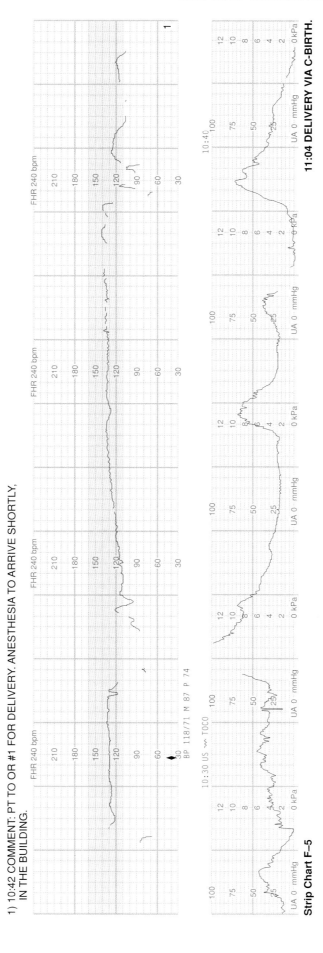

Strip Chart F–5

HX OF PATIENT G: 25 Y.O., G1P0, 39 4/7 WEEKS'. UNREMARKABLE PRENATAL COURSE & HEALTH HISTORY. PRESENTS WITH C/O SROM SINCE 00:30, CONTRACTIONS. BETA STREP NEGATIVE.

1) 03:51 TEMP 97.7.
2) 03:51 DIL: 0.5 EFF: 50 STA: -1.

3) 03:52 NIBP: 129/87, HR: 75.
4) 03:53 COMMENT: CLEAR FLUID NOTED, CONTRACTIONS PALPATE MILD.

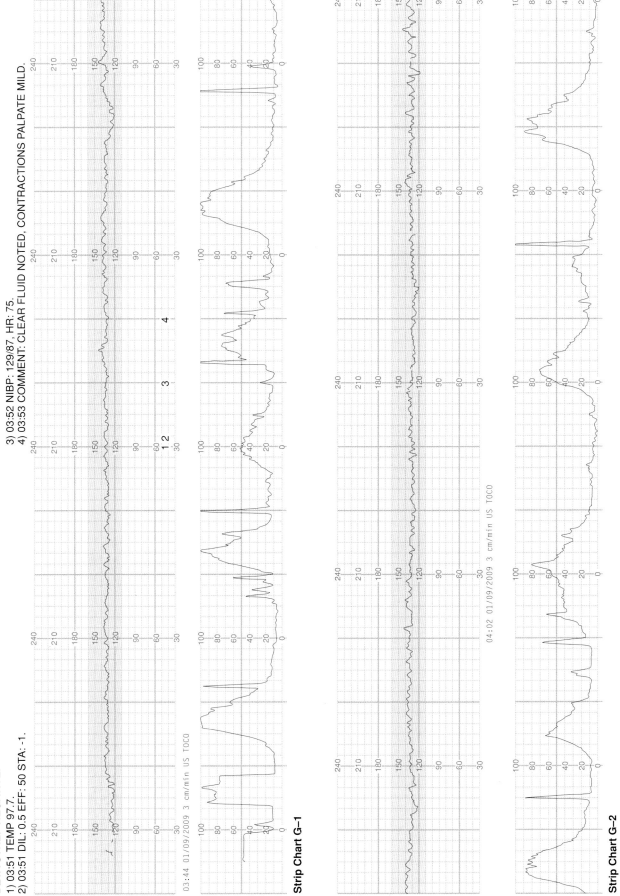

Strip Chart G–1

Strip Chart G–2

~ 1 HOUR LATER.

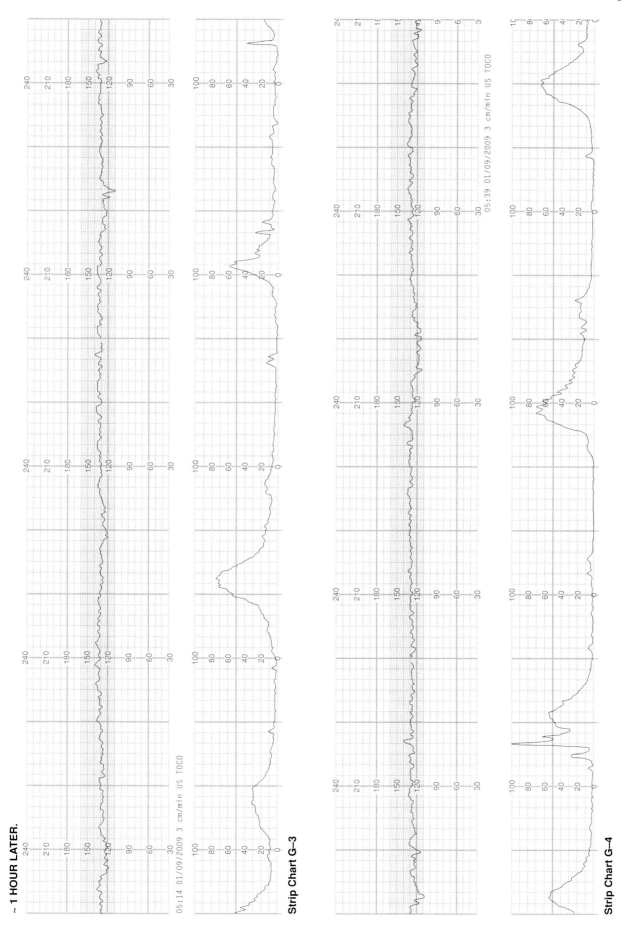

05:14 01/09/2009 3 cm/min US TOCO

Strip Chart G–3

05:39 01/09/2009 3 cm/min US TOCO

Strip Chart G–4

1) 05:42 COMMENT: PT TO L SIDE.

05:50 01/09/2009 3 cm/min US TOCO

Strip Chart G–5

~ 2 HOURS LATER. PT IS OOB FOR COMFORT.
1) 08:15 COMMENT: PT LEANING FORWARD IN ROCKING CHAIR.

2) 08:18 COMMENT: MATERNAL PULSE 90, BY PALPATION.

08:14 01/09/2009 3 cm/min US TOCO

Strip Chart G–6

1) 08:32 COMMENT: IV STARTED IN L HAND.

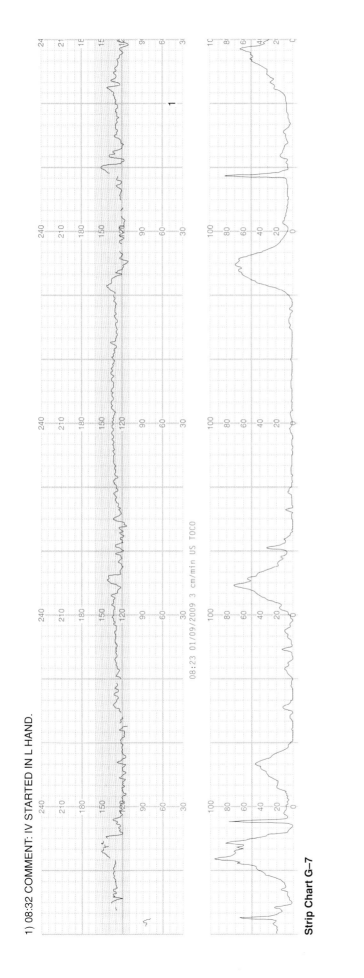

08:23 01/09/2009 3 cm/min US TOCO

Strip Chart G–7

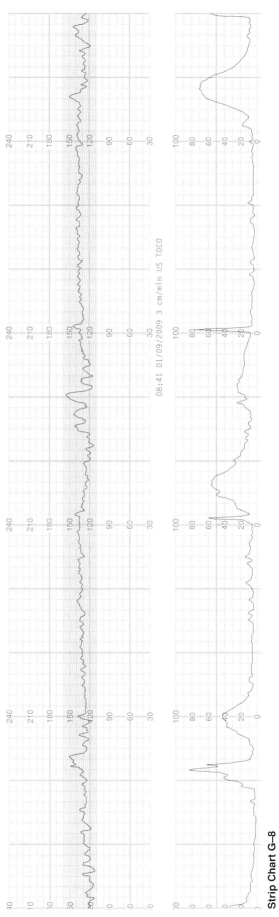

08:41 01/09/2009 3 cm/min US TOCO

Strip Chart G–8

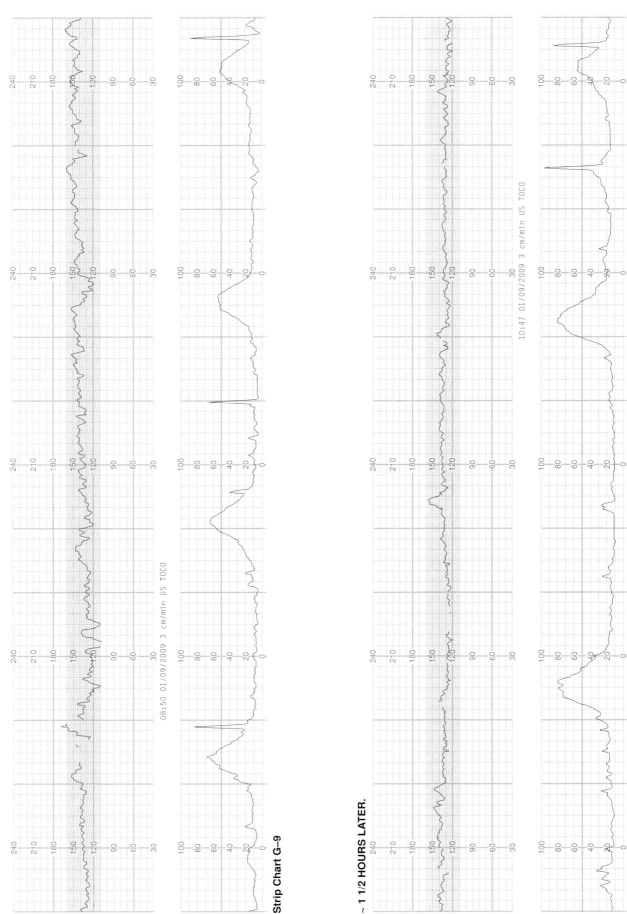

08:50 01/09/2009 3 cm/min US TOCO

Strip Chart G–9

~ 1 1/2 HOURS LATER.

10:47 01/09/2009 3 cm/min US TOCO

Strip Chart G–10

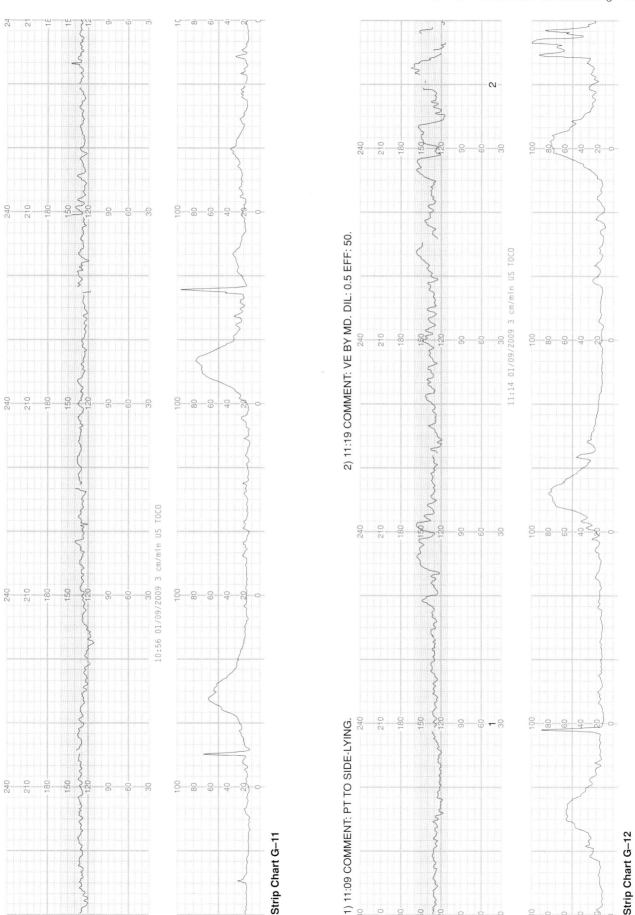

10:56 01/09/2009 3 cm/min US TOCO

Strip Chart G-11

1) 11:09 COMMENT: PT TO SIDE-LYING.

2) 11:19 COMMENT: VE BY MD. DIL: 0.5 EFF: 50.

11:14 01/09/2009 3 cm/min US TOCO

Strip Chart G-12

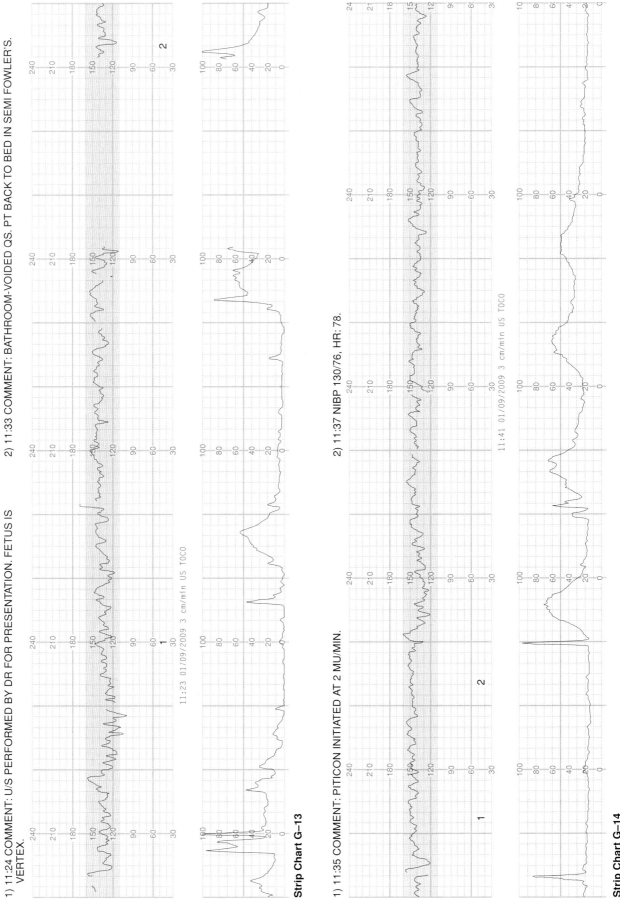

1) 11:24 COMMENT: U/S PERFORMED BY DR FOR PRESENTATION. FETUS IS VERTEX.

2) 11:33 COMMENT: BATHROOM-VOIDED QS. PT BACK TO BED IN SEMI FOWLER'S.

11:23 01/09/2009 3 cm/min US TOCO

Strip Chart G–13

1) 11:35 COMMENT: PITICON INITIATED AT 2 MU/MIN.

2) 11:37 NIBP 130/76, HR: 78.

11:41 01/09/2009 3 cm/min US TOCO

Strip Chart G–14

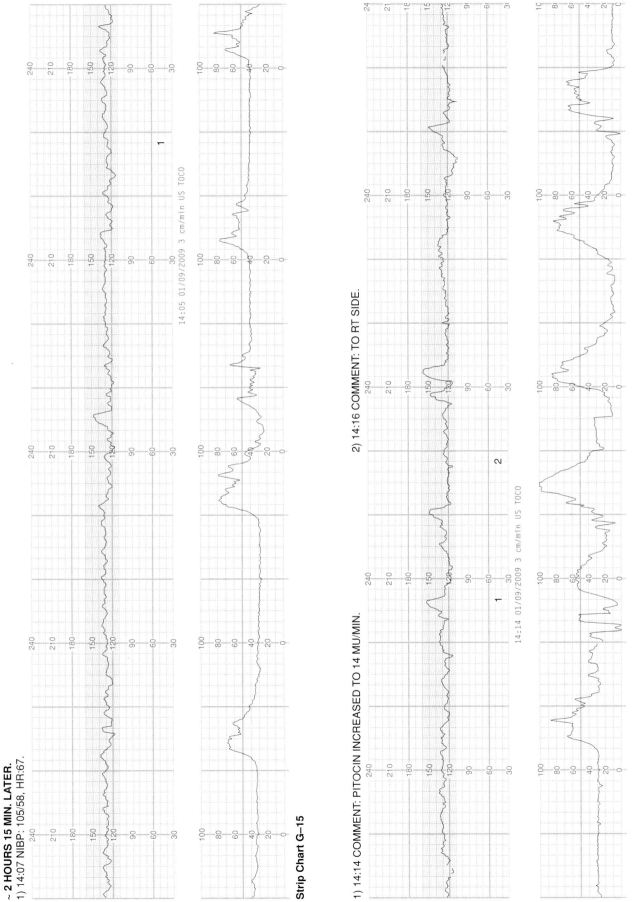

~ **2 HOURS 15 MIN. LATER.**
1) 14:07 NIBP: 105/58, HR:67.

14:05 01/09/2009 3 cm/min US TOCO

Strip Chart G–15

2) 14:16 COMMENT: TO RT SIDE.

1) 14:14 COMMENT: PITOCIN INCREASED TO 14 MU/MIN.

14:14 01/09/2009 3 cm/min US TOCO

Strip Chart G–16

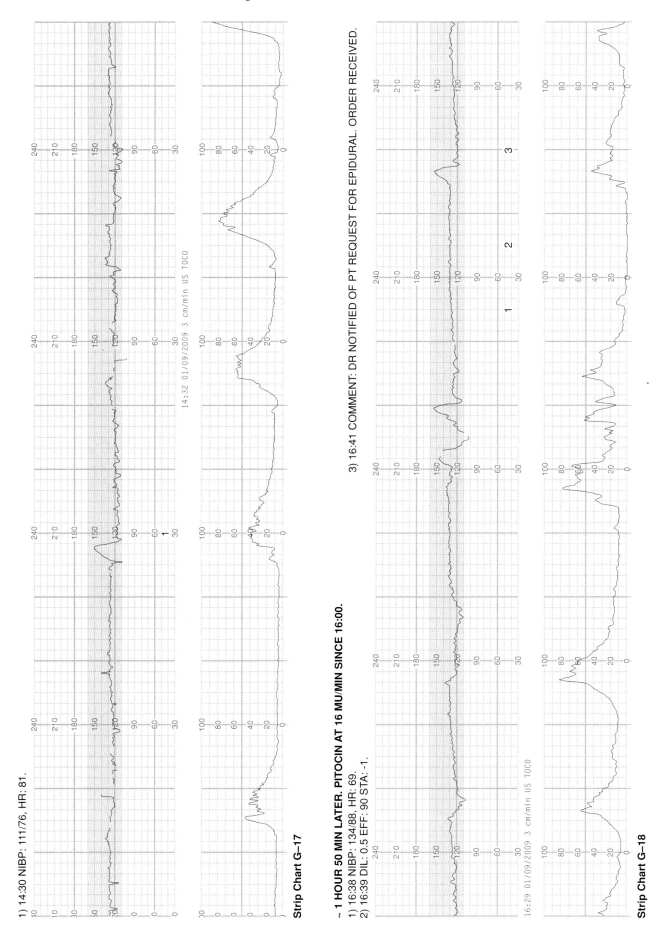

1) 14:30 NIBP: 111/76, HR: 81.

14:32 01/09/2009 3 cm/min US TOCO

Strip Chart G–17

~ 1 HOUR 50 MIN LATER. PITOCIN AT 16 MU/MIN SINCE 16:00.
1) 16:38 NIBP: 134/88, HR: 69.
2) 16:39 DIL: 0.5 EFF: 90 STA: -1.
3) 16:41 COMMENT: DR NOTIFIED OF PT REQUEST FOR EPIDURAL. ORDER RECEIVED.

16:29 01/09/2009 3 cm/min US TOCO

Strip Chart G–18

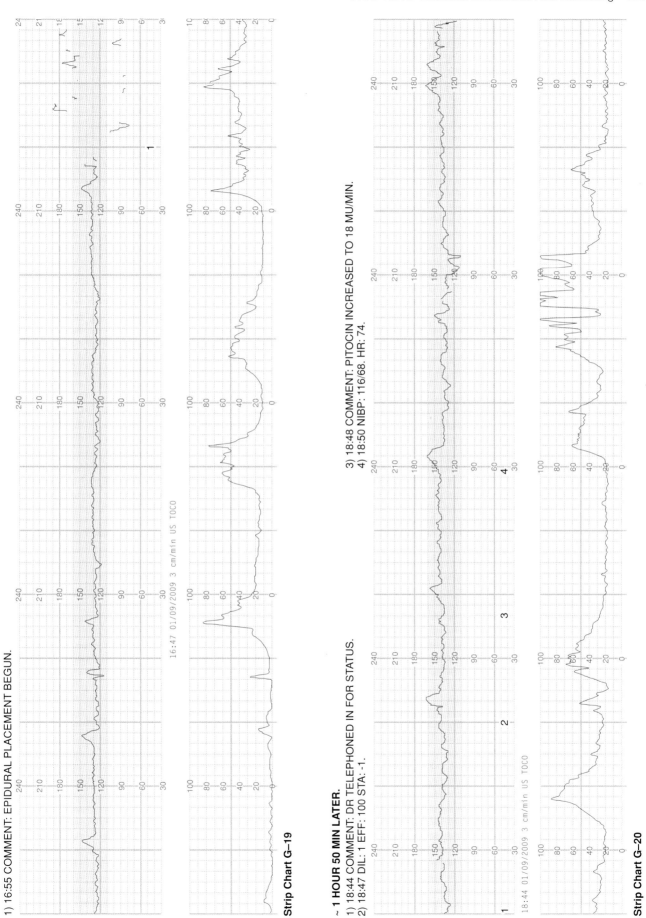

1) 16:55 COMMENT: EPIDURAL PLACEMENT BEGUN.

16:47 01/09/2009 3 cm/min US TOCO

Strip Chart G–19

~ 1 HOUR 50 MIN LATER.
1) 18:44 COMMENT: DR TELEPHONED IN FOR STATUS.
2) 18:47 DIL: 1 EFF: 100 STA: -1.

3) 18:48 COMMENT: PITOCIN INCREASED TO 18 MU/MIN.
4) 18:50 NIBP: 116/68. HR: 74.

18:44 01/09/2009 3 cm/min US TOCO

Strip Chart G–20

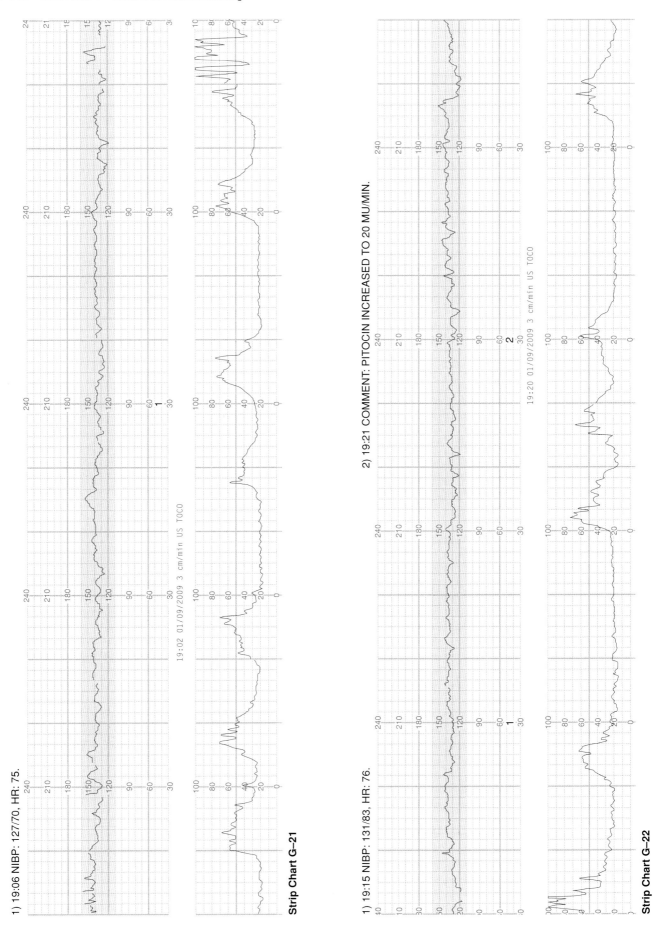

1) 19:06 NIBP: 127/70, HR: 75.

19:02 01/09/2009 3 cm/min US TOCO

Strip Chart G–21

1) 19:15 NIBP: 131/83, HR: 76.

2) 19:21 COMMENT: PITOCIN INCREASED TO 20 MU/MIN.

19:20 01/09/2009 3 cm/min US TOCO

Strip Chart G–22

~ 1/2 HOUR LATER. 19:50 VE 1.5/100/0, PITOCIN TO 22MU/MIN. PT C/O PAIN, EPIDURAL BEING REPLACED.
1) 20:05 COMMENT: EPIDURAL REPLACEMENT.
2) 20:06 NIBP: 133/66, HR: 90.
3) 20:07 COMMENT: EPIDURAL PROCEDURE STARTED BY DR.

4) 20:11 COMMENT: EPIDURAL CATHETER IN PLACE.
5) 20:13 COMMENT: EPIDURAL TEST DOSE.
6) 20:14 COMMENT: EPIDURAL-BOLUS DOSE.

7) 20:17 NIBP: 136/84, HR: 81.
8) 20:18 COMMENT: PITOCIN INCREASED TO 24 MU/MIN.

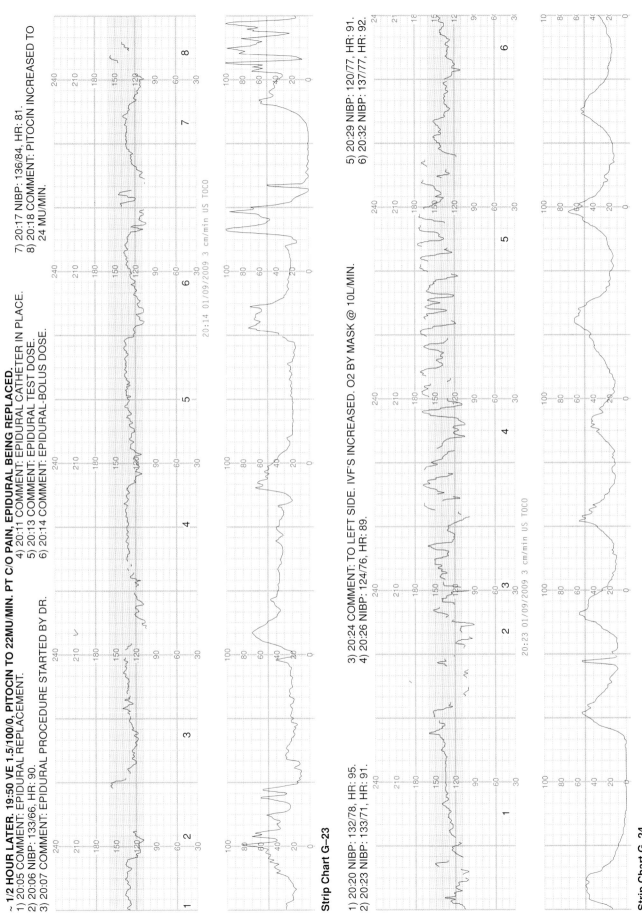

20:14 01/09/2009 3 cm/min US TOCO

Strip Chart G–23

1) 20:20 NIBP: 132/78, HR: 95.
2) 20:23 NIBP: 133/71, HR: 91.

3) 20:24 COMMENT: TO LEFT SIDE. IVF'S INCREASED. O2 BY MASK @ 10L/MIN.
4) 20:26 NIBP: 124/76, HR: 89.

5) 20:29 NIBP: 120/77, HR: 91.
6) 20:32 NIBP: 137/77, HR: 92.

20:23 01/09/2009 3 cm/min US TOCO

Strip Chart G–24

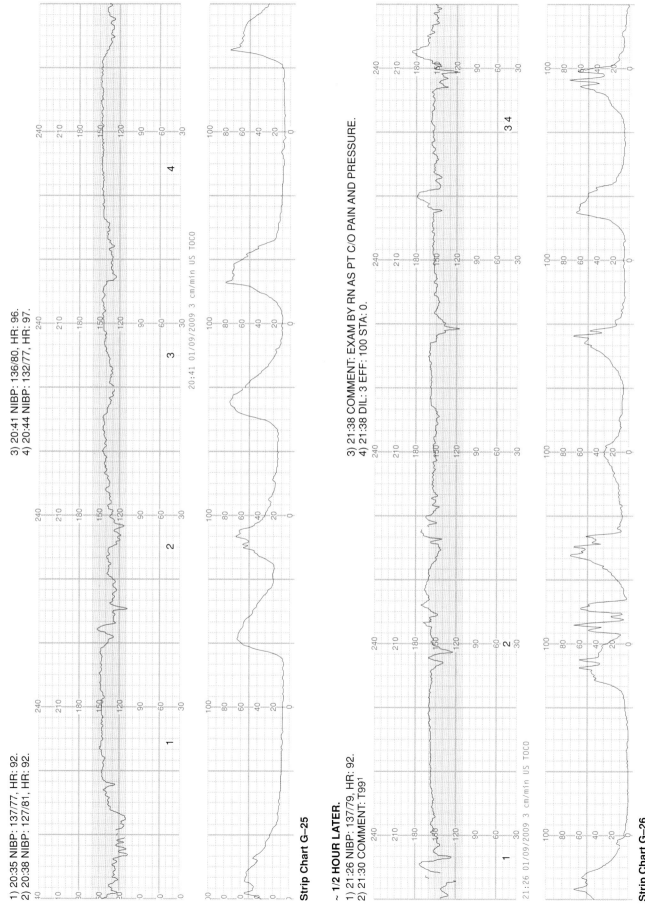

1) 20:35 NIBP: 137/77, HR: 92.
2) 20:38 NIBP: 127/81, HR: 92.

3) 20:41 NIBP: 136/80, HR: 96.
4) 20:44 NIBP: 132/77, HR: 97.

20:41 01/09/2009 3 cm/min US TOCO

Strip Chart G–25

~ 1/2 HOUR LATER.

1) 21:26 NIBP: 137/79, HR: 92.
2) 21:30 COMMENT: T991

3) 21:38 COMMENT: EXAM BY RN AS PT C/O PAIN AND PRESSURE.
4) 21:38 DIL.: 3 EFF: 100 STA: 0.

21:26 01/09/2009 3 cm/min US TOCO

Strip Chart G–26

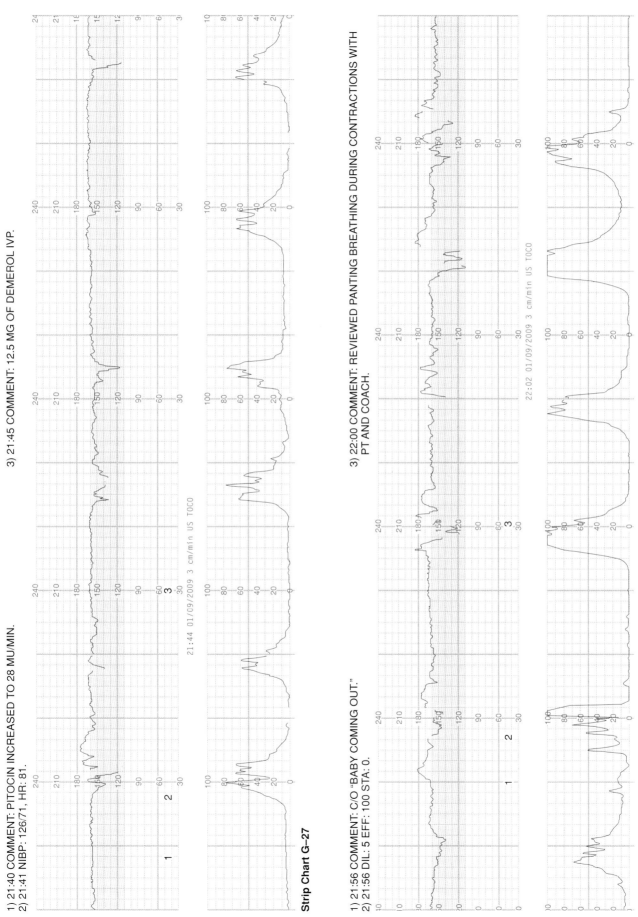

1) 21:40 COMMENT: PITOCIN INCREASED TO 28 MU/MIN.
2) 21:41 NIBP: 126/71, HR: 81.

3) 21:45 COMMENT: 12.5 MG OF DEMEROL IVP.

21:44 01/09/2009 3 cm/min US TOCO

Strip Chart G–27

1) 21:56 COMMENT: C/O "BABY COMING OUT."
2) 21:56 DIL: 5 EFF: 100 STA: 0.

3) 22:00 COMMENT: REVIEWED PANTING BREATHING DURING CONTRACTIONS WITH PT AND COACH.

22:02 01/09/2009 3 cm/min US TOCO

Strip Chart G–28

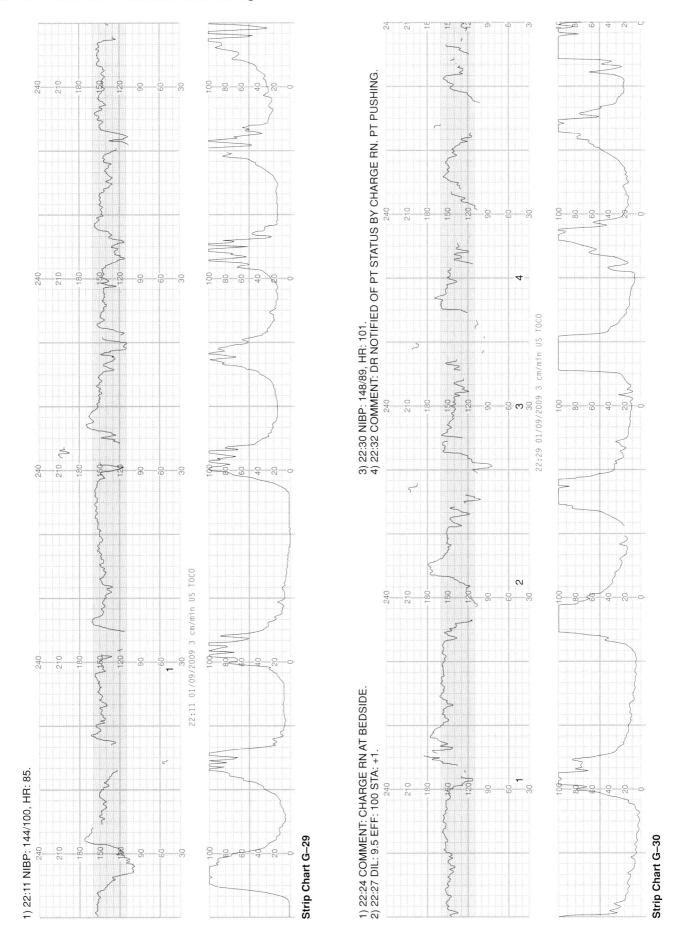

1) 22:11 NIBP: 144/100, HR: 85.

22:11 01/09/2009 3 cm/min US TOCO

Strip Chart G-29

1) 22:24 COMMENT: CHARGE RN AT BEDSIDE.
2) 22:27 DIL: 9.5 EFF: 100 STA: +1.

3) 22:30 NIBP: 148/89, HR: 101.
4) 22:32 COMMENT: DR NOTIFIED OF PT STATUS BY CHARGE RN. PT PUSHING.

22:29 01/09/2009 3 cm/min US TOCO

Strip Chart G-30

1) 22:42 NIBP: 149/89, HR: 116.

2) 22:44 COMMENT: PT PUSHING WELL.

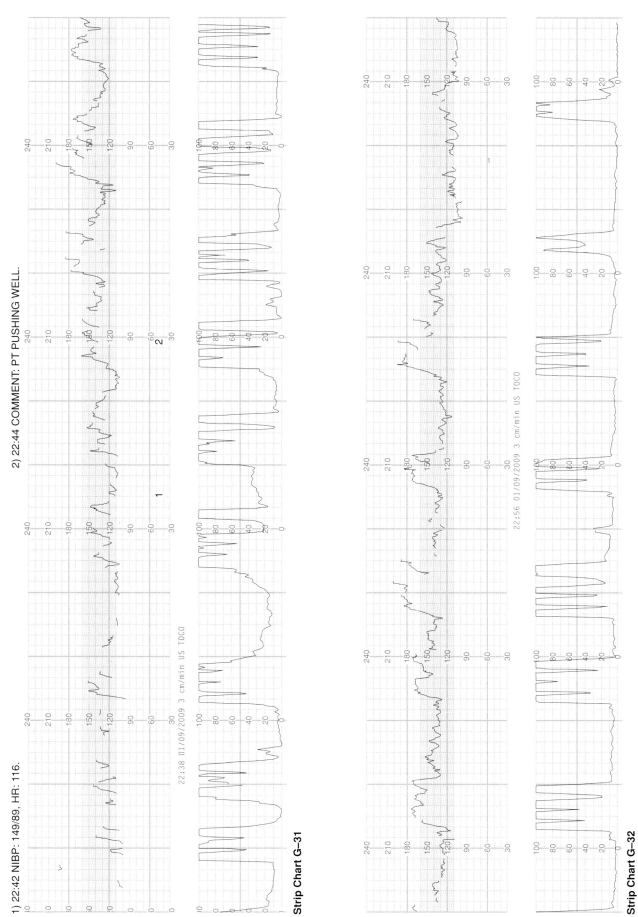

22:38 01/09/2009 3 cm/min US TOCO

22:56 01/09/2009 3 cm/min US TOCO

Strip Chart G–31

Strip Chart G–32

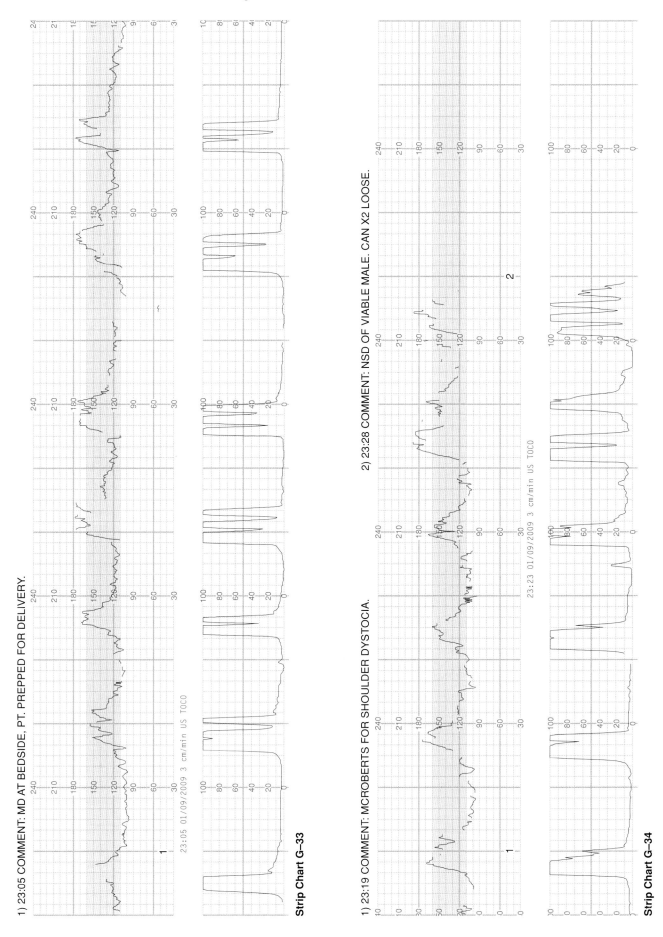

1) 23:05 COMMENT: MD AT BEDSIDE, PT. PREPPED FOR DELIVERY.

23:05 01/09/2009 3 cm/min US TOCO

Strip Chart G–33

1) 23:19 COMMENT: MCROBERTS FOR SHOULDER DYSTOCIA.

2) 23:28 COMMENT: NSD OF VIABLE MALE. CAN X2 LOOSE.

23:23 01/09/2009 3 cm/min US TOCO

Strip Chart G–34

HX OF PATIENT H: 40 Y.O., G1P0, EARLY PRENATAL CARE, NO SIGNIFICANT MEDICAL OR FAMILY HISTORY, NORMAL AFP. FOLLOWED WITH ANTEPARTUM TESTING FOR AMA.

NST AT 36 WEEKS':

1) COMMENT: PT STATES GOOD FETAL MOVEMENT, INSTRUCTED TO PRESS MARKER FOR MOVEMENT FELT.

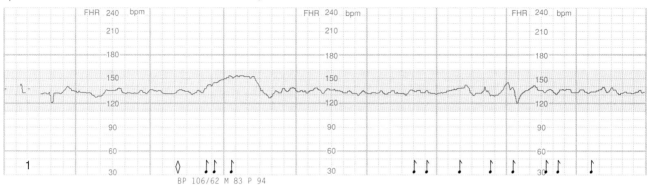

BP 106/62 M 83 P 94

09:40 06/10/2006 US TOCO 3 cm/min

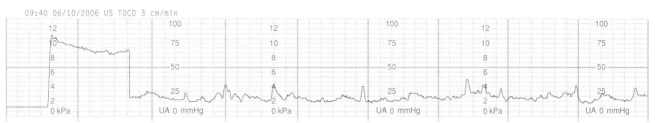

Strip Chart H–1A

PLEASE EVALUATE H-1A AND H-1B TOGETHER AS A UNIT.

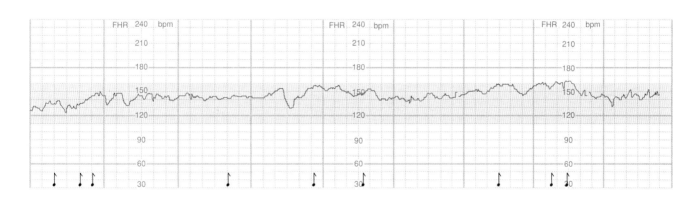

09:50 06/10/2006 US TOCO 3 cm/min

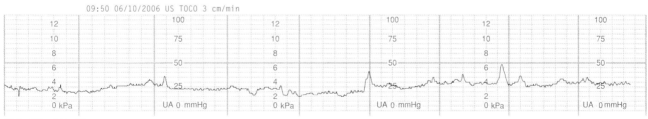

Strip Chart H–1B

NST AT 38 6/7 WEEKS':

1) COMMENT: PT STATES UCS MILD AND DENIES SROM AND BLEEDING. PERFORMING FMC AT HOME, BABY MOVING WELL.

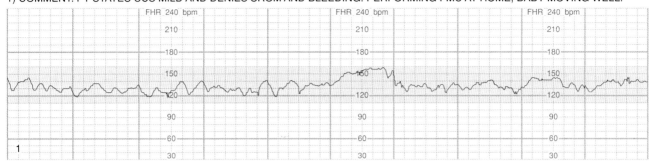

09:00 06/30/2006 US TOCO 3 cm/min

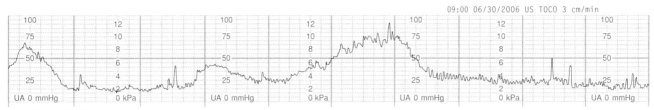

Strip Chart H–2A

PLEASE EVALUATE H-2A AND H-2B TOGETHER AS A UNIT.

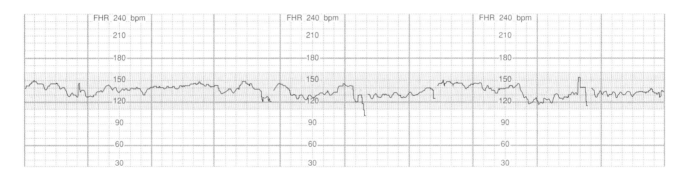

09:10 06/30/2006 US TOCO 3 cm/min

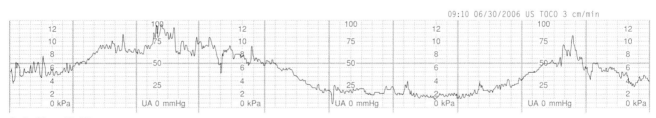

Strip Chart H–2B

NST THE FOLLOWING DAY (39 WEEKS') FOR C/O SPOTTING:

1) COMMENT: PT WOKE UP THIS AM WITH BRIGHT RED SPOTTING, NOW RESOLVED. NOT FEELING UCS. DENIES SROM.

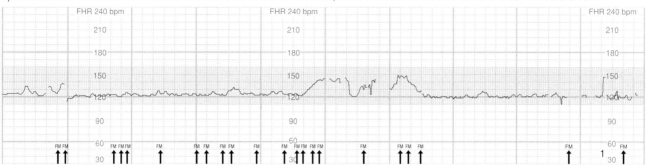

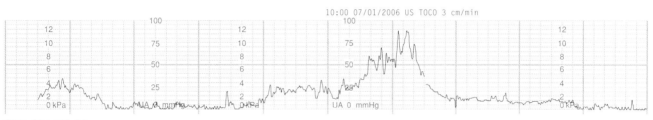

Strip Chart H–3A

PLEASE EVALUATE H-3A AND H-3B TOGETHER AS A UNIT.

1) COMMENT: DISCHARGED TO HOME WITH LABOR WARNINGS, FOLLOW-UP TESTING SCHEDULED.

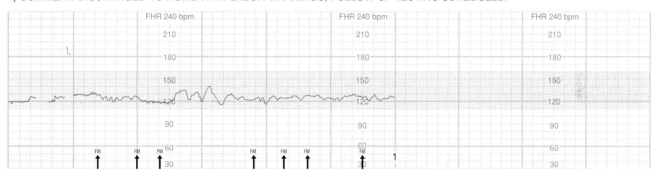

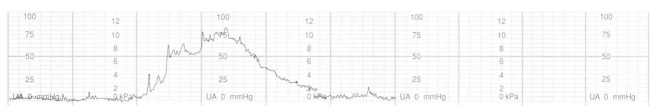

Strip Chart H–3B

FOLLOW-UP NST AT 39 2/7 WEEKS'. BLEEDING RESOLVED.

1) COMMENT: PT STATES FEELNG UCS "MORE TODAY." PALPATE MILD TO MOD, PT BREATHING THROUGH PEAKS OF SOME. STATES BABY MOVING LESS TODAY.

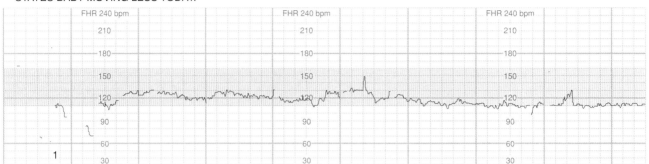

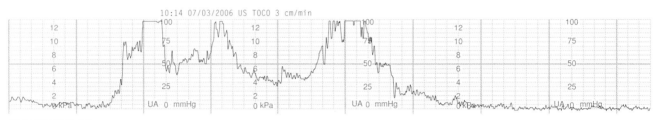

10:14 07/03/2006 US TOCO 3 cm/min

Strip Chart H–4A

*PLEASE EVALUATE H-4A AND H-4B TOGETHER AS A UNIT.

1) COMMENT: VE 1/50/-2, SAME AS IN OFFICE.

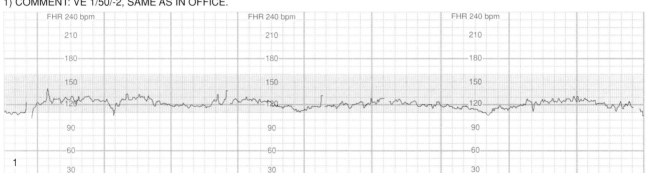

10:22 07/03/2006 US TOCO 3 cm/min

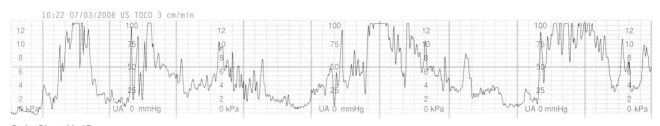

Strip Chart H–4B

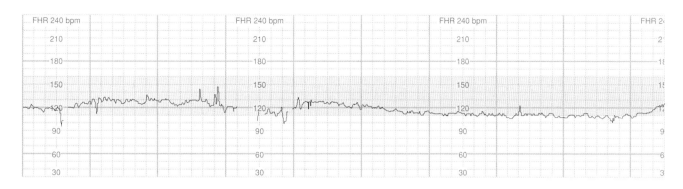

Strip Chart H–4C

*PLEASE EVALUATE H-4C AND H-4D TOGETHER AS A UNIT.

1) COMMENT: TOCO READJUSTED
2) COMMENT: CTXN PER PT
3) COMMENT: PT CHANGED POSITION

4) COMMENT: TOCO READJUSTED
5) COMMENT: PATIENT DISCHARGED HOME WITH LABOR
   WARNINGS.

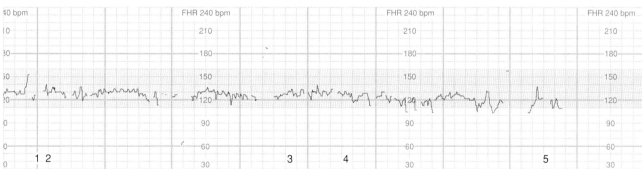

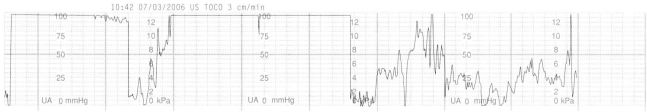

Strip Chart H–4D

Guide to Interpretation

STRIP CHART A–1

Fetal Heart Rate		Uterine Activity	
Baseline:	175 bpm	Frequency:	1–4 minutes
Variability:	Moderate	Duration:	1–2 minutes
Periodic/Episodic Changes:	Variable Decelerations	Strength:	Tocotransducer in place—must palpate
		Resting Tone:	Tocotransducer in place—must palpate
Category:		II	

Discussion: Patient presents with what appears to be a fetal tachycardia. She is not febrile; however, her temperature should be monitored closely in light of this finding. A careful history should be taken, including inquiry about possible drug (OTC or illicit) or herbal use, and consideration to activity level, weather/environment, and nutritional status/hydration prior to admission. IV hydration should be considered promptly.

STRIP CHART A–2

Fetal Heart Rate		Uterine Activity	
Baseline:	175 bpm	Frequency:	2–4.5 minutes
Variability:	Moderate	Duration:	60–90 seconds
Periodic/Episodic Changes:	Variable and Late Decelerations	Strength:	Mild–Moderate
		Resting Tone:	Tocotransducer in place—must palpate
Category:		II	

Discussion: Maternal heart rate and fetal movement are additional parameters that are being recorded on the tracing. It is noteworthy that the portion of the FHR that presently is considered baseline (and demonstrates fetal tachycardia) appears to coincide with fetal movement. It would be helpful to the assessment to have the bedside impression of what is occurring; for example, whether the fetus is heard on the monitor, observed through the abdomen, or noted by the mother to be experiencing a period of excessive movement.

STRIP CHART A–3

Fetal Heart Rate		Uterine Activity	
Baseline:	170 bpm	Frequency:	2.5–5 minutes
Variability:	Moderate	Duration:	1–3 minutes
Periodic/Episodic Changes:	Variable Decelerations	Strength:	Tocotransducer in place—must palpate
		Resting Tone:	Tocotransducer in place—must palpate
Category:		II	

STRIP CHART A–4

Fetal Heart Rate		Uterine Activity	
Baseline:	165 bpm	Frequency:	3–5 minutes
Variability:	Moderate	Duration:	1–2 minutes
Periodic/Episodic Changes:	Variable Decelerations	Strength:	Tocotransducer in place—must palpate
		Resting Tone:	Tocotransducer in place—must palpate
Category:		II	

Discussion: The FHR has taken on a somewhat odd appearance that bears observation. It may be advisable to delay starting oxytocin until this pattern is resolved. Internal FHR monitoring (FECG) with a spiral electrode may also be considered for closer observation.

STRIP CHART A–5

Fetal Heart Rate		Uterine Activity	
Baseline:	165 bpm	Frequency:	1–4 minutes
Variability:	Moderate	Duration:	70–90 seconds
Periodic/Episodic Changes:	Prolonged Deceleration	Strength:	Tocotransducer in place—must palpate
		Resting Tone:	Tocotransducer in place—must palpate
Category:		II	

Discussion: During the optimal portion of this tracing to observe the FHR (the area between the last two contractions), the FHR baseline appears to be 165 bpm. It is logical that during the period of hypercontractility (starting 2 minutes into the tracing and continuing for 6 minutes), the FHR would decelerate. However, once again, it appears that the episodes of tachycardia coincide with period of fetal movement and commentary of bedside observation may provide further clarification.

STRIP CHART A–6

Fetal Heart Rate		Uterine Activity	
Baseline:	125 bpm	Frequency:	2–2.5 minutes
Variability:	Minimal–Moderate	Duration:	2 minutes
Periodic/Episodic Changes:	Accelerations	Strength:	Tocotransducer in place—must palpate
		Resting Tone:	Tocotransducer in place—must palpate
Category:	I		

Discussion: Approximately 2 hours after admission, the FHR is beginning to look quite different. It is always important to compare for changes over time. The baseline is no longer seems to be tachycardic and episodes of fetal movement coincide with what now appear to be accelerations of the FHR. The contraction pattern bears consideration, as contractions are occurring frequently and are lengthy and there does not appear to be adequate (at least 1 minute) uterine rest between them. More information regarding bedside clinical observation would be helpful, including findings of palpation of abdomen during and in between contractions.

STRIP CHART A-7

Fetal Heart Rate		Uterine Activity	
Baseline:	120 bpm	Frequency:	2–3 minutes
Variability:	Minimal–Moderate	Duration:	60–90 seconds
Periodic/Episodic Changes:	Acceleration	Strength:	Tocotransducer in place—must palpate
		Resting Tone:	Tocotransducer in place—must palpate
Category:	I		

STRIP CHART A-8

Fetal Heart Rate		Uterine Activity	
Baseline:	125 bpm	Frequency:	1–3.5 minutes
Variability:	Moderate	Duration:	40 seconds–2 minutes (?)
Periodic/Episodic Changes:	Acceleration	Strength:	Tocotransducer in place—must palpate
		Resting Tone:	Tocotransducer in place—must palpate
Category:	I		

Discussion: During the last 2 minutes of the tracing, the FHR recording takes on an odd appearance (increased variability and higher rate) at the same time that a "coincidence" alert occurs. Some monitors can have the ability to differentiate between two heart rates (FHR and MHR, or between the FHR patterns of twins). This is helpful when both rates are similar. It is likely that this patch of recording reflects a brief period of double counting the MHR, rather than an actual representation of the FHR. It is essential to be familiar with the capabilities and features of the equipment used in your setting in order to fully understand the data presented. UA is difficult to assess as tocotransducer needs adjustment.

STRIP CHART A-9

Fetal Heart Rate		Uterine Activity	
Baseline:	120 bpm	Frequency:	Tocotransducer not recording adequately
Variability:	Moderate	Duration:	Tocotransducer not recording adequately
Periodic/Episodic Changes:		Strength:	Tocotransducer in place—must palpate
		Resting Tone:	Tocotransducer in place—must palpate
Category:	I		

Discussion: It appears that the MHR continues to be erroneously obtained by the ultrasound transducer, producing a recording of double-counting of the MHR during the first half of this tracing. Once the monitor is adjusted, the FHR recording returns. It is necessary that closer attention be paid to monitoring of UA.

STRIP CHART A–10

Fetal Heart Rate		Uterine Activity	
Baseline:	120 bpm	Frequency:	Tocotransducer not recording adequately
Variability:	Minimal–Moderate	Duration:	Tocotransducer not recording adequately
Periodic/Episodic Changes:	Indeterminate	Strength:	Tocotransducer in place—must palpate
		Resting Tone:	Tocotransducer in place—must palpate
Category:	I		

Discussion: In the first half of this tracing, there continues to be a loss of FHR signal acquisition and contractions continue to not be recording. With oxytocin infusing, it is essential to have continuous information about both the FHR and UA. The external monitors need to be adjusted or internal monitoring considered.

STRIP CHART A–11

Fetal Heart Rate		Uterine Activity	
Baseline:	125 bpm	Frequency:	Tocotransducer not recording adequately
Variability:	Moderate	Duration:	Tocotransducer not recording adequately
Periodic/Episodic Changes:	None	Strength:	Tocotransducer in place—must palpate
		Resting Tone:	Tocotransducer in place—must palpate
Category:	I		

STRIP CHART A–12

Fetal Heart Rate		Uterine Activity	
Baseline:	120 bpm	Frequency:	1.5–2 minutes
Variability:	Moderate	Duration:	1–2 minutes
Periodic/Episodic Changes:	None	Strength:	Tocotransducer in place—must palpate
		Resting Tone:	Tocotransducer in place—must palpate
Category:	I		

Discussion: In approximately 7 hours and with 20 mU/min of oxytocin infusing, the patient has progressed 1 cm. Any effects on the FHR from the Stadol (decreased variability) given 2 hours prior should be resolved by this time.

STRIP CHART A–13

Fetal Heart Rate		Uterine Activity	
Baseline:	115 bpm	Frequency:	1.5–2.5 minutes
Variability:	Moderate	Duration:	60–80 seconds
Periodic/Episodic Changes:	None	Strength:	Tocotransducer in place—must palpate
		Resting Tone:	Tocotransducer in place—must palpate
Category:	I		

STRIP CHART A–14

Fetal Heart Rate		Uterine Activity	
Baseline:	110 bpm	Frequency:	1–2.5 minutes
Variability:	Minimal-Moderate	Duration:	60–90 seconds
Periodic/Episodic Changes:	None	Strength:	Tocotransducer in place—must palpate
		Resting Tone:	Tocotransducer in place—must palpate
Category:	I		

Discussion: Although the contraction pattern does not technically qualify as tachysystole (>5 contractions/10 min), it is on the borderline and warrants observation. Internal monitoring (IUPC) could be helpful.

STRIP CHART A–15

Fetal Heart Rate		Uterine Activity	
Baseline:	115 bpm	Frequency:	1–2.5 minutes
Variability:	Minimal	Duration:	60–90 seconds
Periodic/Episodic Changes:	Early Decelerations	Strength:	Tocotransducer in place—must palpate
		Resting Tone:	Tocotransducer in place—must palpate
Category:		II	

STRIP CHART A–16

Fetal Heart Rate		Uterine Activity	
Baseline:	115 bpm	Frequency:	1–3 minutes
Variability:	Minimal	Duration:	80 seconds–2 minutes
Periodic/Episodic Changes:	Early Decelerations	Strength:	Tocotransducer in place—must palpate
		Resting Tone:	Tocotransducer in place—must palpate
Category:		II	

STRIP CHART A–17

Fetal Heart Rate		Uterine Activity	
Baseline:	115 bpm	Frequency:	1.5–3 minutes
Variability:	Minimal	Duration:	80 seconds–2 minutes
Periodic/Episodic Changes:	Early and Late Decelerations	Strength:	Tocotransducer in place—must palpate
		Resting Tone:	Tocotransducer in place—must palpate
Category:		II	

Discussion: In 3 hours, the patient has progressed 1 cm. Since the most recent exam 1.5 hours prior, she progressed 1.5 cm and went from 50% to 100% effacement. The UC pattern continues to push the limits of normal in terms of frequency and duration of contractions and should be evaluated. By now, the effects of the second dose of Stadol on the fetus should be resolved. The actions to implement intrauterine resuscitation are prudent; however, this would warrant greatly decreasing or discontinuing the oxytocin and include administration of oxygen at 10 L/min (via nonrebreather mask), increasing IV fluids (1,000-cc bolus), and having the tracing evaluated by the care provider.

STRIP CHART A–18

Fetal Heart Rate		Uterine Activity	
Baseline:	120 bpm	Frequency:	2–2.5 minutes
Variability:	Minimal	Duration:	90–140 seconds
Periodic/Episodic Changes:	Early Decelerations	Strength:	Tocotransducer in place—must palpate
		Resting Tone:	Tocotransducer in place—must palpate
Category:		II	

STRIP CHART A–19

Fetal Heart Rate		*Uterine Activity*	
Baseline:	115 bpm	Frequency:	60–80 seconds
Variability:	Minimal	Duration:	80 seconds–3 minutes
Periodic/Episodic Changes:	Early Decelerations	Strength:	Tocotransducer in place—must palpate
		Resting Tone:	Tocotransducer in place—must palpate
Category:		II	

Discussion: The UC pattern is tachysystole and should be addressed by turning down or turning off the oxytocin and consulting with the care provider.

STRIP CHART A–20

Fetal Heart Rate		*Uterine Activity*	
Baseline:	120 bpm	Frequency:	1–3 minutes
Variability:	Minimal-Moderate	Duration:	1–2 minutes
Periodic/Episodic Changes:	Early and Late Decelerations	Strength:	Tocotransducer in place—must palpate
		Resting Tone:	Tocotransducer in place—must palpate
Category:		II	

STRIP CHART A–21

Fetal Heart Rate		*Uterine Activity*	
Baseline:	115 bpm	Frequency:	1–2.5 minutes
Variability:	Moderate	Duration:	1–2 minutes
Periodic/Episodic Changes:	Early and Variable Decelerations	Strength:	Tocotransducer in place—must palpate
		Resting Tone:	Tocotransducer in place—must palpate
Category:		II	

STRIP CHART A–22

Fetal Heart Rate		Uterine Activity		
Baseline:	115 bpm	Frequency:	1–3 minutes	
Variability:	Minimal-Moderate	Duration:	50 seconds–2 minutes	
Periodic/Episodic Changes:	Early Decelerations	Strength:	Tocotransducer in place— must palpate	
		Resting Tone:	Tocotransducer in place— must palpate	
Category:	I	II	III	

Discussion: It is difficult to categorize the deceleration pattern (early vs. late) when the UCs are not clearly recorded.

STRIP CHART A–23

Fetal Heart Rate		Uterine Activity		
Baseline:	110 bpm	Frequency:	Indeterminate	
Variability:	Minimal	Duration:	Indeterminate	
Periodic/Episodic Changes:	Prolonged Deceleration	Strength:	Tocotransducer in place— must palpate	
		Resting Tone:	Tocotransducer in place— must palpate	
Category:		II		

Discussion: At this time, with the patient near fully dilated and feeling the urge to push and the tracing with minimal variability and decelerations, decreasing or discontinuing the oxytocin should be considered. The patient is a primip, and the length of her pushing (which puts further stress on the fetus) is unknown. Physiologic pushing (open glottis, pushing with the urge) and pushing on her side could be useful techniques in this instance.

STRIP CHART A–24

Fetal Heart Rate		Uterine Activity		
Baseline:	115 bpm	Frequency:	2–2.5 minutes	
Variability:	Minimal	Duration:	90 seconds	
Periodic/Episodic Changes:	Late and Prolonged Deceleration	Strength:	Tocotransducer in place— must palpate	
		Resting Tone:	Tocotransducer in place— must palpate	
Category:		II		

Discussion: Fortunately, the pushing phase was relatively short (<30 minutes), minimizing the amount of stress on the fetus.

OUTCOME: Female delivered at 09:46. Apgars 9/10, weight 3,062 g (6 lb, 12 oz). Short cord – 28 cm (11 inches) noted.

STRIP CHART B-1

Fetal Heart Rate		Uterine Activity	
Baseline:	105 bpm	Frequency:	Indeterminate
Variability:	Moderate	Duration:	Indeterminate
Periodic/Episodic Changes:	Variable Decelerations (?)	Strength:	Indeterminate
		Resting Tone:	Indeterminate
Category:		II	

Discussion: It is challenging to interpret this portion of tracing. The data that is available, however, warrants close observation, as it does not fall within normal parameters (110–160 bpm). The brief excursions of an FHR >180 could indicate double-counting of a very fetal low heart rate, an issue that can usually be ruled out with use of internal FHR monitoring (FECG), as this mode of monitoring has a greater range (see Chapter 2). With a lower than normal heart rate, information about the maternal pulse is essential. If there is any doubt about which signal (maternal or fetal) is being recorded, it is important to palpate for maternal pulse and simultaneously compare findings with the audible signal from the electronic fetal monitor. Concerns about UA in this segment of tracing include the patient experiencing pain not only with, but also between, contractions and the inability to record contraction data.

STRIP CHART B-2

Fetal Heart Rate		Uterine Activity	
Baseline:	130 bpm	Frequency:	Indeterminate
Variability:	Minimal	Duration:	Indeterminate
Periodic/Episodic Changes:	Late decelerations (?)	Strength:	Indeterminate
		Resting Tone:	Indeterminate
Category:		II	

Discussion: The FHR baseline is difficult to ascertain, primarily as there is no clear UA data against which to evaluate. It is unlikely, however, that the FHR is 115 bpm with accelerations as noted. It would make sense, however, for the maternal heart rate (MHR) to be elevated during contractions in response to increased pain. At this time, it is essential to clarify the UA pattern (monitor internally with an IUPC if an external tracing cannot be maintained). It is concerning that the patient is in pain not only with, but also between contractions, particularly because she is a VBAC (placing her at risk for uterine rupture). Continuous pain is a common symptom of uterine rupture. As the tracing is suspect and the patient's condition not verified, allowing the patient to ambulate would not be advisable at this time.

STRIP CHART B-3

Fetal Heart Rate		Uterine Activity	
Baseline:	125 bpm	Frequency:	Indeterminate
Variability:	Minimal	Duration:	Indeterminate
Periodic/Episodic Changes:	Late decelerations (?)	Strength:	Indeterminate
		Resting Tone:	Indeterminate
Category:		II	

Discussion: Concerns regarding the maternal and fetal condition continue as noted above. Maternal vital signs should be considered within the context of the clinical picture. Although it appears that the tocotransducer has been adjusted numerous times, this essential data continues to not be recorded. With pain medicine now in effect, the "accelerations" (as they are described in the charting) in the heart rate during contractions are no longer present, another piece of evidence consistent with a MHR pattern (the patient is not in as much pain during contractions; therefore, her heart rate is no longer markedly increasing in response).

STRIP CHART B–4

Fetal Heart Rate		Uterine Activity	
Baseline:	125 bpm	Frequency:	Indeterminate
Variability:	Minimal	Duration:	Indeterminate
Periodic/Episodic Changes:	Late decelerations (?)	Strength:	Indeterminate
		Resting Tone:	Indeterminate
Category:		II	

Discussion: Concerns regarding the maternal and fetal condition continue as noted above.

OUTCOME: The fetus is delivered via Cesarean at 16:46 with Apgars of 0/0, diagnosis of uterine rupture confirmed. Resuscitation: A full neonatal code ensued but was not successful. The entire recording was of the MHR. At no time was an FHR acquired or represented on the tracing. Please see Chapter 2 for detailed information about erroneous recording of MHR.

STRIP CHART C–1

Fetal Heart Rate		Uterine Activity	
Baseline:	150 bpm	Frequency:	3–5 minutes
Variability:	Moderate	Duration:	90 seconds–3 minutes
Periodic/Episodic Changes:	Intermittent Late and Variable Decelerations	Strength:	Tocotransducer in place—must palpate
		Resting Tone:	Tocotransducer in place—must palpate
Category:		II	

Discussion: It is important to keep in mind throughout review of this tracing (and certainly as the providers assessing it in real time) that his patient presents as high risk; she is of advanced maternal age, postdates, and attempting VBAC. Additionally, her two children were macrosomic at birth and she had an abnormal 1-hour GTT with this pregnancy, indicators that this fetus also may be large. Many of the decelerations in this case do not precisely demonstrate the characteristics of any one specific type of deceleration per NICHD definitions but, rather, overlaps two classifications (variable decelerations and late decelerations). Therefore, discrepancies in interpretation may occur. Regardless of whether these decelerations are deemed to be variable or late, both types represent diminished oxygenated blood flow to the fetus and should be treated as such. Ultimately, it is a provision of appropriate clinical response that is of paramount importance.

STRIP CHART C–2

Fetal Heart Rate		Uterine Activity	
Baseline:	140 bpm	Frequency:	3–5 minutes
Variability:	Minimal	Duration:	2 minutes
Periodic/Episodic Changes:	Late Decelerations	Strength:	Tocotransducer in place—must palpate
		Resting Tone:	Tocotransducer in place—must palpate
Category:		II	

Discussion: In most other aspects, these decelerations match of the definition of the visual appearance of a variable deceleration; however, they do not reach their nadir in ≥30 seconds. Also, while the timing of variable decelerations in relation to contractions is not a defining component, these decelerations are notably delayed (offset from contractions) in both onset and recovery, a finding that is consistent with late decelerations.

STRIP CHART C–3

Fetal Heart Rate		Uterine Activity	
Baseline:	140 bpm	Frequency:	1–3 minutes
Variability:	Minimal	Duration:	1–2.5 minutes
Periodic/Episodic Changes:	Late Decelerations.	Strength:	25–100 mm Hg
		Resting Tone:	15 mm Hg
Category:		II	

Discussion: With this patient, decelerations seem to be improved with positioning to the left side. Closer observation via internal monitoring was warranted and should assist in determination of fetal status. While this tracing is a Category II, it is pushing the limits of becoming a Category III.

STRIP CHART C–4

Fetal Heart Rate		Uterine Activity	
Baseline:	145 bpm	Frequency:	5 minutes
Variability:	Moderate	Duration:	80 seconds–2 minutes
Periodic/Episodic Changes:	Variable and Late Decelerations	Strength:	30–45 mm Hg
		Resting Tone:	10 mm Hg
Category:		II	

Discussion: After about an hour of no progress with cervical dilation, oxytocin was begun. The fetus is noted to be in a posterior position.

STRIP CHART C–5

Fetal Heart Rate		Uterine Activity	
Baseline:	140 bpm	Frequency:	2–5 minutes
Variability:	Minimal–Moderate	Duration:	90 seconds
Periodic/Episodic Changes:	Variable and Late Decelerations	Strength:	15–55 mm Hg
		Resting Tone:	15–20 mm Hg
Category:		II	

STRIP CHART C–6

Fetal Heart Rate		Uterine Activity	
Baseline:	140 bpm	Frequency:	4 minutes
Variability:	Minimal	Duration:	80–90 seconds
Periodic/Episodic Changes:	Variable and Late Decelerations	Strength:	45–60 mm Hg
		Resting Tone:	10 mm Hg
Category:		II	

Discussion: There has been no cervical change in 2 hours; oxytocin continues to be increased. During the period of time between 00:05–00:07, the episode of rapidly occurring excursions above and below the FHR represent artifact that is usually attributable to interruption in the connection of the spiral electrode at some point between the fetal head and the monitor.

STRIP CHART C–7

Fetal Heart Rate		Uterine Activity	
Baseline:	145 bpm	Frequency:	3.5–5 minutes
Variability:	Minimal–Moderate	Duration:	80 seconds
Periodic/Episodic Changes:	Variable and Late Decelerations	Strength:	55–60 mm Hg
		Resting Tone:	10–20 mm Hg
Category:		II	

Discussion: Decelerations continue to show some response to positioning. With an IUPC in place, consideration could be given to amnioinfusion in an effort to remediate some of the variable decelerations present.

STRIP CHART C–8

Fetal Heart Rate		Uterine Activity	
Baseline:	150 bpm	Frequency:	3–4 minutes
Variability:	Minimal	Duration:	80–90 seconds
Periodic/Episodic Changes:	Variable and Late Decelerations	Strength:	50–55 mm Hg
		Resting Tone:	20 mm Hg
Category:		II	

Discussion: The tracing continues to border on becoming a Category III; however, oxytocin is continued. From the annotations, it seems that the FHR is being closely observed in an institution where medical staff is in house.

STRIP CHART C–9

Fetal Heart Rate		Uterine Activity	
Baseline:	150 bpm	Frequency:	2–4.5 minutes
Variability:	Minimal	Duration:	90 seconds
Periodic/Episodic Changes:	Variable and Late Decelerations	Strength:	55–70 mm Hg (?)
		Resting Tone:	IUPC needs to be adjusted
Category:		II	

STRIP CHART C–10

Fetal Heart Rate		Uterine Activity	
Baseline:	145 bpm	Frequency:	2–5 minutes
Variability:	Minimal–Moderate	Duration:	80 seconds (?)
Periodic/Episodic Changes:	Variable and Late Decelerations	Strength:	IUPC needs to be adjusted
		Resting Tone:	IUPC needs to be adjusted
Category:		II	

Discussion: The patient has progressed 2 cm over the course of 1.5 hours.

STRIP CHART C–11

Fetal Heart Rate		Uterine Activity	
Baseline:	160 bpm	Frequency:	1–2.5 minutes
Variability:	Minimal	Duration:	90 seconds
Periodic/Episodic Changes:	Variable, Late and Early Decelerations	Strength:	70–80 mm Hg (?)
		Resting Tone:	IUPC needs to be adjusted
Category:		II	

Discussion: It is important to note trends in the FHR and this is best accomplished by comparing present data to that which occurred previously, particularly if there is data available from a time prior to any stresses on the fetus. The baseline FHR is slowly rising, which may be an indication of fetal metabolic acidemia or hypoxia. Screening for fetal oxygenation with fetal scalp stimulation would be indicated. And although not technically tachysystole, there is an episode of contractions that occur close together with a simultaneous increase in frequency of decelerations. Contractions that occur too frequently do not allow adequate oxygenation to resume between contractions. Increased UA can also be an indication of uterine rupture or dehiscence and, therefore, requires close attention to the fetal response.

STRIP CHART C-12

Fetal Heart Rate		Uterine Activity	
Baseline:	160 bpm	Frequency:	1.5–5 minutes
Variability:	Minimal	Duration:	IUPC needs to be adjusted
Periodic/Episodic Changes:	Variable and Late Decelerations	Strength:	IUPC needs to be adjusted
		Resting Tone:	IUPC needs to be adjusted
Category:		II	

Discussion: While still technically within normal limits at 160 bpm, the FHR is bordering on tachycardia. This rate represents a change in the FHR suggestive that the fetus' oxygen needs are increasing and raising concern about development of acidemia. The oxytocin should not be increased under these circumstances.

STRIP CHART C-13

Fetal Heart Rate		Uterine Activity	
Baseline:	160 bpm	Frequency:	2–3 minutes
Variability:	Minimal	Duration:	60–80 seconds
Periodic/Episodic Changes:	Variable and Late Decelerations	Strength:	60–75 mm Hg
		Resting Tone:	0 mm Hg
Category:		II	

Discussion: The physician has been notified, which is appropriate. However, the nursing notes do not convey concern over the tracing or imply for the physician to be present at the bedside. While he/she has been notified of the patient's change in status to fully dilated and pushing, the increasing depth and duration of the decelerations should elicit concern about whether the FHR will recover from the successive incidents.

STRIP CHART C-14

Fetal Heart Rate		Uterine Activity	
Baseline:	160 bpm	Frequency:	1–3 minutes
Variability:	Minimal	Duration:	80 seconds–2 minutes
Periodic/Episodic Changes:	Variable, Late, and Prolonged Decelerations	Strength:	Pushing
		Resting Tone:	0 mm Hg
Category:		II	

STRIP CHART C–15

Fetal Heart Rate		Uterine Activity	
Baseline:	160 bpm	Frequency:	1–4 minutes
Variability:	Minimal–Moderate	Duration:	1–2 minutes
Periodic/Episodic Changes:	Variable and Late Decelerations	Strength:	Pushing
		Resting Tone:	0 mm Hg
Category:		II	

Discussion: From the appearance of the UA pattern, it is clear that the patient is pushing with each contraction. With a FHR that is not responding well to the stress of pushing, it can be very helpful to rest through some of the contractions (e.g., push every other, or even every third, contraction) to allow the fetus time for recovery between such attempts. Pushing with the patient in positions other than lithotomy and encouraging physiologic pushing can also be helpful in regard to optimizing perfusion to and minimizing stress on the fetus.

STRIP CHART C–16

Fetal Heart Rate		Uterine Activity	
Baseline:	175 bpm	Frequency:	1.5–2 minutes
Variability:	Minimal–Moderate	Duration:	60–90 seconds
Periodic/Episodic Changes:	Variable and Late Decelerations	Strength:	Pushing
		Resting Tone:	0 mm Hg
Category:		II	

Discussion: It is difficult to assess the FHR baseline due to the frequency of decelerations. However, it is clear that the fetus is now tachycardic, one of the first indicators in the progression of fetal hypoxia. Once again, there is an episode of tachysystole. Oxytocin should be not be infusing.

STRIP CHART C–17

Fetal Heart Rate		Uterine Activity	
Baseline:	180 bpm	Frequency:	2 minutes
Variability:	Absent	Duration:	60–80 seconds
Periodic/Episodic Changes:	Variable, Late, and Prolonged Decelerations	Strength:	60–70 mm Hg
		Resting Tone:	0 mm Hg
Category:			III

Discussion: This tracing is worsening and indicates the need for expedient delivery. The patient has been pushing for 50 minutes, and there has been no descent of the fetal head and the position remains ROP. The decision is made to proceed with operative birth. There is no further recording of the FHR after the EFM is discontinued at the end of this tracing. The impetus for calling the C/S appears to be lack of progress/descent, rather than concern over fetal condition. There is no clear indication from the documentation (in terms of notifications/consultations, interventions, ongoing monitoring, etc.) that the compromised status of the fetus was appreciated appropriately.

OUTCOME: 05:38 Delivery of live male via cesarean, 4,515 g (9 lb, 15 oz). Occult shoulder cord noted. No evidence of uterine rupture or abruption; normally inserted, three-vessel cord. Apgars 0/3/8, full neonatal code performed and to NICU. Cord blood results: arterial pH 6.97, BE –18 and venous pH 7.21, BE –11. Long-term deficits included severe brain damage, cerebral palsy, and spastic quadriplegia, along with related dysfunction of various other organs.

STRIP CHART D–1

Fetal Heart Rate		Uterine Activity	
Baseline:	145 bpm	Frequency:	1–5.5 minutes
Variability:	Moderate	Duration:	40 seconds–2 minutes
Periodic/Episodic Changes:	Accelerations	Strength:	Mild–Moderate
		Resting Tone:	Tocotransducer in place—must palpate
Category:	I		

STRIP CHART D–2

Fetal Heart Rate		Uterine Activity	
Baseline:	145 bpm	Frequency:	2–4 minutes
Variability:	Moderate	Duration:	40–100 seconds
Periodic/Episodic Changes:	Accelerations	Strength:	Tocotransducer in place—must palpate
		Resting Tone:	Tocotransducer in place—must palpate
Category:	I		

STRIP CHART D–3

Fetal Heart Rate		Uterine Activity	
Baseline:	150 bpm	Frequency:	Irregular
Variability:	Moderate	Duration:	Indeterminate
Periodic/Episodic Changes:	Accelerations	Strength:	Tocotransducer in place—must palpate
		Resting Tone:	Tocotransducer in place—must palpate
Category:	I		

STRIP CHART D–4

Fetal Heart Rate		Uterine Activity	
Baseline:	150 bpm	Frequency:	5–6 minutes
Variability:	Moderate	Duration:	2.5–3 minutes
Periodic/Episodic Changes:	Variable and Prolonged Decelerations	Strength:	Mild–Moderate
		Resting Tone:	Tocotransducer in place— must palpate
Category:		II	

Discussion: This tracing represents the FHR approximately 30 minutes after beginning the oxytocin, which is when it begins to take effect. The FHR now has a different appearance than in earlier segments, demonstrating variable and prolonged decelerations. Variability continues to be moderate (indicating an absence of fetal metabolic acidemia), and this would be an optimal time to respond to the deceleration patterns in an effort to resolve them. A change in patient position, IV fluid bolus of 1,000 cc, and discontinuing or decreasing the oxytocin are all reasonable considerations. Most oxytocin protocols would indicate that a dose increase is not appropriate at this time.

STRIP CHART D–5

Fetal Heart Rate		Uterine Activity	
Baseline:	150 bpm	Frequency:	Indeterminate
Variability:	Moderate	Duration:	2.5 minutes
Periodic/Episodic Changes:	Variable and Late Decelerations	Strength:	Tocotransducer in place— must palpate
		Resting Tone:	Tocotransducer in place— must palpate
Category:		II	

Discussion: The patient has been disconnected from EFM to use the bathroom and fetal status is not yet re-established upon her return when the oxytocin dose is increased. With the FHR tracing demonstrating areas of concern (decelerations), it would be prudent to delay the scheduled oxytocin dose increase until more continuous EFM data is obtained. At this time, the patient should be assisted with options to void with continuous EFM in place.

STRIP CHART D–6

Fetal Heart Rate		Uterine Activity	
Baseline:	160 bpm	Frequency:	Irregular
Variability:	Moderate	Duration:	2 minutes
Periodic/Episodic Changes:	Late Decelerations	Strength:	Tocotransducer in place— must palpate
		Resting Tone:	Tocotransducer in place— must palpate
Category:		II	

Discussion: The FHR baseline has increased from the admission tracing and borders on tachycardia. It is important to compare data to that which is previously available, in order to put findings into clinical context. Fetal tachycardia is often one of the earliest indicators of fetal compromise in the progression of fetal hypoxia although, in this particular case at this point in time, the moderate variability indicates the absence of fetal metabolic acidemia. Additionally, late decelerations are present, which can lead to fetal metabolic acidemia. Therefore, it is appropriate to notify the care provider of such findings and avoid any compromise to maternal/fetal blood flow. Although the order is to continue increasing the oxytocin dosage, it is unlikely that such action would be consistent with institutional protocol when these nonreassuring findings are present. This tracing warrants close observation, particularly for any changes in the variability.

STRIP CHART D–7

Fetal Heart Rate		Uterine Activity	
Baseline:	155 bpm	Frequency:	2.5–4 minutes
Variability:	Moderate	Duration:	80 seconds–2.5 minutes
Periodic/Episodic Changes:	Variable and Prolonged Decelerations	Strength:	Moderate
		Resting Tone:	Tocotransducer in place—must palpate
Category:		II	

Discussion: The oxytocin dose is halved at this time. It would be appropriate to discontinue the oxytocin and implement intrauterine resuscitation (position change, IV fluid bolus, oxygen at 10L/min via nonrebreather mask). It is important for the nurse in charge of the unit (charge RN, supervisor, etc.) to know when there is concern about patient/fetal status so that he/she can be prepared to respond in a timely and appropriate manner and provide staffing as needed.

STRIP CHART D–8

Fetal Heart Rate		Uterine Activity	
Baseline:	Indeterminate	Frequency:	Indeterminate
Variability:	Moderate (?)	Duration:	Indeterminate
Periodic/Episodic Changes:	Prolonged Deceleration	Strength:	Tocotransducer in place—must palpate
		Resting Tone:	Tocotransducer in place—must palpate
Category:		II	

Discussion: While the FHR baseline is indeterminate (there is not at least 2 minutes of FHR baseline represented) from just this segment of tracing, the FHR does appear to return to the previously established baseline of 155 during the last minute of this strip. When the FHR baseline is indeterminate, it is necessary to incorporate the most recent information available (if possible and relevant) and also try to obtain useful data as quickly as possible. Without an established FHR baseline and clear UA data, it is not possible to definitively determine periodic/episodic changes; however, it is clear that at least the prolonged decelerations continue. Without an established FHR baseline, it is also difficult to accurately determine FHR variability, although in this case it does appear to continue to be moderate. Oxytocin should not be infusing when fetal status is unknown. Eventually the appropriate actions of discontinuing the oxytocin and notifying the care provider are accomplished. Maternal vital signs may provide additional information.

STRIP CHART D–9

Fetal Heart Rate		Uterine Activity	
Baseline:	160 bpm	Frequency:	2–3 minutes
Variability:	Moderate	Duration:	60–100 seconds
Periodic/Episodic Changes:	Variable and Prolonged Decelerations	Strength:	Tocotransducer in place—must palpate
		Resting Tone:	Tocotransducer in place—must palpate
Category:		II	

Discussion: It would not be appropriate to resume the oxytocin at this time. The only reassuring aspect of this tracing is that the FHR variability is still in the moderate range. However, even that has decreased from what was previously demonstrated and now borders on the minimal range. The care provider's presence is required at the bedside and intrauterine resuscitation should be in progress.

STRIP CHART D–10

Fetal Heart Rate		Uterine Activity	
Baseline:	155 bpm	Frequency:	4 minutes
Variability:	Moderate	Duration:	1–3 minutes
Periodic/Episodic Changes:	Prolonged Decelerations	Strength:	Tocotransducer in place—must palpate
		Resting Tone:	Tocotransducer in place—must palpate
Category:		II	

Discussion: This segment of tracing is a Category II but very closely bordering on a Category III; operative delivery may be immediately required. Scalp stimulation is a technique that can be effective in reassuring providers about fetal status. However, it is neither appropriate nor useful to perform this technique during a FHR deceleration (see Chapters 1 and 3).

STRIP CHART D–11

Fetal Heart Rate		Uterine Activity	
Baseline:	155 bpm	Frequency:	5 minutes
Variability:	Moderate	Duration:	1–2 minutes
Periodic/Episodic Changes:	Variable Decelerations	Strength:	Tocotransducer in place—must palpate
		Resting Tone:	Tocotransducer in place—must palpate
Category:		II	

Discussion: There has been no progress in regard to cervical dilation in the three hours that oxytocin has been infusing and the FHR is not responding well to the stress of induction. It would be appropriate to leave the oxytocin off until the FHR has recovered and then attempt a restart if the induction process is to continue.

STRIP CHART D–12

Fetal Heart Rate		Uterine Activity	
Baseline:	Indeterminate	Frequency:	Indeterminate
Variability:	Indeterminate	Duration:	Indeterminate
Periodic/Episodic Changes:	Indeterminate	Strength:	Tocotransducer in place—must palpate
		Resting Tone:	Tocotransducer in place—must palpate
Category:		II	

Discussion: Without UA data, FHR data cannot be determined. If the process of induction is to continue, closer attention to monitoring UA is necessary; an IUPC should be considered.

STRIP CHART D-13

Fetal Heart Rate		Uterine Activity	
Baseline:	155 bpm	Frequency:	1–6 minutes (?)
Variability:	Moderate	Duration:	1–2 minutes (?)
Periodic/Episodic Changes:	Prolonged Decelerations	Strength:	Tocotransducer in place— must palpate
		Resting Tone:	Tocotransducer in place— must palpate
Category:		II	

STRIP CHART D-14

Fetal Heart Rate		Uterine Activity	
Baseline:	155 bpm	Frequency:	1–6 minutes
Variability:	Moderate	Duration:	1–3 minutes
Periodic/Episodic Changes:	Variable and Prolonged Decelerations	Strength:	Tocotransducer in place— must palpate
		Resting Tone:	Tocotransducer in place— must palpate
Category:		II	

Discussion: Now that the UA pattern is more clearly recorded, elements of the FHR (baseline, variability, and periodic/ episodic changes) can be assessed. Decision to proceed with operative birth is made by these clinicians based on lack of labor progress. Another option may include reassessment of fetal oxygenation with proper use of fetal scalp stimulation and, if absence of fetal metabolic acidemia is confirmed by the elicitation of an acceleration, continuing cautiously with induction under close observation.

STRIP CHART D-15

Fetal Heart Rate		Uterine Activity	
Baseline:	160 bpm	Frequency:	×1
Variability:	Moderate	Duration:	3 minutes
Periodic/Episodic Changes:	Late Deceleration	Strength:	Tocotransducer in place— must palpate
		Resting Tone:	Tocotransducer in place— must palpate
Category:		II	

Discussion: Delivery is noted to occur more than 40 minutes after EFM is discontinued. Although the cesarean was called for lack of progress, it is necessary to remember that the FHR had been a Category II with some concerning aspects and required observation. It is necessary to continue EFM in this interim and store the recorded data with the patient record.

OUTCOME: Live male delivered via Cesarean at 13:13, 3,260 g (7 lb, 3 oz). Apgars 5/7. Resuscitation: tactile stimulation, blow-by O2. Cord pH 7.18, BE –3.

STRIP CHART E-1

Fetal Heart Rate		Uterine Activity	
Baseline:	135 bpm	Frequency:	Indeterminate
Variability:	Moderate	Duration:	60 seconds
Periodic/Episodic Changes:	Accelerations	Strength:	Moderate
		Resting Tone:	Tocotransducer in place—must palpate
Category:	I		

STRIP CHART E-2

Fetal Heart Rate		Uterine Activity	
Baseline:	135 bpm	Frequency:	3 min
Variability:	Moderate	Duration:	60–100 sec
Periodic/Episodic Changes:	Accelerations and Variable Decelerations	Strength:	Tocotransducer in place—must palpate
		Resting Tone:	Tocotransducer in place—must palpate
Category:	I		

Discussion: The occasional variable decelerations noted are mild and not clinically significant at this time.

STRIP CHART E-3

Fetal Heart Rate		Uterine Activity	
Baseline:	135 bpm	Frequency:	Indeterminate
Variability:	Moderate	Duration:	Indeterminate
Periodic/Episodic Changes:	Accelerations	Strength:	Tocotransducer in place—must palpate
		Resting Tone:	Tocotransducer in place—must palpate
Category:	I		

Discussion: UA does not seem to be being recorded. The tocotransducer should be adjusted.

STRIP CHART E–4

Fetal Heart Rate		Uterine Activity	
Baseline:	135 bpm	Frequency:	Irregular
Variability:	Moderate	Duration:	100–140 seconds
Periodic/Episodic Changes:	Accelerations	Strength:	Tocotransducer in place—must palpate
		Resting Tone:	Tocotransducer in place—must palpate
Category:	I		

STRIP CHART E–5

Fetal Heart Rate		Uterine Activity	
Baseline:	135 bpm	Frequency:	Irregular
Variability:	Minimal–Moderate	Duration:	80 seconds–2 minutes
Periodic/Episodic Changes:	Acceleration ×1	Strength:	Tocotransducer in place—must palpate
		Resting Tone:	Tocotransducer in place—must palpate
Category:	I		

STRIP CHART E–6

Fetal Heart Rate		Uterine Activity	
Baseline:	135 bpm	Frequency:	2–3 minutes
Variability:	Minimal–Moderate	Duration:	100–130 seconds
Periodic/Episodic Changes:	Accelerations	Strength:	Tocotransducer in place—must palpate
		Resting Tone:	Tocotransducer in place—must palpate
Category:	I		

Discussion: The episode of four contractions occurring without any break in between bears watching. There should be at least 1 minute of rest between contractions so that the fetus may have a chance to recover. If this type of UA pattern continues, oxytocin should be decreased and the care provider notified.

STRIP CHART E-7

Fetal Heart Rate		Uterine Activity	
Baseline:	Indeterminate	Frequency:	Indeterminate
Variability:	Indeterminate	Duration:	90 seconds (?)
Periodic/Episodic Changes:	Variable Decelerations	Strength:	Tocotransducer in place—must palpate
		Resting Tone:	Tocotransducer in place—must palpate
Category:		II	

Discussion: Although there is not enough data to adequately assess the FHR, it appears that the FHR baseline is likely 125 bpm with moderate variability. The organized group of deflections occurring mostly below the FHR baseline that can be seen during the last minute of this tracing is a FHR dysrhythmia. This is distinguishable from artifact by its visual appearance. Artifact usually occurs rather randomly and has a more erratic appearance, with disorganized deflections above and/or below the baseline of varying heights/depths. The downward deflections in the dysrhythmia pattern represent "dropped" beats and should be further investigated with M-mode ultrasound (see Chapter 3). Maternal BP is hypotensive and should be observed closely; both for the well being of the patient and as this may be causing or contributing to the pattern of fetal dysrhythmia.

STRIP CHART E-8

Fetal Heart Rate		Uterine Activity	
Baseline:	130 bpm	Frequency:	2–3 minutes
Variability:	Minimal–Moderate	Duration:	90–120 seconds
Periodic/Episodic Changes:	Early Decelerations	Strength:	Tocotransducer in place—must palpate
		Resting Tone:	Tocotransducer in place—must palpate
Category:		II	

Discussion: Intermittent episodes of fetal dysrhythmia continue.

STRIP CHART E-9

Fetal Heart Rate		Uterine Activity	
Baseline:	150 bpm	Frequency:	1–2 minutes
Variability:	Minimal	Duration:	60 seconds–2 minutes
Periodic/Episodic Changes:	Early Decelerations	Strength:	20–30 mm/Hg
		Resting Tone:	15 mm Hg
Category:		II	

Discussion: The fetus has not been able to maintain its baseline heart rate at a stable rate, and the FHR baseline is now notably higher than it was previously. These findings, combined with the tachysystole that is occurring, warrant decreasing/discontinuing the oxytocin.

STRIP CHART E-10

Fetal Heart Rate		Uterine Activity	
Baseline:	155 bpm	Frequency:	1–3 minutes (?)
Variability:	Minimal–Moderate	Duration:	Indeterminate
Periodic/Episodic Changes:	Early, Variable, and Late Decelerations	Strength:	Indeterminate
		Resting Tone:	Indeterminate
Category:		II	

Discussion: The IUPC needs to be reset to record properly so that UA can be accurately assessed.

STRIP CHART E-11

Fetal Heart Rate		Uterine Activity	
Baseline:	155 bpm	Frequency:	1–2.5 minutes
Variability:	Minimal	Duration:	Indeterminate
Periodic/Episodic Changes:	Decelerations	Strength:	Indeterminate
		Resting Tone:	Indeterminate
Category:		II	

Discussion: The IUPC continues to require adjustment. Without a clear UA pattern, it makes it difficult to determine the type of decelerations present. Tachysystole is occurring, and the FHR is responding with decelerations.

STRIP CHART E-12

Fetal Heart Rate		Uterine Activity	
Baseline:	Indeterminate	Frequency:	1.5–2 minutes
Variability:	Indeterminate	Duration:	70–100 seconds
Periodic/Episodic Changes:	Variable and Prolonged Decelerations	Strength:	40–60 mm Hg
		Resting Tone:	20 mm Hg
Category:		II	

Discussion: The FHR baseline is indeterminate during this segment of tracing but appears to be attempting to return to its previous 155-bpm baseline. The singular aspect of this tracing that keeps it marginally within Category II at this time is that there appears to be variability present in the brief portions of the tracing that appear to represent a return to baseline.

STRIP CHART E-13

Fetal Heart Rate		Uterine Activity	
Baseline:	150 bpm	Frequency:	1.5–2.5 minutes
Variability:	Minimal	Duration:	70–90 seconds
Periodic/Episodic Changes:	Variable and Prolonged Decelerations	Strength:	40–60 mm Hg
		Resting Tone:	15–20 mm Hg
Category:		II	

STRIP CHART E-14

Fetal Heart Rate		Uterine Activity	
Baseline:	150 bpm	Frequency:	1.5–2.5 minutes
Variability:	Minimal	Duration:	80–90 seconds
Periodic/Episodic Changes:	Early and Variable Decelerations	Strength:	50–70 mm Hg
		Resting Tone:	15–25 mm Hg
Category:		II	

Discussion: Oxytocin is resumed although elements of the FHR that are not reassuring persist and the frequency and length of contractions leave little time for the fetus to recover. The patient should be properly evaluated (at the bedside) at this time.

STRIP CHART E-15

Fetal Heart Rate		Uterine Activity	
Baseline:	165 bpm	Frequency:	1–2 minutes
Variability:	Minimal	Duration:	80–90 seconds
Periodic/Episodic Changes:	Early and Variable Decelerations	Strength:	60 mm Hg
		Resting Tone:	15–20 mm Hg
Category:		II	

Discussion: The FHR is now tachycardic, indicating that the fetus' oxygen needs are increasing and raising concern about development of acidemia. It is unknown how long the fetus will be able to tolerate the stress of contractions. Oxytocin should be discontinued and intrauterine resuscitation implemented. The patient should be evaluated by the care provider.

STRIP CHART E–16

Fetal Heart Rate		Uterine Activity	
Baseline:	165 bpm	Frequency:	1.5–2 minutes
Variability:	Minimal	Duration:	70–90 seconds
Periodic/Episodic Changes:	Early and Variable Decelerations	Strength:	50–65 mm Hg
		Resting Tone:	20 mm Hg
Category:		II	

STRIP CHART E–17

Fetal Heart Rate		Uterine Activity	
Baseline:	175 bpm	Frequency:	1–3 minutes
Variability:	Minimal–Moderate	Duration:	60–70 seconds
Periodic/Episodic Changes:	Variable and Prolonged Decelerations	Strength:	65–80 mm Hg
		Resting Tone:	20–25 mm Hg
Category:		II	

STRIP CHART E–18

Fetal Heart Rate		Uterine Activity	
Baseline:	Indeterminate	Frequency:	1–2.5 minutes
Variability:	Indeterminate	Duration:	60–90 seconds
Periodic/Episodic Changes:	Variable and Prolonged Decelerations	Strength:	50–75 mm Hg
		Resting Tone:	20–30 mm Hg
Category:		II	

Discussion: The FHR is demonstrating difficulty in returning to baseline during this episode of tachysystole. It is not predictable at this time whether the FHR will have the ability to recover. Efforts should be focused on decreasing the stress of contractions (oxytocin should not be running; tocolytics may be employed) and implementing intrauterine resuscitation. The provider should be called to the bedside if not already present. Although there is not enough FHR baseline present to make a determination, it appears as though the FHR baseline is likely 180 bpm.

STRIP CHART E–19

Fetal Heart Rate		Uterine Activity	
Baseline:	Indeterminate	Frequency:	1–2 minutes
Variability:	Indeterminate	Duration:	60–90 seconds
Periodic/Episodic Changes:	Variable and Prolonged Decelerations	Strength:	Pushing
		Resting Tone:	Tocotransducer in place— must palpate
Category:		II	

Discussion: Pushing is likely to further the stress on the fetus, as is the tachysystole. Although there is not enough FHR baseline present to make a determination, the FHR baseline appears to be 170 bpm.

STRIP CHART E–20

Fetal Heart Rate		Uterine Activity	
Baseline:	Indeterminate	Frequency:	1–1.5 minutes
Variability:	Indeterminate	Duration:	80–90 seconds
Periodic/Episodic Changes:	Variable and Prolonged Decelerations	Strength:	Pushing
		Resting Tone:	Tocotransducer in place— must palpate
Category:			III

Discussion: Although there is not enough FHR baseline present to make a determination, the FHR baseline appears to be 175 bpm.

STRIP CHART E–21

Fetal Heart Rate		Uterine Activity	
Baseline:	Indeterminate	Frequency:	Indeterminate
Variability:	Indeterminate	Duration:	Indeterminate
Periodic/Episodic Changes:	Variable and Prolonged Decelerations	Strength:	Strong
		Resting Tone:	Indeterminate
Category:			III

STRIP CHART E–22

Fetal Heart Rate		Uterine Activity		
Baseline:	Indeterminate	Frequency:	Indeterminate	
Variability:	Indeterminate	Duration:	Indeterminate	
Periodic/Episodic Changes:	Variable and Prolonged Decelerations	Strength:	Indeterminate	
		Resting Tone:	Indeterminate	
Category:				III

Discussion: The FHR is now indeterminate because there is no UA data against which to compare; however, the FHR baseline appears to be 185 bpm.

STRIP CHART E–23

Fetal Heart Rate		Uterine Activity		
Baseline:	Indeterminate	Frequency:	Indeterminate	
Variability:	Indeterminate	Duration:	Indeterminate	
Periodic/Episodic Changes:	Variable and Prolonged Decelerations	Strength:	Indeterminate	
		Resting Tone:	Indeterminate	
Category:				III

Discussion: The FHR baseline appears to be 180 bpm.

STRIP CHART E–24

Fetal Heart Rate		Uterine Activity		
Baseline:	Indeterminate	Frequency:	Indeterminate	
Variability:	Indeterminate	Duration:	Indeterminate	
Periodic/Episodic Changes:	Variable and Prolonged Decelerations	Strength:	Indeterminate	
		Resting Tone:	Indeterminate	
Category:				III

Discussion: Monitoring has been inadequate (no UA data) for >45 minutes. The FHR baseline appears to be 180 bpm and has been tachycardic for >3 hours.

OUTCOME: 22:27 delivery of live male, 4,110 g (9 lb, 1 oz), over a midline episiotomy with a second-degree tear. Apgars 2/6/7. Resuscitation: tactile stimulation, PPV, intubated (between the first and second Apgar score; there were no spontaneous respirations), and taken to NICU. Cord pH 7.0, BE –18. Neonatal seizures began within 8 hours.

STRIP CHART F–1

Fetal Heart Rate		*Uterine Activity*	
Baseline:	130 bpm	Frequency:	Irregular
Variability:	Minimal	Duration:	70 seconds–1 minute
Periodic/Episodic Changes:	Prolonged Decelerations	Strength:	Tocotransducer in place—must palpate
		Resting Tone:	Tocotransducer in place—must palpate
Category:		II	

Discussion: This tracing is a Category II bordering on a Category III. The minimal amount of variability that remains present is all that is keeping this tracing within Category II. Closer observation of the FHR with internal monitoring is warranted.

STRIP CHART F–2

Fetal Heart Rate		*Uterine Activity*	
Baseline:	130 bpm	Frequency:	Indeterminate
Variability:	Absent–Minimal	Duration:	Indeterminate
Periodic/Episodic Changes:	Prolonged and Variable Decelerations	Strength:	Mild
		Resting Tone:	Tocotransducer in place—must palpate
Category:			III

Discussion: Intrauterine resuscitation is being initiated, the care provider has been contacted, and the patient is informed of the fetal status. These steps are appropriate and should have been initiated sooner. Although it would be helpful to have a clearer recording of the contraction pattern to better interpret this tracing, it is clear that the fetal status is compromised and intervention is needed.

STRIP CHART F–3

Fetal Heart Rate		*Uterine Activity*	
Baseline:	135 bpm	Frequency:	Indeterminate
Variability:	Absent–Minimal	Duration:	Indeterminate
Periodic/Episodic Changes:	Prolonged and Variable Decelerations	Strength:	Tocotransducer in place—must palpate
		Resting Tone:	Tocotransducer in place—must palpate
Category:			III

Discussion: Patient status is appropriately escalated to the attention of the nurse in charge. It is important that she is aware that the patient presently requires 1:1 care, may need additional assistance depending on changes in status, and that surgical intervention seems likely.

STRIP CHART F–4

Fetal Heart Rate		Uterine Activity	
Baseline:	135 bpm	Frequency:	Irregular
Variability:	Absent–Minimal	Duration:	60 seconds–3 minutes
Periodic/Episodic Changes:	Prolonged, Variable, and Late Decelerations	Strength:	Tocotransducer in place— must palpate
		Resting Tone:	Tocotransducer in place— must palpate
Category:			III

STRIP CHART F–5

Fetal Heart Rate		Uterine Activity	
Baseline:	130 bpm	Frequency:	1.5–4 minutes
Variability:	Absent–Minimal	Duration:	70 seconds–3 minutes
Periodic/Episodic Changes:	Prolonged Decelerations	Strength:	Tocotransducer in place— must palpate
		Resting Tone:	Tocotransducer in place— must palpate
Category:			III

Discussion: Based on the minimal variability, presence of decelerations, and absence of accelerations, this fetus appears compromised from the start of the tracing, which can be consistent with an antepartum fetal brain injury. Also, there does not appear to be a sentinel event or particular incident or instance denoting a marked decline in fetal status during this time of observation. However, there does seem to be a delay in initiation of surgical intervention. It is unknown whether such delay has a negative impact on outcome; however, it may call into question the care provided, as nearly 2 hours elapsed from the time of admission to birth.

OUTCOME: 11:04 live male, 3,317g (7 lb, 5 oz) live male via Cesarean birth. Resuscitation: tactile stimulation; PPV with 21% oxygen and oximetry monitoring, increased to 100% oxygen. Apgars 2/6/8. Seizures noted at 28 hours of life. Cerebral palsy later diagnosed.

STRIP CHART G–1

Fetal Heart Rate		Uterine Activity	
Baseline:	135 bpm	Frequency:	1.5–2 minutes
Variability:	Moderate	Duration:	70–90 seconds
Periodic/Episodic Changes:	(Intermittent) Late Deceleration (?)	Strength:	Mild
		Resting Tone:	Tocotransducer in place— must palpate
Category:		II	

STRIP CHART G-2			
Fetal Heart Rate		*Uterine Activity*	
Baseline:	135 bpm	Frequency:	1.5–4 minutes
Variability:	Moderate	Duration:	1–2 minutes
Periodic/Episodic Changes:	Late Decelerations	Strength:	Tocotransducer in place—must palpate
		Resting Tone:	Tocotransducer in place—must palpate
Category:		II	

STRIP CHART G-3			
Fetal Heart Rate		*Uterine Activity*	
Baseline:	135 bpm	Frequency:	3–5.5 minutes
Variability:	Moderate	Duration:	1–2 minutes
Periodic/Episodic Changes:	Late Decelerations	Strength:	Tocotransducer in place—must palpate
		Resting Tone:	Tocotransducer in place—must palpate
Category:		II	

STRIP CHART G-4			
Fetal Heart Rate		*Uterine Activity*	
Baseline:	130 bpm	Frequency:	5 minutes
Variability:	Minimal–Moderate	Duration:	1.5–2 minutes
Periodic/Episodic Changes:	Late Decelerations	Strength:	Tocotransducer in place—must palpate
		Resting Tone:	Tocotransducer in place—must palpate
Category:		II	

STRIP CHART G–5

Fetal Heart Rate		Uterine Activity	
Baseline:	130 bpm	Frequency:	3–5 minutes
Variability:	Moderate	Duration:	80 seconds–2 minutes
Periodic/Episodic Changes:	Accelerations	Strength:	Tocotransducer in place — must palpate
		Resting Tone:	Tocotransducer in place — must palpate
Category:	I		

Discussion: The FHR appears to respond favorably to a change in position.

STRIP CHART G–6

Fetal Heart Rate		Uterine Activity	
Baseline:	140 bpm	Frequency:	2–3 minutes
Variability:	Minimal–Moderate	Duration:	60–80 seconds
Periodic/Episodic Changes:	Late Decelerations (?)	Strength:	Tocotransducer in place — must palpate
		Resting Tone:	Tocotransducer in place — must palpate
Category:		II	

Discussion: It is helpful to have information about the maternal pulse to differentiate it from the FHR when the data is unclear.

STRIP CHART G–7

Fetal Heart Rate		Uterine Activity	
Baseline:	130 bpm	Frequency:	2–5 minutes
Variability:	Minimal–Moderate	Duration:	50–70 seconds
Periodic/Episodic Changes:	Late Decelerations	Strength:	Tocotransducer in place — must palpate
		Resting Tone:	Tocotransducer in place — must palpate
Category:		II	

STRIP CHART G–8

Fetal Heart Rate		Uterine Activity	
Baseline:	135 bpm	Frequency:	1.5–4.5 minutes
Variability:	Moderate	Duration:	70–90 seconds
Periodic/Episodic Changes:	Late and Variable Decelerations	Strength:	Tocotransducer in place—must palpate
		Resting Tone:	Tocotransducer in place—must palpate
Category:		II	

STRIP CHART G–9

Fetal Heart Rate		Uterine Activity	
Baseline:	140 bpm	Frequency:	3–4 minutes
Variability:	Moderate	Duration:	60–90 seconds
Periodic/Episodic Changes:	Late and Variable Decelerations	Strength:	Tocotransducer in place—must palpate
		Resting Tone:	Tocotransducer in place—must palpate
Category:		II	

STRIP CHART G–10

Fetal Heart Rate		Uterine Activity	
Baseline:	135 bpm	Frequency:	1.5–6 minutes
Variability:	Moderate	Duration:	60–80 seconds
Periodic/Episodic Changes:	Late Decelerations, Acceleration x1	Strength:	Tocotransducer in place—must palpate
		Resting Tone:	Tocotransducer in place—must palpate
Category:		II	

STRIP CHART G–11

Fetal Heart Rate		Uterine Activity		
Baseline:	130 bpm	Frequency:	1–5 minutes	
Variability:	Moderate	Duration:	40–90 seconds	
Periodic/Episodic Changes:	Late Decelerations	Strength:	Tocotransducer in place— must palpate	
		Resting Tone:	Tocotransducer in place— must palpate	
Category:			II	

STRIP CHART G–12

Fetal Heart Rate		Uterine Activity		
Baseline:	135 bpm	Frequency:	1.5–5 minutes	
Variability:	Moderate	Duration:	80 seconds–2 minutes	
Periodic/Episodic Changes:	Late Decelerations, Accelerations	Strength:	Tocotransducer in place— must palpate	
		Resting Tone:	Tocotransducer in place— must palpate	
Category:			II	

Discussion: Late decelerations have been present from the beginning of the tracing, indicating that there is some degree of uteroplacental insufficiency. The extent of this deficit on the fetal condition is defined by the presence moderate variability and accelerations, both of which indicate an absence of fetal metabolic acidemia at the time of their occurrence.

STRIP CHART G–13

Fetal Heart Rate		Uterine Activity		
Baseline:	145 bpm	Frequency:	Indeterminate	
Variability:	Moderate	Duration:	Indeterminate	
Periodic/Episodic Changes:	Indeterminate	Strength:	Tocotransducer in place— must palpate	
		Resting Tone:	Tocotransducer in place— must palpate	
Category:			II	

Discussion: Because the UC pattern is not recording well and there is a gap in data, some parameters cannot be determined at this time.

STRIP CHART G–14

Fetal Heart Rate		Uterine Activity	
Baseline:	145 bpm	Frequency:	Irregular
Variability:	Moderate	Duration:	70 seconds–2 minutes
Periodic/Episodic Changes:	(Intermittent) Late Decelerations	Strength:	Tocotransducer in place—must palpate
		Resting Tone:	Tocotransducer in place—must palpate
Category:		II	

Discussion: The optimal time to initiate oxytocin would be following a clear assessment establishing fetal oxygenation status. In this case, the tracing immediately preceding the start of the oxytocin was indeterminate, followed by a gap in the data, therefore, not supporting the absence of fetal metabolic acidemia.

STRIP CHART G–15

Fetal Heart Rate		Uterine Activity	
Baseline:	130 bpm	Frequency:	1.5–4 minutes
Variability:	Moderate	Duration:	60–80 seconds
Periodic/Episodic Changes:	Late Decelerations, Acceleration ×1	Strength:	Tocotransducer in place—must palpate
		Resting Tone:	Tocotransducer in place—must palpate
Category:		II	

STRIP CHART G–16

Fetal Heart Rate		Uterine Activity	
Baseline:	130 bpm	Frequency:	1–2 minutes
Variability:	Minimal–Moderate	Duration:	60–90 seconds
Periodic/Episodic Changes:	Late Decelerations, (?) Accelerations	Strength:	Tocotransducer in place—must palpate
		Resting Tone:	Tocotransducer in place—must palpate
Category:		II	

Discussion: It is clear that the FHR is, on average, at a lower rate during this run of contractions that borders on tachysystole. An episode of contractions occurring with such frequency makes it difficult to assess the FHR baseline (and, therefore, the variability and periodic/episodic changes). Consequently, accurate assessment of fetal oxygen status is impeded during such episodes.

STRIP CHART G-17

Fetal Heart Rate		Uterine Activity	
Baseline:	130 bpm	Frequency:	2.5–6.5 minutes
Variability:	Minimal	Duration:	80–90 seconds
Periodic/Episodic Changes:	Late Decelerations, Accelerations ×1	Strength:	Tocotransducer in place—must palpate
		Resting Tone:	Tocotransducer in place—must palpate
Category:		II	

STRIP CHART G-18

Fetal Heart Rate		Uterine Activity	
Baseline:	130 bpm	Frequency:	1–3 minutes
Variability:	Minimal	Duration:	60–80 seconds
Periodic/Episodic Changes:	Variable and Late Decelerations	Strength:	Tocotransducer in place—must palpate
		Resting Tone:	Tocotransducer in place—must palpate
Category:		II	

STRIP CHART G-19

Fetal Heart Rate		Uterine Activity	
Baseline:	130 bpm	Frequency:	1–3 minutes
Variability:	Minimal	Duration:	60 seconds–2 minutes
Periodic/Episodic Changes:	Late Decelerations	Strength:	Tocotransducer in place—must palpate
		Resting Tone:	Tocotransducer in place—must palpate
Category:		II	

STRIP CHART G–20

Fetal Heart Rate		Uterine Activity	
Baseline:	140 bpm	Frequency:	1.5–3.5 minutes
Variability:	Moderate	Duration:	70 seconds–2 minutes
Periodic/Episodic Changes:	Late Decelerations	Strength:	Tocotransducer in place—must palpate
		Resting Tone:	Tocotransducer in place—must palpate
Category:		II	

Discussion: The patient has dilated 0.5 cm in approximately 2 hours. There is little information regarding the strength of contractions. The patient has an early epidural in place, which may affect her labor progress. An IUPC would be helpful, as soon as the patient is dilated enough to insert one, especially as she is on a very high dose of oxytocin. It has been 18 hours since SROM. A bedside evaluation by the care provider is appropriate at this time and should be requested.

STRIP CHART G–21

Fetal Heart Rate		Uterine Activity	
Baseline:	140 bpm	Frequency:	1–3 minutes
Variability:	Minimal–Moderate	Duration:	60–90 seconds
Periodic/Episodic Changes:	Late Decelerations	Strength:	Tocotransducer in place—must palpate
		Resting Tone:	Tocotransducer in place—must palpate
Category:		II	

STRIP CHART G–22

Fetal Heart Rate		Uterine Activity	
Baseline:	140 bpm	Frequency:	1–4 minutes
Variability:	Minimal–Moderate	Duration:	60–80 seconds
Periodic/Episodic Changes:	Late and Variable Decelerations	Strength:	Tocotransducer in place—must palpate
		Resting Tone:	Tocotransducer in place—must palpate
Category:		II	

Discussion: 20 mU/min of oxytocin is usually the maximum dose allowed by most protocols without a special care provider order to increase.

STRIP CHART G–23

Fetal Heart Rate		Uterine Activity	
Baseline:	135 bpm	Frequency:	1.5–3 minutes
Variability:	Minimal–Moderate	Duration:	60–100 seconds
Periodic/Episodic Changes:	Late and Variable Decelerations	Strength:	Tocotransducer in place—must palpate
		Resting Tone:	Tocotransducer in place—must palpate
Category:		II	

Discussion: Although it should be decreased or discontinued, the oxytocin continues to be increased to a high dosage.

STRIP CHART G–24

Fetal Heart Rate		Uterine Activity	
Baseline:	135 bpm	Frequency:	1–1.5 minutes
Variability:	Minimal, then Marked	Duration:	60–100 seconds
Periodic/Episodic Changes:	Late and Variable Decelerations	Strength:	Tocotransducer in place—must palpate
		Resting Tone:	Tocotransducer in place—must palpate
Category:		II	

Discussion: Although her BP remains stable following replacement of the epidural, the FHR is clearly affected by the tachysystole that is occurring. It is appropriate that intrauterine resuscitation is implemented; however, optimal efficacy of such interventions cannot be achieved while the oxytocin is infusing (particularly at a high rate). In the presence of the changes in the FHR and the tachysystole, the oxytocin should be decreased or discontinued. The care provider should be informed of the need for bedside evaluation.

STRIP CHART G–25

Fetal Heart Rate		Uterine Activity	
Baseline:	145 bpm	Frequency:	1–4 minutes
Variability:	Minimal	Duration:	80 seconds
Periodic/Episodic Changes:	Late and Variable Decelerations	Strength:	Tocotransducer in place—must palpate
		Resting Tone:	Tocotransducer in place—must palpate
Category:		II	

STRIP CHART G–26

Fetal Heart Rate		Uterine Activity	
Baseline:	160 bpm	Frequency:	1–2 minutes
Variability:	Minimal	Duration:	60–80 seconds
Periodic/Episodic Changes:	Late and Variable Decelerations	Strength:	Tocotransducer in place—must palpate
		Resting Tone:	Tocotransducer in place—must palpate
Category:		II	

Discussion: The FHR baseline has increased and is bordering on tachycardia. Although not technically tachycardic, it is important to remember that the normal rate for this fetus has remained mainly in the 130 range. The increased rate of 160 bpm represents a change in the FHR suggestive that the fetus' oxygen needs are increasing and raising concern about development of acidemia. This tracing is bordering on becoming a Category III.

STRIP CHART G–27

Fetal Heart Rate		Uterine Activity	
Baseline:	160 bpm	Frequency:	1–3 minutes
Variability:	Minimal	Duration:	70 seconds
Periodic/Episodic Changes:	Variable Decelerations	Strength:	Tocotransducer in place—must palpate
		Resting Tone:	Tocotransducer in place—must palpate
Category:		II	

Discussion: Oxytocin should not be infusing at this time. The tracing is progressively worsening and must be evaluated by the care provider. Not only is increasing the oxytocin inappropriate at this time, but the dosage is high. The patient is complaining of pain and pressure. While a cervical exam was done (Strip Chart G–26), the care provider should certainly be notified that the patient requires assessment. With an epidural in place, the patient should not require additional IV pain medication. The effect of meperidine on FHR variability will further complicate assessment of this important indicator of fetal oxygen status. The patient's labor progress continues to be slow; she is now 3 cm and an IUPC could be utilized to quantify the strength of and resting tone between contractions.

STRIP CHART G–28

Fetal Heart Rate		Uterine Activity	
Baseline:	160 bpm	Frequency:	2–3 minutes
Variability:	Minimal	Duration:	70–90 seconds
Periodic/Episodic Changes:	Variable Decelerations	Strength:	Pushing
		Resting Tone:	Tocotransducer in place—must palpate
Category:		II	

Discussion: There is a discrepancy between what the patient is feeling/demonstrating and the results of the cervical exam. This also occurred with the previous exam. It would certainly be time to seek another opinion, preferably from the care provider who should have been notified of the patient/fetal status and present in the room.

STRIP CHART G–29

Fetal Heart Rate		Uterine Activity	
Baseline:	155 bpm	Frequency:	1.5–3 minutes
Variability:	Minimal	Duration:	60–80 seconds
Periodic/Episodic Changes:	Variable and Late Decelerations	Strength:	Pushing
		Resting Tone:	Tocotransducer in place—must palpate
Category:		II	

Discussion: The patient's blood pressure has registered quite high. It may have been taken while pushing but should be reassessed.

STRIP CHART G–30

Fetal Heart Rate		Uterine Activity	
Baseline:	160 bpm	Frequency:	1.5–2.5 minutes
Variability:	Minimal	Duration:	60–90 seconds
Periodic/Episodic Changes:	Variable Decelerations; Indeterminate	Strength:	Pushing
		Resting Tone:	Tocotransducer in place—must palpate
Category:		II	

Discussion: It appears the charge nurse has entered the room to assess the patient. Either the patient progressed very quickly (from 5 cm to 9.5 cm in approximately 30 minutes) or the previously cervical examination(s) was not accurate.

STRIP CHART G–31

Fetal Heart Rate		Uterine Activity	
Baseline:	Indeterminate	Frequency:	1–2 minutes
Variability:	Indeterminate	Duration:	60–90 seconds
Periodic/Episodic Changes:	Decelerations–Prolonged and Indeterminate	Strength:	Pushing
		Resting Tone:	Tocotransducer in place—must palpate
Category:		III	

Discussion: Although the FHR cannot be determined in this segment of tracing, it is clearly very concerning. The FHR baseline is likely represented by the episodes of tachycardia and, although the type may not be clearly represented, decelerations are certainly present. With an FHR that is not responding well to the stress of pushing, it can be very helpful to rest through some of the contractions (e.g., push every other, or even every third, contraction) to allow the fetus time for reoxygenation between such attempts. Pushing with the patient in positions other than lithotomy and encouraging physiologic pushing can also be helpful in regard to optimizing perfusion to and minimizing stress on the fetus. In this case, to minimize stress on the fetus, it may be wise not to push. All methods of intrauterine resuscitation should be employed and the oxytocin should be turned off.

STRIP CHART G–32			
Fetal Heart Rate		**Uterine Activity**	
Baseline:	Indeterminate, then Bradycardia	Frequency:	1.5–2 minutes
Variability:	Indeterminate	Duration:	Indeterminate
Periodic/Episodic Changes:	Decelerations–Prolonged and Indeterminate	Strength:	Pushing
		Resting Tone:	Tocotransducer in place— must palpate
Category:			III

Discussion: It is unclear what type(s) of decelerations are occurring during this period. However, a logical assumption based on the trend of the FHR over the course of this labor would indicate that the FHR baseline is approximately 180 bpm, with a discernible deceleration pattern.

STRIP CHART G–33			
Fetal Heart Rate		**Uterine Activity**	
Baseline:	Indeterminate	Frequency:	1.5–2 minutes
Variability:	Indeterminate	Duration:	Indeterminate
Periodic/Episodic Changes:	Decelerations–Prolonged and Indeterminate	Strength:	Pushing
		Resting Tone:	Tocotransducer in place— must palpate
Category:			III

Discussion: Although the FHR is technically indeterminate, it appears to be 170 bpm with prolonged and indeterminate type of decelerations. It cannot be predicted at this time how much longer the fetus will tolerate this stress.

STRIP CHART G–34			
Fetal Heart Rate		**Uterine Activity**	
Baseline:	Indeterminate	Frequency:	1–1.5 minutes
Variability:	Indeterminate	Duration:	Indeterminate
Periodic/Episodic Changes:	Decelerations– Indeterminate	Strength:	Pushing
		Resting Tone:	Tocotransducer in place— must palpate
Category:			III

Discussion: Although the FHR is technically indeterminate, it appears to be 160 bpm with decelerations.

OUTCOME: 23:28 delivery of live female, 3,855 g (8 lb, 8 oz). McRobert's maneuver for brief shoulder dystocia and midline episiotomy. Nuchal cord ×2, loose. Apgars 2/3/4/4. Resuscitation: tactile stimulation, PPV, intubation, Narcan, volume expanders via umbilical access, to NICU and placed on ventilator. Cord pH 7.26, BE –9.2.

STRIP CHART H–1A AND H–1B

Fetal Heart Rate		Uterine Activity	
Baseline:	140 bpm	Frequency:	None
Variability:	Moderate	Duration:	N/A
Periodic/Episodic Changes:	Accelerations	Strength:	N/A
		Resting Tone:	N/A
Category:	I		

Discussion: Most institutions would regard this nonstress test as *reactive* (≥2 accelerations within 20 minutes). This tracing demonstrates the importance of understanding the equipment and how to use it properly (see Chapter 2). In this instance, the musical note icon erroneously appears in place of the proper "up arrow" icon that should appear on the tracing when the patient presses an event marker to denote her perception of fetal movement. The musical note icon is appearing because the event marker is plugged into the wrong port in the machine. The port in this machine that translates input into a musical note is actually meant for attachment of a fetal acoustic stimulator. To avoid confusion about which accessory is actually in use, it is important to utilize equipment properly.

STRIP CHART H–2A AND H–2B

Fetal Heart Rate		Uterine Activity	
Baseline:	130 bpm	Frequency:	Irregular
Variability:	Moderate	Duration:	60 seconds–4 minutes
Periodic/Episodic Changes:	Accelerations	Strength:	Mild
		Resting Tone:	Tocotransducer in place—must palpate
Category:	I		

Discussion: This is a reactive nonstress test. It is important to note that it is quite comparable to the previous nonstress test performed. When prior data is available, it should be reviewed for comparison. A fetus should perform at least as well as it has previously shown that it is able. It is helpful that fetal movement counting (FMC) was reinforced with the patient by inquiring about it. This can be a good time for review of this technique.

STRIP CHART H–3A AND H–3B

Fetal Heart Rate		Uterine Activity	
Baseline:	125 bpm	Frequency:	Irregular
Variability:	Moderate	Duration:	60 seconds–3 minutes
Periodic/Episodic Changes:	Accelerations	Strength:	Mild
		Resting Tone:	Tocotransducer in place—must palpate
Category:	I		

Discussion: This is a reactive nonstress test. The fetus seems to be active, as noted by the "up arrow" markings on the tracing.

STRIP CHART H–4A AND H–4B

Fetal Heart Rate		Uterine Activity	
Baseline:	115 bpm (?)	Frequency:	Irregular
Variability:	Minimal–Moderate (?)	Duration:	60 seconds–3 minutes
Periodic/Episodic Changes:	Accelerations, Decelerations (?)	Strength:	Mild–Moderate
		Resting Tone:	Tocotransducer in place— must palpate
Category:	I		

Discussion: In the first portion of this tracing (H–4A), it appears that the FHR baseline is 110 bpm, with minimal–moderate variability, and accelerations. Although those finding are not concerning on their own merit, it is important to note that when this tracing is compared to previous nonstress tests, it certainly has a different appearance. It is also significant that the patient states noting a decrease in fetal movement. In the second portion (H–4B), it is difficult to discern the FHR baseline (thereby obstructing interpretation of variability and periodic/episodic changes) due to the lack of a clear UA pattern. It is possible that the FHR is 125 bpm (more consistent with prior testing) and decelerations are present. To facilitate proper interpretation, it is important to adjust the tocotransducer and observe this fetus longer to see what is actually occurring.

STRIP CHART H–4C AND H–4D

Fetal Heart Rate		Uterine Activity	
Baseline:	110 bpm (?)	Frequency:	Irregular
Variability:	Moderate (?)	Duration:	Tocotransducer not recording well—needs adjustment
Periodic/Episodic Changes:	Decelerations (?)	Strength:	Tocotransducer in place— must palpate
		Resting Tone:	Tocotransducer in place— must palpate
Category:	I		

Discussion: These portions (H–4C and H–4D) of tracing certainly have a different appearance from the NST performed the previous day, an important finding that bears closer investigation. In the second portion, it is difficult to discern the FHR baseline (thereby obstructing interpretation of variability and periodic/episodic changes) due to the lack of a clear UA pattern. It is possible that the FHR is 130 bpm and decelerations are present. To facilitate proper interpretation, it is important to adjust the tocotransducer and observe this fetus longer. In any event, this does not represent a reactive NST and should be further investigated at this time.

OUTCOME: The patient returned 2 days later with the complaint of decreased fetal movement. Absence of cardiac activity indicated a fetal demise. Upon delivery, no fetal abnormalities were found; however, there was an "eccentrically inserted cord". Although cord accidents are often not preventable, the fact that there were signs of deteriorating fetal condition on the last NST with no follow-up investigation is problematic.

Electronic Fetal Monitoring and Health Information Technology

Despite controversy, the use of electronic fetal monitoring (EFM) technology in birth is ubiquitous, and obstetric care providers must understand the nature and capabilities of the tools in use. As a technology, EFM is not only a biophysical and electronic engineering tool to capture the fetal heart rate (FHR) signal, but in many cases also the point-of-care (POC) tool linked to a powerful clinical information system. A solid understanding of the information technology capabilities of EFM is necessary for providers to harness the information benefits and use EFM appropriately and effectively for optimum birth outcomes. This chapter provides a brief introduction on how EFM relates to the electronic health record (HER), computerized clinical information systems, and informatics. Clinicians are encouraged to access the chapter references for additional learning.

THE ELECTRONIC HEALTH RECORD AND HEALTH INFORMATION TECHNOLOGY

The Institute of Medicine (IOM) report *Crossing the Quality Chasm* first called for elimination of handwritten data and set a goal to implement a paperless EHR before the end of the decade, citing evidence that the EHR improves health care quality, safety and efficiency.[1] The electronic format provides a record of clinical data that is legible, organized, complete, and accessible by multiple users across sites of care and episodes of care. In addition, the digital record creates a database of clinical information that can be automatically analyzed. This IOM report energized the development of health information technology (HIT) and the application of information processing technology (computer hardware and software) to enable the collection, analysis, storage, retrieval, and sharing of health care data, information, and knowledge for communication and decision-making. In 2009, The American Recovery and Reinvestment

Act (ARRA) and the Health Information Technology for Economic and Clinical Health Act (HITECH Act) created funding and reimbursement incentives for the adoption of EHRs that included expectations for using certified systems (*the right technology*) for standard use (*the right use of technology*), commonly referred to as "meaningful use."[2,3] The Office of the National Coordinator for HIT (ONC) is the complete source for a current list of certified technology products and specific meaningful use criteria (Office of the National Coordinator for Health Information Technology [ONC]).[4] The ARRA goals include improving care coordination through the effective use of HIT and effective health information exchange (HIE), goals that are relevant to obstetric patients and fetal monitoring. Effective use aims to bring key data directly to the frontline providers at the point-of-care, reduce duplicative work, and provide access to clinical data immediately (such as data entry of the mother's expected delivery date that is entered once and flows to all parts of the medical record simultaneously, or immediate access to interpret and document on a fetal tracing). Effective HIE aims to improve interoperable data standards, so information is portable, travels with the patient, and can be shared among providers (such as access to prenatal FHR assessments and diagnostics). Collectively, these strategies will deliver the right information to the right person at the right time.

The transition to an EHR poses education and practice challenges for clinicians. A multidisciplinary summit sponsored by the American Health Information Management Association addressed such training needs and listed specific actions for not only health care workers, but for employers, vendors, educators, and the government to promote workforce competencies.[5] This panel recommended that health care workers themselves self-assess knowledge gaps and seek ongoing professional development. Obstetric clinicians must recognize how the national agenda is shaping EFM practice with clinical information systems and informatics.

Stork Byte

Don't stand by and let the EHR train go by without perinatal riders; jump on board!

ELECTRONIC FETAL MONITORING AND CLINICAL INFORMATION SYSTEMS

Clinical information systems (CIS) are networks of computers that share clinical data in a digital format; these are typically bedside computer workstations connected to a central server. The CIS is the backbone or architecture for the paperless EHR. The use of CIS in obstetrics expanded in the 1990s with "perinatal systems" capable of transmitting and displaying the fetal tracings recorded from all bedside stations in the system on all screens in the system (*surveillance*) and storing the tracings in an electronic format on an optical disk (*archiving*). Networks expanded to include remote transmission of the fetal tracing through an Internet connection or wireless device to and from settings outside the labor and delivery unit, such as antepartum testing units and ambulatory offices, on a desktop or hand-held device. Clinicians began documenting on the computer tracing. Gradually, the monitor paper was used less or turned off. This conversion from the traditional fetal monitor paper to a digital perinatal system challenges and changes clinical workflow and requires substantial staff effort. Clinicians need to see direct benefits from the system. Initially, clinicians were most interested in the risk management benefit of what came to be known as "central monitoring" or the display of all fetal tracings at a centrally located station. With central monitoring, clinicians could monitor tracings when a care provider could not be at the bedside. Quality assurance projects reported less loss of tracings with electronic storage. And soon, clinicians recognized the value of the CIS *database* functions, including documentation or data entry, data analysis (such as aggregation and trending), and data reporting.

Perinatal systems are niche systems, developed to meet the unique clinical needs of a specialty area and are often separate from an organization's enterprise-wide system because the fetal monitor that captures physiologic data is classified differently for device approval.[3] Increasingly, perinatal documentation is being integrated into the enterprise-wide CIS.

Perinatal Information System Functions

State-of-the-art perinatal systems provide a comprehensive and longitudinal EHR, with surveillance, archiving, documentation, and database applications in use across the care continuum, from prenatal primary care, to inpatient birth, newborn and postpartum, and back to postpartum primary care. This overview focuses on the applications, benefits, and limitations to consider in using computerized systems with EFM tracings (Table 6–1).

Surveillance

Effective surveillance, communication, and response to potential risk promote patient safety. The safety goal with EFM is to correctly identify, interpret, communicate, and intervene in response to the FHR tracing. Computerized EFM surveillance systems are intended to promote this safety goal and reduce risk. Computer surveillance can certainly help clinician surveillance, but there are some limitations to consider.

Central displays assist with the surveillance and communication aspects of safety. Although central displays can provide extra "eyes" for clinicians, a commonly voiced concern is the potential for the caregivers to focus their attention on the computer screen and assess the mother and fetus "from the desk" rather than at the bedside. Most perinatal systems have visual or auditory alarm functions to assist with surveillance by notifying the clinician when the FHR is outside preset parameters (such as signal loss or a change in baseline rates). However, when central displays and alarms are used, clinicians must acknowledge and respond for the safety process to be complete.

Clinician interpretation of an FHR tracing is a learned skill built from practicing visual analysis of pattern shapes. So, any distortion in the visual image (the scale or aspect ratio of the grid underlying the fetal waveform or the speed of the grid underlying the fetal waveform) could distort the appearance of the pattern shape and affect interpretation. A chief concern with the use of the digital tracing is the visual match between the traditional monitor paper printout and (1) the computer screen display (for interpreting the tracing during care), (2) the computer paper printout (for interpreting

TABLE 6-1   BENEFITS AND LIMITATIONS OF PERINATAL ELECTRONIC CLINICAL INFORMATION SYSTEMS

Function	Benefit	Limitation
For all functions	Benefits of electronic health record: legible, complete, accessible through digital transmission, federal requirements for privacy and security, improved charge capture and positive financial return on investment; customized for perinatal care	Costs of system implementation and maintenance Computer downtime Challenges interfacing with other systems
Surveillance	Accessibility of fetal tracing on connected workstations and mobile devices provides multiple viewing and from remote locations Effective communication of FHR data promotes safety; rapid identification and response to FHR tracing	Visual appearance of fetal tracing display differences that could result in interpretation differences Remote viewing may replace or reduce assessment at the bedside Computer clock may not be synchronized with wall clocks
Archiving	Less loss of fetal tracing data than with monitor paper and microfiche Federal standards mandate data security (retrievable and reproducible)	Data loss or corruption despite federal mandates Retrieval barriers with older tracings and older technology Long statutes of limitations requirements to retrieve and reproduce the tracings High litigation risk
Documentation & Database	Maternal–fetal–newborn data is entered once and immediately populates the entire record Record is simultaneously accessible to multiple providers, at multiple sites, over time Effective access to clinical data identifies risks and promotes safety Database is available for data analysis, outcomes reporting, quality measures Electronic record can link with other electronic safety technologies (provider order entry, electronic medication administration record, bar code medication administration, decision support, knowledge portals)	Workforce training for documentation Database management analyst needed Documentation time may increase

the tracing generated from a computer printer), and (3) the archived tracing (for interpreting the tracing retrieved later from the archive) (Figure 6–1). In some cases, the computer screen, print-out, or stored pattern was not comparable to the actual monitor paper pattern and suggested different interpretations of the FHR status. The standards of speed and scale must be identical. Presently, there is no agreed-on standard. Additional issues to consider with electronic displays are the clarity of the waveform and grids, the length of the tracing segment visible on the screen at one time, and the ergonomics of viewing the screen (brightness, colors, height, angle, position of the screen, split screens competing for visual attention).

The time stamp on the electronic EFM tracing is the legal medical record and must accurately correspond to the time of interventions. Because computer clocks and wall clocks are seldom synchronized, clinicians must have a clear policy regarding the time source, documentation of time, and documentation of discrepancies.

Archiving

Fetal monitoring tracings are a part of the medical record described as "patient identifiable source data" or data from which interpretations are derived, and these must be stored and retrievable. Many settings that use computer displays and archiving no longer run monitor paper during care or save monitor paper. However, when patient care is documented on the monitor paper tracing, the paper becomes a record of care and must be stored and retrievable. Some settings store both laser and paper records because of concern about retrieving archived tracings. Each organization should have policies and procedures for

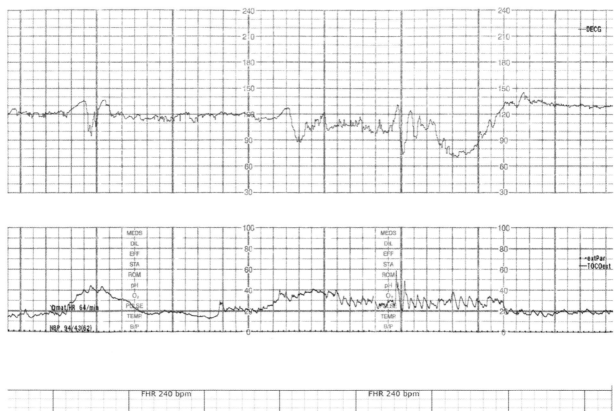

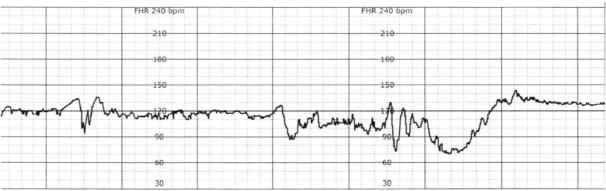

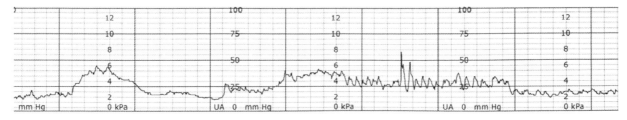

FIGURE 6–1. Comparison of monitor paper tracing (upper) and computer printer tracing (lower).

managing all forms of fetal heart tracing media and records.[6]

The privacy and security of EHRs is now protected by the Health Insurance Portability and Accountability Act (HIPAA) standards (which pertain only to patient data in electronic form; the paper forms do not have this security protection).[3] The security requirements protect electronic records from wrongful access, alteration, and loss through safeguards such as electronic user identification, audit trails of who has accessed a file, and a data back-up plan for network failure. To attain HIPAA compliance, the system must demonstrate that EFM tracings are retrievable and reproducible.

Documentation and Databases

CIS documentation or data entry is done using a variety of user input devices (keyboard, mouse, light pen, touch screen) at a bedside or mobile computer workstation or through wireless devices. Data are also automatically entered from biophysical monitoring devices (EFM, maternal blood pressure, pulse oximeter). With a fully electronic digital record, FHR data and any electronic documentation entered on the tracing will automatically flow to all parts of the EHR, so there is no need for duplicate charting or "double-documenting." Eliminating duplicate documentation reduces the risk of transcription inconsistencies. The computer screens used for documentation (forms) are usually customizable and should be designed to match obstetrical workflow and standard of care. Electronic obstetrical records can improve the accuracy and completeness of data entry and improve the collection of outcome data.

Efficient data analysis and reporting are a necessity in today's data-driven health care system. Collecting and documenting patient data in an EHR database is more efficient for analysis and reporting than the traditional paper-based medical record and unit log book. *Documentation* refers to the actual entry of data in the patient's record, *database* refers to the collected data, and *database management* refers to the software program that performs the analysis of the collected data. All three components are necessary to generate information from collected data. The database software in a CIS facilitates more efficient clinical data collection, analysis, and reporting. The perinatal database software can store, aggregate, and analyze the individual patient data, such as FHR, labor events, and birth outcomes. However, clinical experts must be involved with the design of the database so that relevant perinatal data elements are defined and collected and meaningful analysis is accomplished. Data definitions must be clear, quantifiable, and agreed-on. Standardized terminology should be used so that data entries are consistent and can be compared over encounters and settings (such as standardized terminology for FHR tracing interpretation, as described by the National Institute of Child Health and Human Development (NICHD).[7,8]

A major benefit of perinatal database management is outcomes reporting. A well-designed database can generate reports (paper printouts of data tables, graphs, tracking, trends, audits, summaries) tailored to obstetric department needs, such as census, monthly and vital statistics, performance improvement, quality measures, national standards compliance, and regulatory agency requirements. Specific obstetrical data can be part of the larger agency-wide database if the perinatal system interfaces or is compatible with the larger health care system.

A carefully planned database can be searched to answer clinical research questions about FHR, interventions, and birth outcomes. A retrospective analysis of the database of one unit's records (log books) provided evidence to guide staffing decisions.[9] Individual patient data from the operational live care record can flow to a "read-only" clinical data repository (CDR) that captures and shares data for clinicians and to a larger repository of clinical data (data warehouse) where investigators can analyze the aggregated data using a research technique called *data mining*.[10]

Perinatal System Life Cycle

CIS implementation is best described as a phase in the overall system life cycle. As a phase, implementation is not an independent task but part of an ongoing process that links to the other phases. Informaticists illustrate the system life cycle with various models, but the typical phases include needs assessment, system selection, implementation, and maintenance (Figure 6–2). The system life cycle is a process that is never completed, especially as the expected lifespan of hardware and software grows shorter. Although any one implementation phase is occurring, there may be other technology implementations occurring or competing priorities that interrupt or delay implementation. Too often, a perinatal clinical specialist or manager without previous informatics education or experience is assigned to lead the implementation of an FHM CIS. Sound, systematic project management is essential for successful implementation. The project leader can optimize the process for all stakeholders and avoid trial-and-error implementation by reading the literature, attending conferences, and networking with colleagues.[3] Hunt, Sproat, and Kitzmiller provide practical general nursing strategies for accomplishing each phase of the life cycle.[11] Unfortunately, not enough perinatal systems managers publish about their work.[12,13] Generally, the information systems (IS) staff provides support through the system life cycle, but this is less common with specialty niche systems like EFM.

Stork Byte

Don't reinvent the wheel; read the literature on CIS implementation.

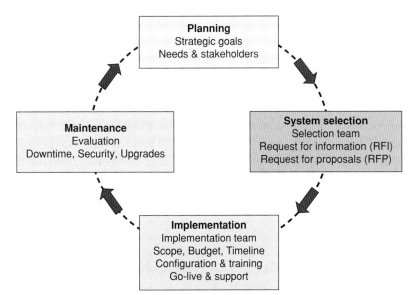

FIGURE 6–2. Perinatal clinical information system life cycle.

Planning

The needs assessment begins with executive commitment to resources and strategic planning with primary stakeholders participating. The overall vision, goals, and information needs must be clear and agreed on throughout all phases. A clear description of the organization's needs will focus the selection phase.

System Selection

The system vendor becomes a strategic business partner for the duration of the use of the system and must be carefully selected. The selection process should involve frontline clinicians and use tools for assessments tailored to perinatal care during demonstrations and site visits.[3] The selection team should be multidisciplinary, with representation from management, information systems, and frontline users. Team members must collectively reflect the organization, possess sound knowledge about the organization and clinical practice, and demonstrate strong communication skills. One of the major causes for implementation failure is a lack of user involvement and ownership. The team is responsible for completing the request for information (RFI) (general information about the product and the vendor), the request for proposal (RFP) (detailed information about the vendor), vendor product demonstrations, site visits, product decision, and contract negotiation.

Implementation

Implementation may include the initial installation of computerized EFM surveillance and archiving or expansion of a current system to include documen-

tation, barcode medication administration, computerized provider order entry (CPOE), or other meaningful use requirements. Barnes[12] uses a case study to illustrate in detail how seven key implementation factors were considered in a project to add intrapartum nursing documentation (admission assessment, delivery summary, labor, recovery, and triage flow sheets) to an existing EFM surveillance and archiving system. The implementation team is lead by the project manager and should represent stakeholders, especially frontline users. This team is responsible for focusing the scope of the project, clarifying and monitoring the budget, and projecting the timeline. The team must identify goals that are precise and measurable for evaluation. A comprehensive assessment is done on the documentation systems, workflow analysis, and training needs. Documentation screens and data reports may need to be customized or configured by the IS design team. Trainers and super-users (staff not assigned to patient care who serve as a point-of-care resource for clinicians) are identified. An individualized work plan for training and the actual start date (go-live date) is determined based on the assessments. Successful implementation depends on a sound plan that is effectively communicated. Common challenges with implementation are the user learning curve and provider order management with CPOE. Leadership and help center support for the staff is critical. Productivity will initially slow down during the learning curve, and additional staffing will be needed. Providers often rely on nurses for assistance during their learning curve. Clinicians need to see tangible benefits (such as not having to enter gravidity and parity repeatedly on forms) and have an efficient process for submitting questions, issues, and change requests.

Maintenance

Key components of the maintenance phase are evaluation, optimization, downtime processes, data security, and implementation of upgrades. Evaluation includes analysis of implementation issues, measuring outcomes against original goals, and identifying any unintended consequences. Technology-related adverse events can occur when safe workflow processes are not maintained post-implementation or by the failure to quickly fix technology when it becomes counterproductive.[14] Many clinicians are not aware of or do not take advantage of the full range of system functionalities. Optimization of the system is increased with continued post-implementation training and skill development. System configuration changes or expansion with new software versions are likely because health care processes, standards, and information needs are dynamic. System vendors may offer maintenance contracts for software patches for viruses and security upgrades. Investment in maintenance can ensure the performance of the system. Vendor-specific user groups offer electronic mailing lists and conferences with valuable information to answer questions and generally help clinicians to optimize the use of their system.

Stork Byte

Don't be an island; reach out and network with other perinatal CIS users.

INFORMATICS AND ELECTRONIC FETAL MONITORING KNOWLEDGE TOOLS

The use of informatics concepts and knowledge tools with computerized information systems can inform decision-making and promote quality clinical care. These informatics concepts and specialty tools can support, not replace, human decision-making with EFM.

Informatics

Health care informatics integrates clinical practice, information science, and computer technology to manage and communicate data, information, knowledge, and wisdom in clinical practice.[15] This information science *knowledge hierarchy* consists of *data* (raw data, or an objective measurement of a variable), *information* (structured data, or an interpretation of organized data with meaning), *knowledge* (domain knowledge, a synthesis of information with the clinician's knowledge base to make a decision), and *wisdom* (value knowledge, an appropriate decision among choices) (Table 6–2).[16] With EFM, the goal is to effectively interpret fetal tracings and respond with appropriate interventions (intrauterine resuscitation). Computers can assist human skill in this process by improving *data* collection (FHR tracing recording and surveillance), improving objective interpretation *information* from collected data (consistent objective pattern analysis of the FHR data), and improving *knowledge* resources for the clinician (guidelines and knowledge portals).

TABLE 6–2 INFORMATICS AND LEVELS OF COMPUTER ANALYSIS OF FHR

Informatics Concept	Informatics Definition	EFM	Clinical Example
Data	An objective measurement of a variable	Electronic or paper tracing of the FHR signal	Recording of the FHR at a specific bpm rate, e.g., 110 bpm
↓	↓	↓	↓
Information	An interpretation of organized data	FHR pattern interpretation, per standardized definitions	Recognition that this 110 bpm rate is an abrupt decrease from the baseline FHR (occurring in <30 seconds) and interpretation of this change as a variable deceleration
↓	↓	↓	↓
Knowledge	A synthesis of information with a clinical knowledge base to make a decision	Synthesis of FHR interpretation, electronic knowledge tools, and the clinician's knowledge base for decision making and planning care	Decision-making and planning interventions

Human interpretation of the FHR tracing and subsequent decisions about care are augmented with information technology tools of clinical decision support (CDS) and FHR pattern analysis.

Clinical Decision Support

A CDS tool is a software program that integrates rules (algorithms, flow charts, decision trees) with the collected patient data in the computer system; it is sometimes called a "smart chart" "intelligent EHR," or "expert system." Some expert systems use an information processing technique called a neural network, rather than rules. The neural network is built from evidence, guidelines, clinician input, and thousands of clinical cases. CDS facilitates the interpretation of data to produce information, provides resources for knowledge-based decisions, and is widely recognized as an application to improve perinatal patient safety.[17,18]

The CDS might provide interpretation of patient data and trigger an alarm or alert when patient data entered into the system are outside normal parameters (FHR alarms), prompt the user for missing clinical data (gestational age) or guide what documentation is needed (request for maternal BP during epidural administration), bring reference resources to the point-of-care (FHR monitoring policy during oxytocin infusion or epidural administration), recommend standard treatments, and generally reduce reliance on memory and the opportunity for clinical error. The CDS tool or resource can be automatically presented to the user or be optional to the user. Automatic tools (called *"push"* technology that pushes information to the user) include alarms, alerts, reminders, prompts, or recommendations. Optional tools are tools the user must go to (*pulls* information to the user) and include links to references, such as an online library (knowledge portals).

Resource content for either approach can consist of practice standards from professional organizations, evidence-based clinical guidelines, policies, treatment protocols, procedures, an online library or Internet links for references, a drug library, and calculation tools. These expert knowledge-base resources are constructed from the input of clinical experts, practice standards (NICHD tracing definitions), research evidence, or the statistical analysis of a large volume of clinical cases (as in computer analysis of FHR tracings). The expert knowledge base generates or recommends the decision an expert would make, but does not execute a decision.

The benefits of CDS include safer care with expanded and enhanced surveillance, standardized data for interpretation, real-time alerts that warn of a change in patient condition or a possible error, reminders for care that is needed, and immediate access to up-to-date references right at the point-of-care. Reminders for complete documentation may increase compliance with documenting quality measures that are now required for meaningful use, increase charge capture and organization revenue, and reduce overall risk for the organization. However, there is a growing concern about clinician alarm fatigue. "Alarm fatigue" occurs when a clinician becomes desensitized to an alarm and either ignores, overrides, or has a delayed response to an alarm.[19] Computer decision support alert (or pop-up) fatigue is a type of alarm fatigue. Management strategies for reducing alarm-related safety events can be applied to computer screen alerts also.[20]

Computer Analysis of the FHR Tracing

Computer analysis of the FHR tracing is a CDS software tool that processes FHR data to produce interpretation information for the clinician. The objective and electronically quantified computer interpretation of the FHR tracing aids the subjective and visually limited human interpretation. Computer analysis can promote patient safety through improved standardization and consistency of interpretation, less variation in practice, and improved communication among clinicians.[21] A number of computer analysis software programs have been developed for antepartum and intrapartum tracings, are being used patient care and research, and are commercially available. The FHR software contains rules that detail the pattern features to detect, measure, and interpret. Some rules may include patient characteristics such as gestational age. Some rules can be customized by the user. The computations are developed and tested from archives of thousands of tracings and clinical cases. Computer output may be an auditory or visual alarm when the FHR is outside normal parameters, or a printout of the measurement and interpretation. These systems use standardized definitions, such as those by the NICHD,[8] to process FHR data into interpretation information. The clinician confirms the interpretation and initiates clinical decision-making. A recent international review of 10 central fetal monitoring systems in clinical use that use computer analysis of the FHR tracing (computerized cardiotocography) detailed commercial names, country of use, data analyzed, displays, available real-time alerts, use of definition guidelines, and research evaluating the analysis functions.[22]

Reliability of clinician FHR tracing interpretation, even among experts, is lacking. Numerous studies through the years have reported low rates of both interobserver and intraobserver agreement among all clinicians—nurses, midwives, and physicians.[23] One limitation in the earlier clinician interpretation study designs has been the absence of standardized, quantified, or sometimes even identified FHR pattern definitions. However, even with the development and use of standardized FHR tracing terminology, reported clinician agreement rates are still inconsistent.[23,24]

Both consensus statements produced by the NICHD recommend research on computer analysis and interpretation.[7,8] Publications by clinical experts identify computer analysis of FHR tracings as a potential strategy to improve reliable interpretation.[25–27] Generally, studies measuring clinician and computer interpretation show similar agreement.[28,29] Some studies have measured clinician interpretation with or without computer analysis assistance. Clinicians who were shown a tracing with computer analysis of the FHR tracing demonstrated more agreement and were more accurate in predicting newborn umbilical artery pH than were clinicians who did not see an analysis.[30]

Because computer analysis is an objective and reliable measure, the technology has been used frequently in research on relationships between clinical variables and FHR response. Early analysis criteria were used in what are now classical studies on FHR characteristics.[31,32] Researchers from a number of countries continue to use existing computer analysis systems to investigate relationships between FHR and clinical conditions[33,34] or investigate novel analysis methods.[35,36]

Computer analysis of FHR characteristics can assist clinicians in processing EFM data, information, and knowledge. Standardized computer analysis can provide an objective measurement tool for research. The unique qualities of and relationship between human intelligence and machine intelligence must continue to be debated, researched, and distinguished.

BALANCING HEALTH INFORMATION TECHNOLOGY

Obstetric clinicians must understand the informatics concepts, benefits, and limitations of the EHR, perinatal systems, and knowledge tools if they are to lead integration in care and advocate for women.

Clinicians must ensure that information technology supports care during labor and birth and does not interfere or introduce unintended risk.

REFERENCES

1. Institute of Medicine. (2001) *Crossing the Quality Chasm: A New Health System for the 21st Century*. Washington, DC: National Academy Press; 2001.
2. McCartney P. Meaningful use and certified electronic health records. *Am J Mater Child Nurs*. 2011a;36(2): 137.
3. McCartney P, Barnes J. (2012) *Perinatal nursing informatics guide for clinical health information technology*. 2012. Retrieved from http://www.awhonn.org/awhonn/store/productDetail.do?productCode=PNIG-12
4. Office of the National Coordinator for Health Information Technology (ONC). *HealthIT.gov*. 2013. Accessed September 1, 2013 from http://www.healthit.gov/
5. American Health Information Management Association. *Building the Workforce for Health Information Transformation*. 2006. Accessed September 1, 2013 at http://www.amia.org/reports/building-work-force-health-information-transformation
6. Association of Women's Health, Obstetric and Neonatal Nurses. *Fetal Heart Monitoring* (Position Statement). Washington, DC: Author; 2009.
7. National Institute of Child Health and Human Development Research Planning Workshop (NICHD). Electronic fetal heart rate monitoring research guidelines for interpretation. *Am J Obstet Gynecol*. 1997;177(6): 1385–1390.
8. Macones GA, Hankins GD, Spong CY, et al. The 2008 National Institute of Child Health Human Development workshop report on electronic fetal monitoring: Update on definitions, interpretations, and research guidelines. *Obstet Gynecol*. 2008;112:661–666; and *J Obstet Gynecol Neonat Nurs*. 2008;37:510–515.
9. Ivory C. Finding buried treasure in unit log books: Data mining. *AWHONN Lifelines*. 2005;9(1):62–66.
10. McCartney P. Clinical databases: EHR and repositories. *Am J Mater Child Nurs*. 2013;38(3):186.
11. Hunt E, Sproat S, Kitzmiller R. *The Nursing Informatics Implementation Guide*. New York: Springer-Verlag; 2004.
12. Barnes J. Implementing a perinatal clinical information system: A work in progress. *J Obstet Gynecol Neonat Nurs*. 2006;35(1):134–140.
13. Kelly CS. Perinatal computerized patient record and archiving systems: Pitfalls and enhancements for implementing a successful computerized medical record. *J Perinat Neonat Nurs*. 1999;12(4):1–14.
14. The Joint Commission *Safely implementing health information and converging technologies. Sentinel Event Alert* 42. 2008. Accessed September 1, 2013 at http://www.jointcommission.org/sentinel_event_alert_issue_42_safely_implementing_health_information_and_converging_technologies/
15. American Nurses Association (ANA). *Nursing Informatics: Scope and Standards of Practice*. Silver Spring, MD: American Nurses Association; 2008.

16. Rowley J. The wisdom hierarchy: Representations of the DIKW hierarchy. *J Info Sci.* 2007;33(2):163–180.

17. McCartney P. Clinical decision support systems. *Am J Mater Child Nurs.* 2007;32(1):58.

18. Provost C, Gray M. Perinatal clinical decision support system. *Nurs Women's Health.* 2007;11(4):407–410.

19. McCartney P. Clinical alarm management. *Am J Mater Child Nurs.* 2012;37(3):202.

20. The Joint Commission. *Medical device alarm safety in hospitals.* (Sentinel Event Alert No. 50). 2013. Accessed September 1, 2013 at http://www.jointcommission.org/sea_issue_50/

21. McCartney P. Computer fetal heart rate pattern analysis. *Am J Mater Child Nurs.* 2011b;36(6):397.

22. Nunes I, Ayres-de-Campos D, Figueredo C, Bernardes J. An overview of central fetal monitoring systems in labour. *J Perinat Med.* 2013;41:93–99.

23. Blackwell SC, Grobman WA, Antoniewicz L, et al. Interobserver and intraobserver reliability of the NICHD 3-Tier Fetal Heart Rate Interpretation System. *Am J Obstet Gynecol.* 2011;205:378.e1–5.

24. Tongsong T, Iamthongin A, Wanapirak C, et al. Accuracy of fetal heart-rate variability interpretation by obstetricians using the criteria of the National Institute of Child Health and Human Development compared with computer-aided interpretation. *J Obstet Gynecol Res.* 2005;31(1):68–71.

25. Bernardes J. Poor reliability of visual analysis of fetal heart rate tracings: What should be done about it? *Am J Obstet Gynecol.* 2012;206(6):e6.

26. Hamilton E, Wright E. Labor pains: Unraveling the complexity of OB decision making. *Crit Care Nurs Q.* 2006;29(4):342–353.

27. Santo S, Ayres-de-Campos D. Human factors affecting the interpretation of fetal heart rate tracings: an update. *Curr Opin Obstet Gynecol.* 2012;24:84–88.

28. Parer J, Hamilton E. Comparison of 5 experts and computer analysis in rule-based fetal heart rate interpretation. *Am J Obstet Gynecol.* 2010;203:451.e1–7.

29. Weiner S. Independent validation of a fetal heart rate pattern recognition software. *Am J Obstet Gynecol.* 2013;208(1 Suppl):S316–17.

30. Costa A, Santos C, Ayres-de-Campos D, et al. Access to computerised analysis of intrapartum cardiotocographs improves clinicians' prediction of newborn umbilical artery blood pH. *BJOG.* 2010;117(10):1288–1293.

31. Dalton KJ, Dawes GS, Patrick JE. The autonomic nervous system and fetal heart rate variability. *Am J Obstet Gynecol.* 1983;146(4):456–462.

32. McCartney P. Computer analysis of the fetal heart rate. *J Obstet Gynecol Neonat Nurs.* 2000;29(5):527–536.

33. Hamilton E, Warrick P, O'Keeffe D. Variable decelerations: Do size and shape matter? *J Matern Fetal Neonat Med.* 2012;25(6):648–653.

34. Nemer D, Nomura R, Ortigosa C, et al. Computerized cardiotocography in pregnancies complicated by maternal asthma. *J Matern Fetal Neonat Med.* 2012;25(7):1077–1079.

35. Roemer VM, Walden R. Fetal heart rate patterns during delivery complicated by hypoxia and acidosis: A computer-aided analysis. *Zeitschrift fur Geburtshilfe und Neonatologie.* 2013;217(1):28–34.

36. Wolfberg AJ, Derosier DJ, Roberts T, et al. A comparison of subjective and mathematical estimations of fetal heart rate variability. *J Matern Fetal Neonat Med.* 2008;21(2):101–104.

CHAPTER 7

Electronic Fetal Monitoring Competence Validation

Nursing competence can be defined as possession of the requisite knowledge and technical skills related to a specific area of professional clinical practice. Validation of competence implies both an evaluation of the nurse's level of knowledge and verification of his or her clinical skills. For many reasons that will be discussed in this chapter, many methods of competence validation intended to evaluate nurses who use electronic fetal monitoring (EFM) fall short of achieving these goals.

Traditional testing methods may be useful in determining whether the nurse has the appropriate knowledge of a specific clinical practice area but provide little or no information about technical expertise. Possession of even a thorough knowledge base does not necessarily mean that the nurse has the ability to translate that information into safe and effective clinical practice. It is particularly important when evaluating EFM skills to examine the nurse's competence beyond his or her didactic understanding and assess his or her ability to utilize critical thinking to appropriately implement this routine method of screening in the clinical setting. This includes evaluating, responding to, and communicating findings as part of the overall competence validation process.[1] Traditional skills checklists are commonly used to document clinical expertise. However, this method gives no indication whether the technically expert nurse has the ability to think critically and consider the implications of the clinical intervention. Verification of clinical skills is only one component of the competence validation process.

A more complex issue is whether competent nurses will consistently use their knowledge and clinical skills over time for each patient interaction. Multiple factors, including nurse-to-patient staffing ratios,[2] fatigue, interpersonal stress, and communication and interactions with other care providers[3,4] influence the ability of competent nurses to provide safe and effective perinatal care on a routine basis. The purpose of this chapter is to review the pros and cons of various methods of competence validation for nurses who use EFM and propose an alternative

approach to this process that has the potential to provide more accurate information. No one method will address all of the issues involved in competence validation, nor can any single method ensure that the competent nurse will provide safe and effective care in every interaction. However, some available methods work better than others. If the goal of competence validation is to enhance the likelihood that nurses will provide safe and effective care to all women in labor, a thorough evaluation and discussion of these methods is worthwhile.

PROS AND CONS OF TRADITIONAL APPROACHES

Written Examination

Pros: Written tests (including both traditional paper and pencil and computerized) about EFM content are relatively easy to develop and can be administered to many nurses in a short time frame. Knowledge about key principles of fetal heart rate (FHR) pattern interpretation, physiology, and appropriate nursing interventions can be evaluated by the use of multiple choice, fill-in-the-blank, and matching items. Most of the basic concepts can be covered in 25 to 50 test questions. Examination scoring can be accomplished easily and quickly. A minimum score can be established, and those who achieve the minimum passing score can be designated as possessing the minimum knowledge about EFM required for clinical practice. Written examination appears, at least on the surface, to provide objective data about the nurse's knowledge base. Regulatory agencies such as the Joint Commission accept this method as evidence that the institution has made an appropriate effort to validate competence.[5]

Cons: Although devising test questions may seem easy, few nurses have been educated in the rigorous process of test item writing and examination development. Production of a psychometrically sound examination requires that those writing items are familiar with the process and have significant practice and experience in analyzing individual test items and the examination as a whole. Without reliability and validity data about items that are used on the written examination, few sound conclusions can be drawn from the examination results. Obtaining such data through the use of psychometric techniques is costly, time consuming, and beyond the scope of expertise of most nurses who develop EFM examinations in the institutional setting. Use of a poorly developed written examination as a method to validate competence can provide a false sense of assurance to the institution that the nurses who have achieved a passing score are indeed competent to provide intrapartum nursing care. Further degrading this method of competence validation is the unfortunate common practice of reusing the same examination. Although this may be done to conserve resources and time, another possible explanation for repeating the same examination each year is the limited content area of EFM. Test developers are challenged with the limits of incorporating the same, relatively small amount of content into new, meaningful questions. Thus, in many institutions, perinatal nurses find themselves taking the same poorly developed written examination each year, while administrators remain under the impression that these nurses have participated in a meaningful process to validate competence in EFM.

Recommendations: If an institution chooses written examination as the preferred method for evaluation of requisite knowledge of EFM, the best approach is to use an examination that has been shown to be psychometrically sound and legally defensible. There should be reliability and validity data for individual items and the examination as a whole. The examination should be developed by clinicians who are experts in the areas of both EFM content and item writing. Items should be pretested before inclusion on the examination and continuously evaluated after each examination administration. A rigorous approach to examination development should provide assurance that the successful candidate does possess appropriate level and depth of knowledge in EFM content. At present, the only EFM examination that meets these criteria is that developed by a team of content experts through the National Certification Corporation for the Obstetric, Gynecologic and Neonatal Nursing Specialties (NCC). Eligibility for this examination requires candidates to demonstrate that they are currently working in a clinical practice setting where EFM is used. The test is applicable for multidisciplinary competence validation and may be taken by nurses, physicians, and midwives. Use of the NCC examination can save considerable time for the person in the institution who is responsible for EFM examination development, allowing them to pursue more valuable educational objectives. One of the added benefits of choosing NCC is the requirement for continuing education that is part of the maintenance process. Fifteen contact hours specific to EFM content are required every 3 years to maintain this NCC credential. There is the implied commitment to maintaining current knowledge of EFM principles by those who are credentialed through the NCC examination process. Thus, this examination evaluates knowledge using a rigorous process and promotes multidisciplinary participation in continuing education programs.

It is important to be circumspect in regard to ascribing to programs offered by individuals and companies who award a "certification" following completion of an examination they have prepared and that includes requirements to take their course and use their book. Not only are psychometric testing factors an issue, there also seems to be an inherent conflict that can affect the quality of the process when an examination is geared to course content. If an institution is committed to utilizing written examination, the best use of financial resources is to participate in an examination developed and supported by a national organization with expertise in the examination process.

Skills Checklists

Pros: Skills checklists are an excellent method of ensuring that all expected skills are covered during the orientation process and that accuracy in implementing these skills has been observed. Refer to the AWHONN *Clinical Competencies and Education Guide: Antepartum and Intrapartum Fetal Heart Monitoring*[1] for a list of suggested clinical skills for nurses who use EFM. These can be adapted and revised based on institutional or unit practices. Comprehensive, well-developed skills checklists serve as a reference to guide the preceptor during orientation and provide the orientee with a defined set of clinical expectations. Direct observation of accurate implementation of the designated technical skills should be criteria for completion of orientation and assumption of primary responsibility for patient care. Regulatory agencies will accept skills checklists as evidence that the institution has attempted to verify clinical skills for professional nurses.

Cons: Technical skills associated with use of EFM are not overly complex. Once nurses have been observed performing all expected technical skills several times with accuracy, it can be assumed those skills are maintained if the nurse is providing such patient care on a routine basis (unless some evidence arises to suggest otherwise). Nurses who have difficulties with the technical aspects of EFM are usually quickly identified by peers or through clinical situations where their deficiencies become apparent. These situations can be addressed with remediation strategies designed for the individual nurse.

Verification of skills for experienced nurses should focus on consistency rather than a baseline evaluation. Use of skills checklists for annual clinical skills verification for experienced perinatal nurses are not helpful in truly assessing whether the nurse consistently applies technical expertise to every clinical interaction. Observer bias presents a confounding issue because adherence to unit policies and appropriate nurse–patient interactions are likely to be at the highest level when one is being knowingly observed. Therefore, this method does not provide information about routine nursing interventions when an observer/evaluator is not present. Use of skills checklists for experienced nurses provides a false sense of assurance that the nurse under observation gives technically competent care on a routine basis.[6]

Recommendations: Skills checklists are useful for orientation of new nurses only, as a reference to ensure that expected technical skills have been demonstrated by the orientee before primary responsibility for patient care is assigned. Use of skills checklists for experienced nurses should be avoided.

EFM Case Studies with Strip Reviews

Pros: EFM strip review is a popular method of competence validation because the questions posed are associated with a specific clinical case and a graphic display of the FHR pattern. In many cases, single test items on written examinations provide scarce detail of the clinical scenario related to the question posed. Participants may find this frustrating, and they often try to fill in the missing information on their own. Such assumptions can lead to incorrect responses. Many nurses are visual learners and find it easier to relate to a picture of the FHR pattern, rather than narrative descriptions, when attempting to answer questions regarding appropriate clinical interventions. A case study approach is inherently more interesting to the adult learner because it is closer to his or her daily experiences in the clinical setting. Responses to case study questions are more likely to germinate from critical thinking and interpretation than with single-topic examination items. Thus, information from a case study approach to competence validation is more valuable than scores on written examinations.[6] Regulatory agencies such as the Joint Commission accept this method as evidence that the institution has made an appropriate effort to validate competence.[5]

An additional benefit of using case studies with EFM strips is the knowledge gained by those who participate in the development process. A committee of staff nurse volunteers can be recruited to develop case studies from interesting strips of actual patients. A group process can be used to review the expected responses, appropriate interpretations, and related interventions. This discussion can lead to an increased knowledge of EFM principles for all involved. Not all participants need be nurse experts with many years of clinical experience. A willingness to volunteer can be the criterion for participation. This is an excellent opportunity to mentor nurses with less experience and develop collegial relationships.

The most effective approach to case study is to actively seek participation from physician and nurse midwife colleagues. Any opportunity for collaboration between disciplines jointly responsible for FHR pattern interpretation and clinical interventions should be encouraged. The process of developing and reviewing case studies is an ideal avenue for clarifying ongoing clinical issues and coordinating the interpretation and expectations of provider groups. For example, a physician may expect a series of responses or interventions for specific FHR or uterine activity (UA) pattern that is not in tandem with current nursing practice at the institution. Disagreement about the course of clinical management in the presence of tachysystole as the result of oxytocin administration is a common issue. When the FHR remains reassuring, nurses may still routinely decrease the oxytocin dosage or discontinue the infusion completely, according to their knowledge base or even institutional policy. Physician colleagues may believe the nurses are overreacting by adjusting the oxytocin when the FHR is not yet showing signs of deterioration. An open discussion of the rationale based on physiologic principles, current research, and standards of care may lead to less conflict in the clinical setting.[7]

Another common area of disagreement is description of FHR patterns. Development of case studies and accurate responses can lead to a common understanding of FHR pattern nomenclature that is mutually agreed upon and routinely used by all providers. If not already in place, this is an opportunity to suggest adoption of a common set of definitions for FHR pattern interpretation and medical record documentation initially recommended by the National Institute of Child Health and Human Development (NICHD) Research Planning Workshop in 1997 and then further defined and updated in 2008.[8,9] These definitions are supported by the American College of Obstetricians and Gynecologists[10] and AWHONN.[1] It is important to adopt a standard set of definitions so that all providers are speaking the same language in both oral communication and written documentation in the medical record.[5] A clear definition of fetal well-being should guide the majority of unit operations and can be used to simplify communication between nurses and physicians.[11] The presence of fetal well-being is the criterion for maternal discharge, maternal medications, and use of oxytocin and epidural anesthesia in most clinical situations. Absence of fetal well-being necessitates direct physician evaluation, with written documentation of further clinical management.[11] Coming to agreement on definitions can be a significant outcome of joint development of and participation in EFM case study review. It is possible that interdisciplinary collaboration will have a positive spillover effect on daily clinical operations.[7]

Cons: EFM case studies with strip reviews have the potential to provide valuable information about core knowledge and expected clinical skills. However, at times, the case studies are poorly developed and the questions evaluate content not provided in the patient history. Nurses are educated to assess the overall clinical picture including maternal history and previous and ongoing fetal status. If a case study provides minimal maternal data and only a brief snapshot of the FHR pattern, this approach can be frustrating to the participant and does not approximate clinical reality. Unless the question is "What are the appropriate interventions based on this 15-minute admission strip?" a single 15-minute strip is not enough for a realistic case study presentation. In the clinical practice setting, if a nurse noted an FHR pattern that was not definitively predictive of normal fetal acid–base status (e.g., Category 2), one of the initial actions would be a quick review of the previous EFM strip and consideration of maternal factors. Thus, for case studies to be of value, enough information should be

provided to simulate an actual clinical situation. Additionally, case studies should be de-identified whenever possible, so that participants are not privy to either patient or provider information. Essential to the success of case review is that discussions do not disintegrate into reproach of the clinicians involved.

Recommendations: Develop comprehensive case studies with adequate maternal history and EFM data to represent the clinical scenario. Use items that go beyond simple interpretation. Evaluate appropriate interventions and discuss possible outcomes. Use EFM case studies as an opportunity to mentor inexperienced nurses, strengthen relationships between nurses and physicians, clarify ongoing clinical issues, and promote collaboration and communication.

It is also important to consider that, for a variety of reasons, it may be more feasible for a particular institution to consider purchasing an electronic strip review course rather than developing its own case study review. This can be a valuable option when utilized for the important purposes just described, including multidisciplinary education and preparation for standardized testing. Although it lacks some of the benefits of collaboration inherent to creating a case study review, such an approach can be helpful in engaging other disciplines since online course work can be completed at one's own pace and convenience. If resistance or barriers to multidisciplinary collaboration exist, this can be a useful initial step toward common ground by introducing standardized terminology, definitions, and management approaches.

ALTERNATIVE APPROACHES TO COMPETENCE VALIDATION

Medical Record Audits

Guidelines and standards of care from professional organizations such as AWHONN, ACOG, and the Joint Commission provide a useful framework for validating the competence of nurses who use EFM. Institutional policy and procedures, protocols, care plans, and clinical pathways should reflect practice parameters outlined in publications by these professional organizations. Therefore, it is reasonable to use this approach to develop a tool for competence validation.[6] The first step in the process is a thorough review of published practice guidelines and standards of care. An added benefit of assembling and reviewing all pertinent literature is the assurance that institutional policies and procedures, protocols, care plans, and clinical pathways are consistent with current guidelines and standards of care.[12,13] Some institutions have policies for frequent assessments and routine interventions that are not based on evidence or guidelines and standards of care. These policies result in unnecessary, time-consuming practices that do not contribute to optimal maternal–fetal outcomes.[7] The medical record audit development process can serve as an opportunity to streamline clinical care and promote evidence-based practice. Fortunately, for most clinical issues, there is no need to develop policies independently, since professional organizations have publications that can serve as a useful framework. Consistency with published guidelines and standards of care can decrease liability, should the institution be involved in litigation related to care during childbirth.[11]

Advantages of Using Medical Record Audit Tools

Medical record audits can be designed to cover both aspects of the competence validation process, providing substantial data regarding both the requisite knowledge base and the clinical skills essential to intrapartum nursing practice. A retrospective comparison of the FHR and UA data as documented in the medical record to the actual EFM tracing provides valuable, objective information about the nurse's ability to accurately interpret the patterns depicted. Medical record audits effectively eliminate the confounding factor of observer bias inherent in the skills checklist approach.

Nursing interventions documented in the medical record related to the FHR and UA displayed on the EFM tracing provide evidence of the nurse's knowledge of maternal–fetal physiology and can be used to verify clinical skills. For example, periods of tachysystole with concurrent increases in oxytocin dosage administration may indicate that the nurse is unaware of the clinical signs of tachysystole, the institutional policy on oxytocin administration, the pharmacokinetics of oxytocin, or the appropriate nursing interventions when there is excessive uterine activity during oxytocin administration. Prolonged periods on the EFM tracing where the FHR or UA is absent or uninterpretable may indicate that the nurse needs more information and further demonstration about Leopold's maneuvers and correct transducer placement. Inaccurate notations in the medical record about FHR patterns could be

evidence that the nurse needs more practice in FHR pattern interpretation. Correct interpretations of FHR patterns that are not predictive of normal fetal acid-base status that are documented without notation of subsequent nursing interventions suggest that the nurse may benefit from additional clinical preceptorship and more education regarding appropriate response to FHR patterns. Notations about FHR patterns that are not predictive of normal fetal acid–base status, accompanied by entries that the physician or certified nurse midwife (CNM) is aware and not responding, with no further interventions noted, may indicate that the nurse needs to review the unit chain of command algorithm.

A well-documented medical record that is comparable with the EFM tracing and includes appropriate nursing interventions at frequencies reasonably consistent with institutional policies provides evidence that the nurse has a solid knowledge base about the physiology of FHR pattern interpretation, labor and birth, and institutional policies and standards of care and is able to apply that knowledge in clinical practice. Selected parameters can be used to develop a medical record audit tool to review nursing care related to EFM during labor and birth.

Validation of Competence Before Completion of Orientation

Before completion of orientation, randomly selected medical records and EFM strips can be reviewed with the orientee, as both a learning exercise and as part of the competence validation process. The person responsible for orientation can use this session to reinforce accuracies in interpretation, documentation, and appropriate nursing interventions. This process can build confidence for nurses new to the specialty and allow a nonthreatening opportunity for the orientee to ask questions and seek clarification. This exercise can help identify those who need further education and/or clinical practice experience before completion of orientation.

Annual Ongoing Competence Validation

When medical record audits are used as a component of annual competence validation for all nurses, nurse members of a unit practice committee are ideal candidates to coordinate the program. Three or more medical records, complete with EFM strips, can be selected at random for review by committee as previously described. A nurse who is found to need further education and clinical practice experience can be identified and provided close supervision. In this instance, a follow-up audit should be done to validate competence before the nurse resumes independent responsibility for care. Reviewing at least three randomly selected medical records that reflect varying instances of care provided by each nurse evaluated contributes to overall accuracy of the data collected.

Adaptation to Specific Clinical Issues

An added benefit to use of the medical record audit for verification of individual clinical competence is that specific quality care issues pertinent to the entire perinatal unit may also be discovered and addressed. The tool should be designed based on individual unit needs. For example, if particular issues are suspected or identified, such as incomplete admission assessments, inaccuracies in documentation as compared to the EFM strip, inappropriate increases in oxytocin, etc., the tool can be developed to evaluate these specific practice areas and gather data for feedback as needed. Heightened awareness of the importance of accurate medical record documentation and the peer review process can be incentives to enhance quality. Audits also can be useful in developing medical record forms that are more user-friendly and provide cues or prompts to enter the required data. Areas for noting aspects of nursing care that are often provided but infrequently documented, such as comfort measures during labor and interactions with the woman's support persons, can be added to written or electronic flow sheets.

Perinatal Unit Evaluation

Medical record audits provide significant information about unit practices and adherence to unit policies. The practice culture of the unit can be identified through evaluation of randomly selected medical records over a designated time period. For example, an audit of women who receive oxytocin for labor induction may reveal that tachysystole, excessive oxytocin dosage, and nonintervention during FHR patterns that are not definitively predictive of normal fetal acid–base status are characteristics of care providers, rather than individual nurses. Quality and frequency of communication between nurses and providers can also be evaluated by way of medical record audits. Trends in appropriate interventions or lack of interventions are also easily identified in this manner.

Inconsistencies or inaccuracies in FHR interpretation can be determined. Based on medical record audits, programs can be designed to close any gaps in education and enhance safe practice, and information can be provided to alert care providers of ongoing clinical issues that may contribute to unsafe care and potential patient injuries. Periodic unit evaluation through the use of medical record audits is an ideal method to verify that competent care providers are providing competent care on a routine basis.

Guidelines for Designing a Medical Record Audit Tool

Selected medical records of women during labor can be reviewed and compared to the electronic FHR tracings. Overall accuracy, consistency with established institutional policies and procedures and AWHONN and ACOG guidelines, interpretability, and clinical practice issues can be evaluated during the intrapartum period using some of the following parameters. (See Box 7–1 for suggested components of a medical record audit tool.)

Benefits of Using Medical Record Audits to Validate Competence

- Medical record audits can be used for both knowledge base evaluation and clinical skills verification.
- Medical record audits are objective and comprehensive while avoiding the observer bias inherent in using skills checklists.
- The process works well when used before completion of orientation to reinforce knowledge and clinical skills and can build confidence for nurses new to the specialty.
- The process can be incorporated into the unit's annual competence validation program for all nurses and can allow identification of nurses who could benefit from additional education and clinical practice experience.
- Tool development can be useful in ensuring that institutional policies, procedures, protocols, care plans, and clinical pathways are consistent with published guidelines and standards of care from professional organizations.
- Audit processes can lead to redesign and enhancements of current medical record forms.
- Feedback can heighten awareness of the importance of accurate documentation on the medical record.

BOX 7-1 | Suggested Components of a Medical Record Audit

- Are the times noted on the Admission Assessment, Labor Flow Chart, and initial electronic fetal monitoring (EFM) strip chart reasonably consistent?
- If elective labor induction, is gestational age of at least 39 weeks' confirmed?
- Is there documentation of physician notification of admission within the time frame outlined in the policies and procedures?
- Is fetal well-being established on admission?
- Is fetal well-being established prior to ambulation?
- Is fetal well-being established prior to medication administration?
- Does the fetal heart rate (FHR) baseline rate noted on the fetal strip chart match the FHR baseline documented?
- Does the FHR baseline variability match the FHR baseline variability documented?
- If there is evidence of absent or minimal FHR variability, is it documented?
- If there is evidence of absent or minimal FHR variability, are appropriate interventions documented?
- If there are FHR decelerations on the EFM strip, are they correctly documented?
- Are appropriate interventions documented in response to FHR patterns that do not meet Category I criteria?
- Is there documentation of physician or nurse-midwife notification in response to FHR patterns that do not meet Category I criteria?
- If FHR accelerations are documented, are they represented on the fetal strip chart?
- Are maternal assessments documented according to policy?
- If there is evidence of a FHR pattern that does not meet Category I criteria, how is the oxytocin subsequently managed?
- If there is evidence of tachysystole, are appropriate interventions documented?
- If there is evidence of adequate labor, is oxytocin dosage increased?
- If there is evidence of tachysystole, is oxytocin dosage increased or decreased?
- Does the frequency of uterine contractions on the fetal strip chart match what is documented?
- Is the uterine activity monitor (tocotransducer or intrauterine pressure catheter [IUPC]) adjusted to maintain an accurate UA baseline?

- Are oxytocin dosage increases charted when there is an inaccurate or uninterpretable uterine baseline or uterine activity tracing?
- Are oxytocin dosage increases charted when there is an inaccurate or uninterpretable FHR tracing?
- Is the physician/nurse-midwife's documentation of fetal status consistent with the nurse's?
- Is the automatically generated data from the blood pressure device accurate?
- Does documentation continue throughout the second stage of labor?
- Are women in the second stage of labor encouraged to push before they feel the urge?
- Are women in the second stage of labor encouraged to push with contractions when the FHR is not definitively predictive of normal fetal acid–base status (Category II or III)?
- When the FHR is not definitively predictive of normal fetal acid–base status during the second stage of labor (Category II or III), is pushing discontinued or encouraged with every other or every third contraction to maintain a stable baseline rate and minimize decelerations?
- If the FHR is not clearly predictive of normal fetal acid–base status during the second stage of labor (Category II or III), is oxytocin discontinued?
- Are uterine contractions continuously monitored during the second stage of labor via tocotransducer or IUPC?
- Does the time of birth on the medical record match the time of birth noted at the end of the fetal strip chart?
- If the woman had regional analgesia/anesthesia, is a qualified anesthesia provider involved in the decision to discharge from postanesthesia care unit (PACU) care?
- If the woman had regional analgesia/anesthesia, is the discharge from PACU care scoring evaluation documented?
- Are maternal assessments documented during the immediate postpartum period every 15 minutes for the first hour?
- Are newborn assessments documented during the transition to extrauterine life at least every 30 minutes until the newborn's condition has been stable for 2 hours?

Data from Simpson, Kortz, Knox, 2009.[20]

- Results can be used as part of the unit quality improvement process.
- Improvements in documentation and clinical practice can lead to decreased institutional liability.[12]

Simulation-Based Training

With the growing use of computerized simulators for nursing/medical education, there is increasing opportunity for practice and competence validation prior to patient contact. A benefit to this approach is that the new clinician will begin patient care duties with some experience, rather than learning on the job. For the experienced clinician, this may be a good way to validate mastered skills, depending on the variety and level of situational experiences offered by the simulator. Although use of a fetal simulator for competence validation has not specifically been widely studied, simulation-based training has shown merit in regard to improving performance of both individuals[14] and the dynamic functioning of an obstetric multidisciplinary team.[15–17]

COMPLEX ISSUES RELATED TO COMPETENCE VALIDATION

Professional Responsibility

Maintaining and validating competence is a shared responsibility. Regulatory agencies such as the Joint Commission mandate periodic competence validation for care providers.[5] The institution, as the employer, has a responsibility to make a reasonable attempt to validate competence of its professional nursing staff. Areas of clinical competence are outlined by professional organizations such as AWHONN and ACOG and can be used as a framework for developing comprehensive programs. Institutions also have a responsibility for providing continuing education programs so nurses can have the opportunity to review basic concepts and learn about new trends and techniques.

Nurses have an individual responsibility to maintain competence in clinical practice. Most states' nurse practice acts have statements or standards that address requirements for nurses to keep current in nursing practice. AWHONN's *Standards and Guidelines for Professional Nursing Practice in the Care of Women and Newborns*[18] delineates expectations for achieving and maintaining competence. If the nurse believes the institution's programs fall short in providing continuing education programs that promote knowledge about current practice, there is a responsibility to seek outside educational opportunities while advocating for improvements in institutional programs.

Clinical Errors by Competent Care Providers

Perinatal care providers are expected by their communities, patients, and society in general to provide competent care. Perinatal units are expected to operate essentially without clinical errors or mistakes over long periods.[11] A clinical error during labor and birth can be devastating to the infant and family. Competent care providers do make clinical errors that lead to adverse maternal–fetal outcomes. One of the limitations of even the most comprehensive and rigorous competence validation programs is the

inability to ensure that competent care providers will give competent care to every patient every day. Although clinical judgment disagreements can also lead to adverse patient outcomes, basic clinical errors should not occur and are not well-tolerated by patients or society in general, especially when they result in patient injury.

Clinical errors by competent care providers are common. Most errors are the result of faulty systems and poorly designed processes that set providers up to make mistakes by putting them in situations where errors are more likely to be made.

Perinatal units are prone to error due to multiple factors.[11] Unit operations are routine and usually successful in achieving good patient outcomes. However, successful operations are potentially dangerous because success leads to oversimplification, shortcuts, and a "normalization of deviance."[19] The concept of normalization of deviance is important in understanding the potential for error in perinatal unit operations. In Vaughan's[19] analysis of the Challenger disaster, she concluded that all work groups continually redefine risk in the context of accidents that do not occur. Competent care providers can unknowingly let professional and technical standards degrade over time. Incrementally, the unit culture can become less safe over time because "they get away with it."[19] For example, in some units, understaffing is the routine. On most days, nurses may be responsible for more than two women in active labor receiving oxytocin. Nurses may be mandated to work extra shifts, resulting in fatigue, stress, and burnout. After months of not having adequate nurses to care for women in labor with no adverse outcomes, administrators may begin to believe that this is a cost-effective way of doing business. Another example of normalization of deviance is the desensitization to tachysystole patterns related to oxytocin use.[13] Since the healthy fetus can usually tolerate this stress for a period of time before demonstrating an FHR pattern that is not predictive of normal fetal acid–base status, nurses and physicians may not take an appropriate proactive approach and adjust the oxytocin dosage. Aggressive pushing techniques during which the fetus demonstrates decelerations with each contraction are many times the norm, since most healthy fetuses can tolerate this stress temporarily. Use of a vacuum for operative vaginal birth when the fetus is too high for forceps does not usually result in fetal injury. A consistent problem with physicians not being present during birth may be accepted because most babies do well when they are born into the hands of experienced labor nurses. Ongoing conflict between nurses and physicians in a culture where the expected behavior is to comply with physician orders without initiating the chain of command when appropriate may be tolerated because of the negative implications for nurses who try to change the system. All of these are common examples that lull otherwise competent clinicians into patterns of normalization of deviance.

Most childbearing women are healthy and most fetuses are resilient to iatrogenic stress; thus, most errors do not result in patient injury. Because injuries are rare, there is no immediate or apparent consequence for not strictly adhering to policies or protocols designed to prevent adverse outcomes. Because there are usually good outcomes, even in the case of errors, near-misses are frequently not viewed by competent care providers as opportunities to learn or improve unit behavior. Given the predominance of good outcomes and overall normality of perinatal practice, perinatal units are especially prone to normalizing deviance.[11] Competent care providers who are new to a particular unit are sometimes amazed at what, from their fresh perspective, appear as glaringly, potentially unsafe practices and routines. Having an experienced new staff member is an ideal opportunity to reevaluate unit practice. Unfortunately, what often happens is that these same professionals are later just as amazed when another newcomer questions the safety of the same practices to which they themselves have now grown accustomed.[11] In this manner, unsafe clinical practices can become accepted by those designated as competent, due to unit cultural factors and the fact that most errors do not result in adverse outcomes; not because these staff members are lacking appropriate knowledge and clinical skills.

Where Do We Go from Here?

The goal of any competence validation program is to ensure that competent caregivers will consistently provide competent care. However, competence validation of individual nurses is only one component of safe and effective perinatal nursing care. Characteristics of units that promote safe care and minimal patient injuries have been described in the literature.[11] Unit culture contributes to the ability of competent nurses to consistently provide safe care. Nurse-to-patient ratios, nurse–physician interactions, and routine practices not based on evidence or standards and guidelines for care are important factors.[12] The future of competence

validation should be directed toward evaluating the consistent competence of teams of perinatal care providers and reviewing adverse outcomes related to clinical errors. Currently, the only method for this type of approach is an analysis of claims data from perinatal units. But there are inherent flaws in a simple claims analysis approach because of data to suggest that six patient injuries occur for every one claim filed.[20] More research is needed to develop effective methods of validating clinical competence and promoting safe patient care. For now, the best approach is use of medical record audits to evaluate individual care providers and to analyze the overall unit practices and culture that contribute to the best possible outcomes for childbearing women.

REFERENCES

1. Association of Women's Health, Obstetric and Neonatal Nurses. *Clinical Competencies and Education Guide: Antepartum and Intrapartum Fetal Heart Rate Monitoring.* 5th ed. Washington, DC: Author; 2011.
2. Association of Women's Health, Obstetric and Neonatal Nurses. *Guidelines for Professional Registered Nurse Staffing for Perinatal Units.* Washington, DC: Author; 2010.
3. Joint Commission on Accreditation of Healthcare Organizations. *Behaviors That Undermine a Culture of Safety.* Sentinel Event Alert No. 40. Oak Park, IL: Author; 2008.
4. Joint Commission on Accreditation of Healthcare Organizations. *Comprehensive Accreditation Manual for Hospitals.* Oak Park, IL: Author; 2013.
5. Joint Commission on Accreditation of Healthcare Organizations. *Preventing Infant Death and Injury During Delivery.* (Sentinel Event Alert No. 30). Oak Brook, IL: Author; 2004.
6. Simpson KR. Using guidelines and standards from professional organizations as a framework for competence validation. In: KR Simpson, PA Creehan, eds. *AWHONN's Competence Validation for Perinatal Care Providers: Orientation, Continuing Education and Evaluation.* Philadelphia: PA: Lippincott-Raven; 1998.
7. Simpson KR, James DC, Knox GE. Nurse-physician communication during labor and birth: Implications for patient safety. *J Obstet Gynecol Neonat Nurs.* 2006; 35(4):547–556.
8. National Institute of Child Health and Human Development Research Planning Workshop. Electronic fetal heart rate monitoring: Research guidelines for interpretation. *J Obstet Gynecol Neonat Nurs.* 1997;26(6):635–640.
9. National Institute of Child Health and Human Development Research Planning Workshop. Report on electronic fetal monitoring: update on definitions, interpretations, and research guidelines. *J Obstet Gynecol Neonat Nurs.* 2008;37(5):510–515.
10. American College of Obstetricians and Gynecologists. *Intrapartum Fetal Heart Rate Monitoring:*

Nomenclature, Interpretation, and General Management Principles (Practice Bulletin No. 106; 2009, Reaffirmed 2013). Washington, DC: Author; 2013.

11. Knox GE, Simpson KR, Townsend KE. High reliability perinatal units: Further observations and a suggested plan for action. *J Healthc Risk Mgt.* 2003;23(4): 17–21.

12. Simpson KR, Knox GE. Common areas of litigation related to care during labor and birth: Recommendations to promote patient safety and decrease risk exposure. *J Perinat Neonat Nurs.* 2003;17(1):94–109.

13. Simpson KR, Miller L. Assessment and optimization of uterine activity during labor. *Clin Obstet Gynecol.* 2011;54(1):40–49.

14. Daniels K, Arafeh J, Clark A, et al. Prospective randomized trial of simulation versus didactic teaching for obstetrical emergencies. *Simul Healthc.* 2010 Feb;5(1):40–45.

15. Fisher N, Bernstein PS, Satin A, et al. Resident training for eclampsia and magnesium toxicity management: simulation or traditional lecture? *Am J Obstet Gynecol.* 2010 Oct;203(4):379.

16. Dadiz R, Weinschreider J, Schriefer J, et al. Interdisciplinary simulation-based training to improve delivery room communication. *Simul Healthc.* 2013 Oct;8(5): 279–291.

17. Association of Women's Health, Obstetric and Neonatal Nurses. *Standards and Guidelines for Professional Nursing Practice in the Care of Women and Newborns.* 7th ed. Washington, DC: Author; 2009.

18. Vaughan D. *The Challenger Launch Decision: Risky Technology, Culture and Deviance at NASA.* Chicago, IL: University of Chicago Press; 1996.

19. Localio AR, Lawthers AG, Brennan TA. Relation between malpractice claims and adverse events due to negligence: Results of the Harvard Medical Practice Study III. *NEJM.* 1991;325:245–251.

20. Simpson KR, Kortz CC, Knox GE. A comprehensive perinatal safety program to reduce preventable adverse outcomes and costs of liability claims. *Joint Comm J Qual Patient Safety.* 2009;35(11):565–574.

SUGGESTED READINGS

Association of Women's Health, Obstetric and Neonatal Nurses. *Fetal Heart Monitoring Principles and Practices.* 4th ed. Washington, DC: Author; 2009.

Joint Commission on Accreditation of Healthcare Organizations. *Revisions to LD.03.01.01 (Behaviors That Undermine a Culture of Safety).* Sentinel Event Alert No. 40). Oak Park, IL: Author; 2012.

Robertson B, Schumacher L, Gosman G, et al. Simulation-based crisis team training for multidisciplinary obstetric providers. *Simul Healthc.* 2009 Summer;4(2):77–83.

Ultrasound in Women's Health Care and Pregnancy

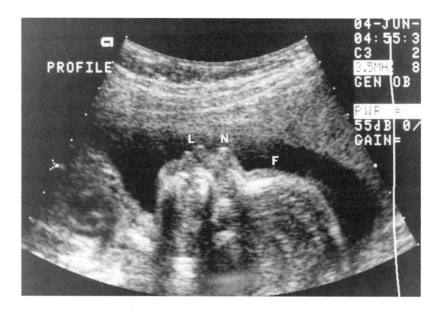

Point-of-Care Sonography in Women's Health and Pregnancy

While this book was in press, several applicable publications and updated guidelines emerged, including an executive summary of a joint Eunice Kennedy Shriver National Institute of Child Health and Human Development, Society for Maternal-Fetal Medicine, American Institute of Ultrasound in Medicine, American College of Obstetricians and Gynecologists, American College of Radiology, Society for Pediatric Radiology, and Society of Radiologists in Ultrasound Fetal Imaging workshop. This document offered recommendations specific to fetal imaging. This summary outlined the indications for ultrasound and MRI in pregnancy, the recommended timing and intervals for fetal imaging, and the identification of research opportunities. Commentary regarding how these recommendations may differ slightly from content in the book is detailed on http://solution.lww.com.

As nurses, midwives, nurse practitioners, and physician assistants take on more responsibility in providing first-line care to women, the need to incorporate sophisticated technology as an adjunct to clinical assessment has become greater. These same clinicians are often the first to provide bedside assessment of maternal and fetal conditions. In the case of an advanced nurse practitioner (ANP), he or she may be the only clinician evaluating and treating a woman from adolescence through the postmenopausal years. As a result, gaining knowledge and acquiring skill with advanced technologies such as sonography has become paramount.

The point-of-care (POC) assessment and complementary treatments encompass many skills, but the focus of this section is on point-of-care sonography. Utilizing sonography in the diagnostic process provides immediate assessment and improves safety and quality of care. POC ultrasound is performed in direct response to a woman's physical signs or symptoms, such as to evaluate vaginal bleeding in pregnancy. Nurses and advanced practice nurses have been recognized as the logical clinicians to incorporate ultrasound into clinical practice based on their basic knowledge of anatomy, physiology, obstetrics, and gynecology. Prior to adding sonography into clinical practice, however, it is necessary to enhance didactic and clinical knowledge encompassing practice-specific sonography content (e.g., gynecologic ultrasound for the assisted reproductive nurse specialist).

This section of the book on maternal and fetal assessment provides some of the educational foundations and resources for POC sonography. Competency must be established prior to performing POC ultrasound, as in any new clinical procedure or practice. Achieving clinical competency requires patience and practice, in conjunction with having an established system of consultation and collaboration.

Point-of-Care Sonography in Women's Health Care: Indications and Guidelines

During the past decade, the use of sonography has become an integral tool in all aspects of health care, including emergency medicine, orthopedics, anesthesiology, critical care, urology, and trauma. Due to its diagnostic value in maternal/fetal assessment in pregnancy, as well as all aspects of women's health care, it has become an essential device for most women's health practices. Because of the ultrasound machine's portability and ease of operation, sonography is available in all areas of the hospital, in clinics, and in private offices, as well as in remote areas such as military battle sites or rural communities. Sonography is now being offered as first-line "ultrasound first" assessment in the diagnosis and treatment of many health care issues.[1] And because sonography has become such an integral part of health care, it is now being taught in many medical schools throughout the country beginning with the first year's curriculum.[2] As a result, the implementation of sonographic assessment has become a critical skill not only for specialized physicians, but also for all health care providers including nurses, midwives, advanced nurse practitioners (APN), and physician assistants (PA).

Specific to women's health care and pregnancy, sonography is the imaging modality of choice for the evaluation of many signs and symptoms, such as determining the cause of vaginal bleeding in all trimesters, locating intrauterine devices, assessing for residual urine in the postpartum woman, and evaluating the endometrium in peri- and postmenopausal women. In many hospitals, labor room nurses are expected to have the minimum sonographic skills necessary to determine fetal presentation during labor when a physician or midwife is unavailable.

The majority of sonographic exams performed by nonsonographers are performed during a specific encounter in which the information obtained by ultrasound will immediately benefit the patient, thus avoiding delay in treatment. This type of assessment-specific ultrasound has been termed "point-of-care"

(POC) and described by the American Institute of Ultrasound in Medicine in 2010[3] as ultrasound use during a specific encounter or procedure to:

- Enhance patient care,
- Diagnose critical conditions,
- Provide immediate care, and
- Improve safety and effectiveness of invasive procedures.

Thus, POC ultrasound may be practiced in a variety of settings and utilized by a diverse set of health care providers. For the purposes of this book, the phrase "point-of-care" sonogram will be used according to this definition but will also encompass those ultrasound examinations previously referred to as "limited ultrasound."

The increasing use of ultrasound by health care professionals other than sonologists (physician sonographers), sonographers, perinatologists, or radiologists has justifiably generated concern by professional organizations. Improperly trained personnel using sonography may lead to increases in the incidence of misdiagnoses and medical errors. For example, there have been both official and unofficial reported cases of clinicians performing sonograms for fetal presentation during labor and missing the presence of a second twin, the absence of cardiac activity, or a placenta previa. In part to establish minimal educational criteria, several professional organizations, such as the American Congress of Obstetrics and Gynecologists (ACOG), the American College of Nurse Midwives (ACNM), and the Association of Women's Health, Obstetric and Neonatal Nurses (AWHONN) have published guidelines or position statements for the education and training of their members who wish to incorporate sonography into clinical practice.[4–6]

Additionally, before incorporating sonography into clinical practice, it is important to investigate the individual state's Nurse Practice Act or appropriate state laws to determine the feasibility of adding

| BOX 8-1 | Indications for Ultrasound During Pregnancy[7–9] |

1st Trimester	2nd and 3rd Trimester
Confirm the presence of intrauterine pregnancy	Evaluate gestational age
Evaluate pelvic pain	Evaluate fetal condition in late registrants for prenatal care
Evaluate for suspected ectopic pregnancy	Evaluate fetal growth
Determine source of vaginal bleeding in pregnancy	Evaluate vaginal bleeding
Estimate gestational age	Evaluate cervical insufficiency
Diagnose or evaluate multiple gestations	Evaluate abdominal and pelvic pain
Confirm cardiac activity	Determine presenting part
Provide guidance for chorionic villus sampling, embryo transfer, or localization and removal of intrauterine device	Evaluate for suspected multiple gestation
	Assess need for adjunct to amniocentesis and external cephalic version
Assess for certain fetal anomalies	Assess size–date discrepancy
Evaluate maternal pelvic or adnexal masses or uterine abnormalities	Evaluate for pelvic mass, suspected hydatidiform mole, suspected ectopic pregnancy, uterine anomaly
Screen for fetal aneuploidy	Evaluate for suspected fetal demise
Evaluate suspected hydatidiform mole	Evaluate fetal well-being
	Evaluate amniotic fluid abnormalities, suspected placental abruption or previa
	Evaluate for premature ROM or labor
	Evaluate for abnormal biochemical markers, follow-up of fetal anomaly, or history of prior congenital anomaly, screen for anomalies and findings that may increase the risk of aneuploidy

Adapted from U. S. Department of Health and Human Services, *Diagnostic ultrasound in pregnancy,* NIH Publication No. 84-667, 1984; American College of Radiology (ACR), *Practice guidelines for the performance of obstetrical ultrasound,* 2007:1025–1033; and American College of Obstetricians and Gynecologists (ACOG), *Ultrasonography in pregnancy,* Practice bulletin #101, 2009.

sonography to current practice. Once this has been achieved, hospital policies and procedures may be developed to address the minimal educational content, methods for measuring clinical competency, and risk management concerns pertaining to the implementation of sonography into clinical practice.

The purpose of this chapter is to describe the various sonography practice guidelines pertinent to pregnancy and women's health care. The guidelines begin with the indications for sonographic exams, along with the details of the "standard" exams performed by a sonographer or radiologist. This is followed by guidelines for the application of specific components of the standard sonogram that may be used during a POC assessment and performed by a nonsonographer.

INDICATIONS FOR DIAGNOSTIC ULTRASOUND IN OBSTETRICS

In 1984, the National Institutes of Health[7] formed a committee of obstetric and sonography experts to generate a list of indications for ultrasonography during pregnancy. These indications were updated by the American College of Radiology (ACR)[8] and the American College of Obstetrics and Gynecology (ACOG),[4] as shown in Box 8–1. Based on these guidelines, it should be noted that routine sonography for every pregnant woman is not an indication in itself.

PROFESSIONAL ORGANIZATION GUIDELINES

Traditionally, the vast majority of obstetric and gynecologic sonograms have been performed by sonographers, radiologists, and other physicians with specialized training in ultrasound. Professional organizations, such as the ACR and the American Institute of Ultrasound in Medicine (AIUM), published guidelines that set general recommendations for what should be included for each type of complete sonogram.

The American Institute of Ultrasound in Medicine

The AIUM is a multidisciplinary professional organization whose membership includes physicians, sonographers, and others from all medical specialties involved in sonography. Their primary goal is to promote the safe and effective use of ultrasound through education, research, and guideline publications; as well as through the accreditation of facilities where ultrasound is performed. The AIUM also works in conjunction with other medical and nursing specialties to develop joint clinical guidelines that pertain to a specific type of practice. The AIUM Guideline for the Performance of Obstetric Ultrasound Examinations, written in conjunction with ACOG, is an example of this collaborative work.

AIUM Practice Guideline for the Performance of Obstetric Ultrasound Examinations

In 2007, the AIUM revised its obstetric guidelines in conjunction and collaboration with ACOG and the ACR. Personnel requirements and other aspects specific to the area of specialization (i.e., obstetrician vs. radiologist) are addressed by the individual professional organization. Additionally, this document stresses that fetal ultrasound should only be performed in response to a valid medical indication while utilizing the lowest possible exposure settings.

One of the major changes in this document from prior publications was the recategorization of the various types of sonograms, terms that were then adopted by other professional organizations. The new sonographic classifications include (1) the *standard* first-trimester ultrasound examination, (2) *standard* second/third trimester examinations (formerly referred to as the basic scan), (3) *limited* examination, and (4) *specialized* examinations (formerly referred to as the comprehensive or targeted scan).[9] Because ACOG not only coauthored this guideline but also adopted this classification system for its own 2009 guideline, the details for each classification are described later, along with other content from the ACOG obstetric guideline.[4]

The AIUM guideline also provides information pertaining to the anatomic landmarks needed for each specific fetal measurement and stands as an excellent document to use during the clinical practicum. Members of AIUM have access to an online enhanced version of this guideline that shows images of each anatomic landmark with proper cursor placement.[9]

AIUM Practice Guideline for the Performance of the Ultrasound Examination of the Female Pelvis

As with obstetric ultrasound, AIUM recommends that scanning of the female pelvis should only be performed when there is an indication or a valid medical reason for the procedure. These indications may include pelvic pain, menstrual disorders, postmenopausal bleeding, abnormal pelvic examination, localization of an intrauterine device, and evaluation and monitoring of infertility treatments. Please refer to the guideline for a complete list of indications, as well as a description of the specific landmarks for measurement and evaluation.[10] Further description of the sonographic evaluation of the female pelvis is detailed in Chapter 10.

AIUM Practice Guideline for the Performance of Ultrasonography in Reproductive Medicine

Ultrasound is an integral part of the evaluation and treatment of women with infertility issues. Whenever possible, AIUM recommends that a transvaginal approach be used for the evaluation of each organ and anatomic structure in the female pelvis. A comprehensive examination should first be performed to rule out pelvic pathology. If all necessary images cannot be obtained with the transvaginal approach, then the transabdominal scan should be done. Also, if there is any question of a pelvic mass, a transabdominal transducer can be used.

Under certain circumstances, a *limited* pelvic ultrasound may be performed based on a specific indication. Examples of a limited pelvic ultrasound include a folliculogram, which is used to monitor ovarian stimulation; and other procedures in reproductive medicine, such as an ultrasound-guided follicular puncture for egg retrieval with in-vitro fertilization and embryo transfer.[11]

This document also delineates recommendations as to appropriate documentation. For example, when a limited folliculogram is performed, documentation should include (1) the number of ovarian follicles in each ovary and (2) endometrial thickness and endometrial morphologic appearance.[11]

American Society for Reproductive Medicine

The American Society for Reproductive Medicine (ASRM) also provides guidelines for registered nurses (RNs) who have had specific training and supervision to perform ultrasound examinations in gynecologic and reproductive medicine. These guidelines do not stand alone; they are intended to be used in conjunction with other nursing guidelines, state laws, and institutional policy that address nursing practice in these areas of nursing. A limited ultrasound examination in gynecology and reproductive medicine performed by nurses would include determining the number and size of developing follicles and the measurement of endometrial thickness and appearance.[11,12]

The American College of Obstetricians and Gynecologists

In 2009, ACOG, in conjunction with AIUM, published a technical and educational bulletin pertinent to sonography performed by obstetricians and gynecologists.[4] This publication updated all components and parameters for the obstetric ultrasound examination and included the three categories of ultrasound examinations established by AIUM in 2007[9]: (1) the limited examination, (2) the standard examination in all trimesters, and (3) the specialized examination.

A *limited ultrasound* is a less extensive examination that may be dictated by the clinical situation requiring investigation. Indications may include assessment of amniotic fluid, presence or absence of cardiac activity, confirmation of the fetal presenting part, interval growth, evaluation of the cervix, and placenta localization. Limited sonography may be performed by sonographers or specially trained personnel. A limited examination does not replace a standard examination.

A *standard ultrasound examination* (formerly referred to as "basic," "complete," "formal," or "level-one ultrasound") generally is performed by sonographers or sonologists in the radiology or ultrasound department as a prescheduled, planned evaluation during all trimesters of pregnancy. The *first-trimester standard sonogram* may be performed by either the transabdominal or transvaginal approach. If a transabdominal examination is not definitive, a transvaginal or transperineal scan should be performed. Although this differs from the AIUM guideline, the intent is the same: if all parameters cannot be visualized with one approach, then the alternate approach should be utilized. Per ACOG, the parameters for a first-trimester ultrasound examination include:

- Evaluation of the uterus, cervix, and adnexa for the presence of a gestational sac
- Documentation of the presence, size, and location of uterine and adnexal masses (such as leiomyomas)
- Assessment of the anterior and posterior cul-de-sac for presence or absence of fluid
- Localization of the sac
- Assessment for presence or absence of cardiac activity

- Assessment of fetal number
- Assessment for presence of a sac but the absence of a definite embryo or yolk sac (which may indicate a pseudogestational sac that may be consistent with an ectopic pregnancy; transvaginally, an embryo should be visible with a mean gestational sac diameter greater than or equal to 20 mm)
- Assessment of fetal anatomy according to gestational age
- Measurement of nuchal translucency at a specific gestational age and in conjunction with serum biochemistry in patients requesting individual risk assessment for aneuploidy

In the second and third trimesters, the standard obstetrical sonogram includes:

- Evaluation of the uterus, adnexal structures, and cervix (when appropriate)
- Evaluation of presentation
- Measurement of amniotic fluid volume
- Assessment of cardiac activity, including abnormal heart rate or rhythm
- Assessment of fetal number; with multiple gestation, the exam includes chorionicity, amnionicity, fetal sizes, estimation of fluid volume, and fetal genitalia
- Evaluation of placental location, appearance, and relationship to cervical os
- Assessment of fetal biometry for fetal gestational age and weight
- Performance of an anatomic survey; each component of the anatomic survey has been specified by the AIUM.[9]

A *specialized sonogram* (formerly referred to as "comprehensive" ultrasound) examination is recommended when an anatomic abnormality is suspected on the basic scan or based on prior maternal obstetric history. The specialized sonogram generally is interpreted or performed by a perinatologist (sonologist) or radiologist who examines the suspicious anatomic feature or abnormality. This category also includes fetal Doppler studies, biophysical profiles, amniotic fluid assessment, fetal echocardiography, or additional biometric measurements.

Overlap among the categories is inevitable. For instance, evaluation of amniotic fluid falls under all three categories. Also, more extensive studies, such as assessing interval fetal growth, was included in the comprehensive category but now falls under the limited ultrasound study. As a result of the creation of these new categories, AWHONN opted to eliminate the descriptor *limited* from its clinical guideline to avoid confusion and miscommunication.[5]

Overlap also is noted between the descriptors "limited" ultrasound and "point-of-care" ultrasound; however, the meaning is similar. They both are defined as an ultrasound exam that is performed to gain specific information warranted by the clinical symptoms at the time of evaluation.

Association of Women's Health, Obstetric and Neonatal Nurses

In 1993, AWHONN issued a specific educational and competency guideline for RNs performing what was then termed "limited sonography." The document described the basic training, educational content, clinical practicum, and competencies needed by experienced OB/GYN nurses who wish to perform limited sonography. The document was updated in 1998 and 2004.

However, following AIUM's 2007 and ACOG's 2009 changes in terminology, the term "limited sonography" was no longer an accurate description for ultrasound exams performed by nurses. Because nurses were performing some components included in each of the new categories, AWHONN opted to update and expand its professional guideline in 2010. The new guideline, *Ultrasound Examinations Performed by Nurses in Obstetric, Gynecologic, and Reproductive Medicine Settings: Clinical Competencies and Education Guide* (3rd ed.), describes the appropriate clinical settings for nurses who perform ultrasound, as well as the recommended didactic component and clinical practice for all types of sonography.[5]

The AWHONN didactic education recommendation is to obtain at least 8 hours of didactic content and instruction specific to the type of ultrasound the nurse will be performing. For example, the didactic focus would be on gynecologic ultrasound for the RN who is working in an infertility setting. There would be no need for such a specialized nurse to learn, for example, the components of a biophysical profile.

The clinical application of ultrasound is a separate educational experience that is performed under the direct supervision of an experienced sonographer, nurse, or physician who is trained in sonography. The precise number of scans a nurse needs to perform to be considered competent cannot be quantified because competency in ultrasound is an individual skill.[13]

The educational competency and clinical practicum provide the basic skills needed for performing ultrasound examinations. Evaluation of learning can be by written examination, verbal exercises, one-on-one tutorials, image reviews, or case studies. Knowledge of hospital protocols and procedures and the appropriate lines of communication should also be validated.[5]

Box 8–2 defines the components of obstetric and gynecologic ultrasound. Once the sonogram has been completed, the nurse documents the findings and reports them to the supervising physician or midwife.

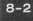 **BOX 8-2** | **Association of Women's Health, Obstetric and Neonatal Nurses (AWHONN)[5]**
Components of Ultrasound Examinations (2010)

Obstetric Ultrasound Examination	Gynecologic Ultrasound	Reproductive Medicine Ultrasound Examination
Determine intra- vs. extrauterine pregnancy	Measure endometrial thickness	Identify uterine position
Assess fetal number	Identify and locate IUD	Measure endometrial thickness
Measure yolk sac	Assess postvoid residual urine	Assess uterine size and position
Measure gestational sac		Locate and measure ovarian follicles
Estimate fetal age (biometry)		Assess components of obstetric first-trimester ultrasound
Estimate fetal weight (biometry)		
Assess fetal cardiac activity		
Assess fetal presentation		
Locate placenta		
Assess amniotic fluid volume		
Assess fetal well-being		
Assess for adjunct ultrasound-guided procedures		
Measure cervical length		

Data from Association of Women's Health, Obstetric and Neonatal Nurses (AWHONN).

AIUM Training Guidelines for Physicians Who Evaluate and Interpret Diagnostic Abdominal, Obstetric, and/or Gynecologic Ultrasound Examinations

For the non–radiology-trained physician, AIUM has published recommendations pertaining to sonography education and training.[14] Key points include:

- Completion of an approved residency program, fellowship, or postgraduate training that includes the equivalent of at least 3 months of diagnostic ultrasound training in the area(s) in which they practice, under the supervision of a qualified physician(s)*, during which the trainees will have evidence of being involved with the performance, evaluation, and interpretation of at least 300** sonograms.
- In the absence of formal fellowship or postgraduate training or residency training, documentation of clinical experience could be acceptable, providing the following could be demonstrated:
  1. Evidence of 100 American Medical Association (AMA) PRA Category 1 Credits™ dedicated to diagnostic ultrasound in the area(s) in which the physicians practice, and,
  2. Evidence of being involved with the performance, evaluation, and interpretation of the images of at least 300** sonograms within a 3-year period. It is expected that, in most circumstances, examinations will be performed under the supervision of a qualified physician(s)*. These sonograms should be in the specialty area(s) in which the physicians are practicing.

At this time, no research study has been able to conclusively determine how many scans in each category a clinician needs to perform in order to be considered clinically competent,[15] and, therefore, no professional organization has set a specific number of sonograms necessary to demonstrate competency in POC sonography. However, AIUM has determined that at least 300 cases were needed to acquire sufficient experience and proficiency with sonography as a *diagnostic* modality and to gain a base understanding of normal and abnormal features. For those physicians utilizing ultrasound in subspecialty applications, the number of cases required by the AIUM is at least 500.

As for annual competency maintenance, the AIUM recommends a minimum of 170 diagnostic obstetric and 170 diagnostic gynecologic ultrasound examinations in order to maintain physician skills. Thirty hours of continuing education specific to OB/GYN every 3 years is also recommended.

American College of Nurse Midwives

In 2012, the ACNM published a position statement that it is within the scope of midwifery practice for midwives to incorporate obstetric and gynecologic sonography into clinical practice. However, when electing to perform ultrasound exams, midwives need to follow the Standards of Practice for Midwifery, which specifies the requirements for expanding midwifery practice beyond core educational competence.[6] Midwives can obtain the necessary sonography education and skills through midwifery educational programs or on a continuing education basis. Once this is accomplished, the midwife should then be eligible for financial reimbursement for those ultrasound examinations performed. Additionally, state regulations, licensing, and facility credentialing should be satisfied.

The ACNM's position statement also directs midwives to the education and training guidelines established by AWHONN, ACOG, and AIUM. Clinical competency can be established during the clinical practicum supervised by an experienced sonographer or other professional competent in the specific type of ultrasound examination being performed. Once again, as with other professional organizations, the recommendation for a minimum number of clinical education hours or number of performed examinations was not established due to individual learning needs; therefore, the determination of clinical competency is left to the discretion of the supervising sonographer.

According to this 2012 position statement, midwives need not be proficient in all aspects of ultrasound but may tailor education and training to the specific exams being performed. For example, if the midwifery clinical practice only requires the ability to perform biophysical profiles, the education and training may be limited to the specific procedure. However, should a competency or credentialing exam become available in the future, midwives may need to be proficient in a greater range of sonography skills.

As it stands at this time, the ACNM position statement delineates specific minimum didactic content that should be included regardless of the type of ultrasound to be performed (Box 8–3).

Additionally, a system for consultation, collaboration, and referral for abnormal findings must

BOX 8-3 | Recommended Didactic Education in Sonography

Didactic content may be incorporated into midwifery educational program curriculum or obtained as an added skill. Minimum recommended educational content:

1. Physics and instrumentation relevant to type of exam to be performed (e.g., physics of ultrasound, proper use of machine and transducer selection, ALARA principle)
2. Required elements and components as described by AIUM for specific exam to be performed (e.g., imaging parameters for each trimester)
3. Required anatomic landmarks defined by AIUM pertinent to type of exam to be performed (e.g., landmarks for biometry)
4. Indications for exam (e.g., indications for POC versus the Standard Examination)
5. Clinical implications of normal and abnormal findings (e.g., documentation, communication, consultation)
6. Ultrasound safety (e.g., output, frequency, length of exams)
7. Components of a complete ultrasound report (e.g., orientation of image, documentation)
8. Client education (e.g., explanation of procedure, communication of results)
9. Additional didactic content can be specific to type of sonograms to be performed (e.g., first-trimester dating vs. cervical length)

Specialized examinations are performed by clinicians with additional experience, education, and expertise.

Adapted from American College of Nurse Midwives (ACNM), *Position statement: midwives' performance of ultrasound in clinical practice*, 2012; American College of Obstetricians and Gynecologists, *Ultrasonography in pregnancy*, Practice bulletin #101, 2009; American Institute of Ultrasound in Medicine (AIUM), Training guidelines for physicians who evaluate and interpret diagnostic abdominal, obstetric, and/or gynecologic ultrasound examinations, 2013.

be established and incorporated into midwifery guidelines. The ACNM also recommended that any midwife who plans to perform fetal anatomic examinations should consider becoming fully credentialed in OB/GYN sonography by the American Registry of Diagnostic Medical Sonographers (ARDMS) (see below).[6] Performing a full fetal anatomic survey requires a greater depth of knowledge, education, and training than POC ultrasound and therefore requires credentialing equivalent to that skill level.

However, the vast majority of midwives will be performing POC imaging and not fetal anatomic surveys. The ACNM has recognized a need for midwifery ultrasound practice standardization and is working with established, nationally recognized credentialing organizations to develop an appropriate proficiency examination that may begin as early as 2015.

American Registry of Diagnostic Medical Sonographers

The ARDMS is an independent, nonprofit organization that credentials qualified sonographers. It was established in 1975 for the sole purpose of administering certification examinations in all specialties of sonography. The ARDMS credentials include the Registered Diagnostic Medical Sonographer (RDMS), the Registered Diagnostic Cardiac Sonographer (RDCS), and the Registered Vascular Technologist (RVT). The obstetrics and gynecology specialty exam is included in the RDMS category.[16]

There are several benefits to successfully completing the certifying examination,[15] particularly for midwives and nurse practitioners. It provides verification of competency at a skill level beyond core competencies. It also increases scope of practice and allows for more thorough, timely assessments, particularly in the triage unit. In addition, some insurance companies will only reimburse for ultrasound examinations performed by a certified or registered sonographer.

The specific eligibility prerequisites for nurses, midwives, nurse practitioners, and other allied health professionals who wish to take the examination to become certified by the ARDMS are listed in Box 8–4. Once an individual has fulfilled the required prerequisites, all applicants must pass the physics and instrumentation examination, as well as the examination for the specialty area, such as OB/GYN. After successful completion of these two examinations, the allied health care provider then becomes RDMS certified. To maintain certification, all individuals must complete 30 hours of ARDMS-accepted continuing education in ultrasound every 3 years.[14]

As of 2012, the ARDMS has been working in conjunction with other professional organizations to develop competency examinations for those who perform specific types of ultrasound examinations but do not meet the requirements for becoming a registered diagnostic medical sonographer. Because of this rapidly changing area of competency/proficiency examination, refer to the ARDMS website ardms.org to determine testing availability for specific practitioners.

Society of Diagnostic Medical Sonographers

The membership of the Society of Diagnostic Medical Sonographers (SDMS) is composed primarily of sonographers and other allied health professionals who perform diagnostic ultrasound. The SDMS issues guidelines and opinions on many aspects of

BOX 8-4 | **American Registry of Diagnostic Medical Sonographers Eligibility Requirements for Allied Health Professionals (Prerequisite 1)**

Education: Two-year allied health education program that is patient care–related. Allied health occupations include, but are not limited to, diagnostic medical sonographer, radiologic technologist, respiratory therapist, occupational therapist, physical therapist, and registered nurse.

PLUS
Required Clinical Ultrasound/Vascular Experience:
12 months full-time (35 hours per week, at least 48 weeks per year).

PLUS
Required Documentation:
Official school transcript and
Education program certificate or license and
Original letter from supervising physician and/or supervising sonographer/technologist or educational program director indicating a minimum of 12 months of full-time clinical experience including exact dates of ultrasound experience/successful completion of sonography program and
Original signed and completed clinical verification form for each appropriate specialty areas

Adapted from American Registry of Diagnostic Medical Sonographers, RDMS SPI requirement and general prerequisites, 2012.

sonography. A major function of the SDMS is educational, including local, regional, and national meetings providing ongoing continuing education. The SDMS has advocated for national licensing rather than licensing on a state-by-state basis, but it supports licensing of sonographers, nonetheless.[17] Prior to 2009, individual states did not require licensing of sonographers. The first state to enact a law was New Mexico on April 6, 2009.[18]

CLINICAL COMPETENCY IN SONOGRAPHY

Obtaining clinical competency in obstetric sonography is a challenge experienced by most nonsonographers for several reasons. To achieve clinical competency, one needs to be able to (1) scan under the supervision of a qualified and experience person, (2) have access to pregnant women as models, and (3) limit exposure time to the pregnant models. Most of these issues have been addressed by various professional organizations; however, obtaining sufficient clinical experience is still an obstacle for many clinicians.

Safety in Training and Research

Diagnostic ultrasound has been in use since the late 1950s. There are no confirmed adverse biological effects on patients resulting from this usage. No hazard has been identified that would preclude the prudent and conservative use of diagnostic ultrasound in education and research. Additionally, experience from normal diagnostic practice relevant to extended exposure times and altered exposure conditions is inconclusive. However, it is considered appropriate to make the recommendation that when examinations are carried out for purposes of training or research, the subject should be informed of the anticipated exposure conditions and how these compare with normal diagnostic practice.[15]

Guidelines for Hands-On Scanning in Pregnant Subjects

Additionally, the AIUM has addressed the appropriate use of ultrasound in education with emphasis on safety for human models[19] during AIUM-sponsored training sessions.

- Subject participation should require appropriate informed consent. The primary obstetrician providing prenatal care should be informed of patient participation.
- The subjects should be prescreened to attempt to avoid unexpected findings.
- There should be a plan to address unexpected findings should they be observed during the educational course.
- There should be no first-trimester examinations.
- Exposure time (i.e., duration of "hands-on" teaching session) should not exceed 1 hour per subject.

COMPETENCY AND COST

The didactic course content for learning ultrasound has been clearly established.[5] It is recommended that midwives[6] utilize the established guidelines of both ACOG[4] and AIUM.[9] Acquiring the clinical skills is a more daunting task because clinical sites are limited. In a study of family medicine residents, Dresang et al.[13] found that clinical competency in performing fetal biometry and fetal anatomic surveys was achieved within 25–50 supervised scans. However, a minimum number of ultrasounds under supervision to achieve clinical competency has not been determined for nurses and/or midwives. Attaining clinical competence is learner dependent.

Whenever nurses, nurse practitioners, or midwives implement a new procedure into practice, the issue of training and cost needs to be addressed. In a study performed by Stringer et al.[15] at the University of Pennsylvania Medical Center and School of Nursing, it was determined that nurses were able to acquire competency in *limited* ultrasound at a reasonable cost. In this study, the nurses completed 12 hours of didactic education and a clinical practicum consisting of 6–9 hours and approximately 15 ultrasound examinations resulting in a mean time of 7.5 hours. The cost per nurse was $1,037.55 (in 2003 dollars). This cost can be further reduced by utilizing home study programs for the 12 hours of recommended (at the time of the study) didactic education as compared with paying lecturers to present the information on an individual basis (12 hours at $41.28/hour) as in Stringer's study.[15]

DOCUMENTATION AND RETRIEVAL

After an ultrasound examination has been completed, a record of the sonogram needs to become part of the maternal chart.[4–6,9] The sonogram needs to be documented with appropriate still images or video or secured in an archival system in the event that the sonogram needs to be revaluated or compared at a later date. The permanent copy of the examination should be labeled, and the results should be documented in the patient's medical record. For instance, if an ultrasound examination is done in the emergency room, the indication for the ultrasound examination, along with the findings and plan of management, should be documented. After consultation and/or discussion with a provider, further studies may be indicated. If the patient is not compliant or unable to be compliant with follow-up appointments, a method for follow-up and documentation specific to this issue should be established by institutional procedures and protocols as well.[4–6,9]

ULTRASOUND FOR NONDIAGNOSTIC PURPOSES

The use of ultrasound for pure entertainment and/or psychosocial reasons is discouraged by many organizations including the U.S. Food and Drug Administration (FDA)[7] and AIUM.[9] The AIUM advocates for the responsible use of diagnostic ultrasound for medical benefits only. As stated in their

document, "Prudent Use in Obstetrics," the AIUM advocates "the responsible use of diagnostic ultrasound and strongly discourages the non-medical use of ultrasound for entertainment purposes. The use of ultrasound without a medical indication to view the fetus, obtain a picture of the fetus or determine the fetal gender is inappropriate and contrary to responsible medical practice. Ultrasound should be used by qualified health professionals to provide medical benefit to the patient."[20]

When the AIUM receives information that a practice, company, or individual is offering or promoting ultrasound for entertainment or nonmedical use, the AIUM first verifies the complaint, notifies the FDA, and then notifies the alleged offender that they have been reported to the FDA.[21]

Keepsake Fetal Imaging

In the past, for many reasons, hospitals or practices have refused to give to the parents hard copies of the fetal images as a keepsake. One of the side effects of this rule was that "keepsake video imaging" companies began to spring up. For a fee, a two- or three-dimensional (2D/3D) sonogram would be performed and the parents could purchase videos, DVDs, or photographs of the fetus. One of the concerns of such easily available unregulated services is that any pregnant woman could have a nonmedically indicated sonogram in addition to her medically indicated sonogram, thus increasing the fetal ultrasound exposure time.

In response to this concern, the AIUM published a statement recognizing that fetal sonography may have an impact on parental–fetal bonding. And, for this reason, parents may desire to have a sonogram performed to acquire a permanent copy of the images. To support this belief and to diminish the number of nonmedically indicated sonograms, the AIUM (1) supports providing images or video clips to the parents during medically indicated ultrasound examinations and recommends (2) that these sonograms be performed by appropriately trained and credentialed medical professionals (physicians, registered sonographers, or sonography registry candidates) who have received specialized training in fetal imaging.[19]

CONSENT FOR ULTRASOUND

The issue of obtaining a written informed consent prior to performing a POC sonogram is still being debated. Often the circumstances requiring a POC ultrasound make it difficult to obtain a written informed consent prior to performing the scan. Although it may be institution- or practice-dependent as to whether a written informed consent is needed, it may be beneficial, at a minimum, to verbally inform the woman why the POC sonogram is being performed and what structures or organs are to be imaged. It may be of equal importance to add that the POC ultrasound is a specific exam being performed to assess a specific complaint and will not include all fetal structures or assessment for anomalies.

CONCLUSION

Nurses, midwives, nurse practitioners, and PAs working in obstetrics, gynecology, and/or assisted reproductive technologies are incorporating ultrasound skills into their everyday practice. Many clinical situations encountered are ideal for the application of ultrasound.

These same clinicians possess the ideal assessment skills required for obstetric and gynecologic triage. Knowledge and skill in sonography can only serve to enhance the success of triage, expedite evaluation and diagnosis, and decrease patient anxiety, as well as decrease waiting time.

Sonography requires the acquisition of specific didactic information and the demonstration of clinical competence. Once the skills are acquired, continuing educational competence must go hand in hand with continued practice. A realistic concern among radiologists is that untrained personnel will utilize ultrasound. Dr. Roy Filly predicted in 1988 that ultrasound would become the new stethoscope. He said, "As we look at the proliferation of ultrasound instruments in the hands of untrained physicians, we can only come to the unfortunate realization that diagnostic sonography truly is the next stethoscope: poorly utilized by many but understood by few."[22] Only proper training and education can prevent this from continuing.

REFERENCES

1. Minton K, Abuhamad A. 2012 Ultrasound first forum proceedings. *J Ultrasound Med.* 2013;32:555–566.
2. Hoppmann R, Cook T, Hunt P, et al. Ultrasound in medical education: a vertical curriculum at the University of South Carolina School of Medicine. *J SC Med Assoc.* 2006;102:330–334.
3. American Institute of Ultrasound in Medicine. Point-of-care ultrasound: emerging applications, emerging users. September, 2011. http://www.aium.org/publications/soundWavesWeekly/article.aspx?aId=89&iId=20100916. Accessed February 15, 2012.
4. American College of Obstetricians and Gynecologists. *Ultrasonography in pregnancy.* Practice bulletin #101. Washington, DC: ACOG; 2009.
5. Association of Women's Health, Obstetric, and Neonatal Nurses (AWHONN). 2010. *Ultrasound examinations performed by nurses in obstetric, gynecologic, and reproductive medicine settings: clinical competencies and education guide* (3rd ed.). Washington, DC: AWHONN; 2010.
6. American College of Nurse Midwives (ACNM). *Position statement: midwives' performance of ultrasound in clinical practice.* Silver Springs, MD: ACNM; 2012.
7. U.S. Department of Health and Human Services. *Diagnostic ultrasound in pregnancy.* NIH Publication No. 84-667. Bethesda, MD: National Institutes of Health; 1984.
8. American College of Radiology (ACR). *Practice guidelines for the performance of obstetrical ultrasound.* Washington, DC: ACR; 2007:1025–1033.
9. American Institute of Ultrasound in Medicine. AIUM practice guideline for the performance of obstetric ultrasound examinations. *J Ultrasound Med.* 2013;32:1083–1101. doi:10.7863/ultra.32.6.1083.
10. American Institute of Ultrasound in Medicine. *AIUM practice guideline for the performance of pelvic ultrasound examinations.* Laurel, MD: AIUM; 2009.
11. American Institute of Ultrasound in Medicine. *AIUM practice guideline for the performance of a focused reproductive endocrinology and infertility scan.* Laurel, MD: AIUM; 2012.
12. American Institute of Ultrasound in Medicine (AIUM) and the Society for Reproductive Endocrinology and Infertility (SREI), an affiliate of the American Society of Reproductive Medicine (ASRM). AIUM practice guideline for ultrasonography in reproductive medicine. Laurel, MD: AIUM; 2008.
13. Dresang LT, MacMillan RW, Dees J. Teaching prenatal ultrasound to family medicine residents. *Fam Med.* 2004 Feb;36(2):98–107.
14. American Institute of Ultrasound in Medicine (AIUM). Training guidelines for physicians who evaluate and interpret diagnostic abdominal, obstetric, and/or gynecologic ultrasound examinations. Laurel, MD: AIUM; April 10, 2013. http://aium.org/officialStatements/47. Accessed December 8, 2013.
15. Stringer M, Miesnik SR, Brown LP, Menei L, Macones GA. Limited obstetric ultrasound examinations: competency and cost. *J Obstet Gynecol Neonatal Nurs.* 2003; 32:307–312.
16. American Registry of Diagnostic Medical Sonographers. RDMS SPI requirement and general prerequisites. 2012. http://www.ardms.org/files/downloads/Prerequisite_Chart.pdf. Accessed December 8, 2013.
17. Society for Diagnostic Medical Sonographers (sdms.org).
18. Oregon House Bill (HB 2014) Related to Medical Imaging. http://www.leg.state.or.us/13reg/measpdf/hb2100.dir/hb2104.en.pdf

19. American Institute of Ultrasound in Medicine (AIUM). *Guidelines for hands-on scanning in pregnant subjects during AIUM-sponsored educational activities.* Laurel, MD: AIUM; 2005. http://aium.org/officialStatements/30. Accessed December 8, 2013.

20. American Institute of Ultrasound in Medicine (AIUM). *Prudent use of ultrasound.* Laurel, MD: AIUM; 2012.

21. American Institute of Ultrasound in Medicine (AIUM). *Keepsake fetal imaging.* Laurel, MD: AIUM; 2012. http://aium.org/officialStatements/31. Accessed December 8, 2013.

22. Filey R. http://www.diagnosticimaging.com/articles/luminaries-make-pledge-recapture-lost-sonography, 2006.

CHAPTER 9

Image Acquisition

ULTRASOUND PHYSICS

Ultrasound is "sound" that is at a frequency above the range that can be heard by the human ear. Ultrasound is defined as an acoustic oscillation or sound wave with a frequency greater than 20,000 Hertz (Hz) or 2 megahertz (MHz).[1] For diagnostic purposes, ultrasound energy is transmitted into the human body with the returning echoes forming an image. The returning signals are referred to as being *echogenic* (producing echoes), *hypoechogenic* (producing low levels of returning echoes), or *hyperechogenic* (producing high levels of returning echoes).

The transmission of ultrasound energy from one place to another is termed *propagation*. The speed at which ultrasound energy moves is its *propagation speed*. Propagation speed is dependent on the type of substance through which the energy is transmitted. Sound waves propagate through matter by causing the vibration of molecules; the stiffness, elasticity, and density of the matter (i.e., liquid, tissue, bone) that the molecules make up determine how fast the sound waves move. Generally speaking, the stiffer the matter, the higher the velocity of movement of the sound (sound propagation). For example, when comparing water to bone, bone is denser and will produce a greater vibration of molecules and a higher propagation speed.

The frequency of sound allows for the differentiation of instruments into certain categories. Frequency is defined as the number of vibrations that occur per unit of time; it is expressed in MHz: the greater the number of vibrations that occur, the higher the frequency (in MHz); the lower the number of vibrations that occur, the lower the frequency.

Frequency also impacts how sound waves will be transmitted: the higher the frequency, the shorter the sound wave (wavelength) and the better the resolution or image acquisition. But the frequency also determines the depth through which sound can penetrate structures, tissues, and organs. Therefore, with higher frequency transducers, the image obtained will have higher resolution. The downside of the high-frequency transducer is that the depth of imaging ability will be compromised, and deeper structures cannot be visualized. With lower transducer frequency, the sound wave is longer (wavelength), allowing it to achieve greater depth of transmission; the downside is that the resolution is decreased.

The ultrasound transducer is a device that transmits and receives energy. It is responsible for converting electrical energy to mechanical energy within the ultrasonic frequency range as it sends the ultrasound signal through the body. It then converts the returning mechanical energy back into electrical energy, which then displayed as an image.

The piezoelectric element within the transducer converts one form of energy into another. The piezoelectric element is comprised of ceramic material. When electrical voltage is supplied to the piezoelectric element, it causes vibration at the element's resonant (operating) frequency. This resonant frequency depends on the element's thickness: the thinner the element, the higher the resonant frequency of the transducer and vice versa. Transducers are manufactured with different thicknesses of piezoelectric elements, which then determines the resonant or operating frequency.

SONOGRAPHY DISPLAY MODES

There are two display modes for the sound waves that are being returned to the machine: A-mode and B-mode. A-mode represents amplitude modulation, which is a single dimension display consisting of a horizontal baseline. The baseline represents time or distance upward deflections that indicate the different acoustic interfaces.

Sonography in obstetrics and gynecology utilizes B-mode, or brightness mode, meaning that each echo returned to the transducer provides a "brightness-modulated" display. B-scans are B-mode displays that provide a cross-section of objects in real time. In the early days of sonography, the B-mode machines only provided static or frozen images. Modern machines allow movement to be visualized; these scans are termed "real-time" scans.

M-mode is a graphic B-mode display in a single dimension that represents the motion of an object, such as cardiac activity. M-mode measures distance over time, allowing the calculation of fetal heart rate. M-mode is primarily used in fetal echocardiography.

The echoes returning from tissue and bone have different degrees of reflection that produce the shades of gray in the image seen on the monitor or in the film or print. The denser the tissue, the greater amount of returning echoes, and the whiter or brighter appearing image. Fluid-filled organs lack the necessary density to reflect echoes back to the transducer; the majority of the echoes pass right through. Therefore, fluid appears black. Such structures are referred to as being anechoic or hypoechoic.

DOPPLER ULTRASOUND TRANSDUCER OPERATION

There are two basic types of Doppler transducer operation in medical ultrasound: continuous-wave Doppler and pulsed-wave Doppler. Continuous-wave systems detect both the transmission and reception of sound wave simultaneously. Both continuous- and pulsed-wave Doppler studies are used to detect the presence and direction of blood flow through vessels. This is referred to as the *Doppler shift,* which measures the difference in the frequency of the reflected sound compared to the frequency of the transmitted sound. Doppler shift depends on the *insonating frequency,* the velocity of moving blood, and the angle between the sound beam and the direction of the moving blood. If the sound beam is perpendicular to the direction of blood flow, there will be no Doppler shift and therefore no display of flow in the vessel. The angle of the sound beam should be less than 60 degrees at all times.

Pulsed transducers or pulse-echo ultrasound transducers send short bursts of sound energy into the imaged area. Return echoes are produced by the different characteristics or densities of the material being studied.

Color Flow Doppler Ultrasound

Color flow Doppler is a form of pulsed-wave Doppler in which the energy of the returning echoes is displayed as an assigned color. By convention, echoes representing flow toward the transducer are typically seen as shades of red, and those representing flow away from the transducer are seen as shades of blue. Color Doppler ultrasound (also referred to as color flow ultrasound) is a technique for visualizing the direction or presence of motion (typically blood flow) within an image plane. The color display is superimposed on the B-mode image, thus allowing simultaneous visualization of anatomy and flow dynamics.

Spectral Doppler Ultrasound

Spectral Doppler is a form of ultrasound image display in which the spectrum of flow velocities is represented graphically on the Y-axis with time displayed on the X-axis; both pulsed-wave and continuous-wave Doppler are displayed in this way.

Duplex Doppler Ultrasound

Duplex Doppler is an image display in which both spectral and color flow are used simultaneously. This facilitates accurate anatomical location of the blood flow under investigation.

Transducers

The choice of which transducer should be used depends on the depth of the structure being imaged. The higher the frequency of the transducer crystal, the less penetration it has but the better the resolution and vice versa.

All transducers have an indicator ridge, button, or arrow that distinguishes orientation. The indicator ridge on the transducer corresponds with the indicator on the monitor (upper left of the image, sometimes the corporate logo) so that the operator can determine which side of the body is being imaged. Ultrasound images are typically displayed as a mirror image. Depending on transducer orientation, when facing the monitor, the left side of the screen in the image is the patient's right (in the transverse plane) or the patient's head (longitudinal plane). (Refer to scan plane section for additional information.) The top of the screen is where the transducer is located on the body. It is recommended that the operator hold the ridge under the thumb so as to not confuse direction during scanning. If the monitor doesn't have an indicator mark, generally, the left side of screen corresponds to the side of transducer under the thumb (Figure 9–1A). Figure 9–1 (B–H) demonstrates the visual progression as the transducer receives the image and how it will then appear to the operator.

Each transducer has an inherent frequency that is a function of its crystal composition and shape. Many of the newer probes offer several frequencies within one probe. The frequency of the probe is determined by the propagation speed of the transducer material

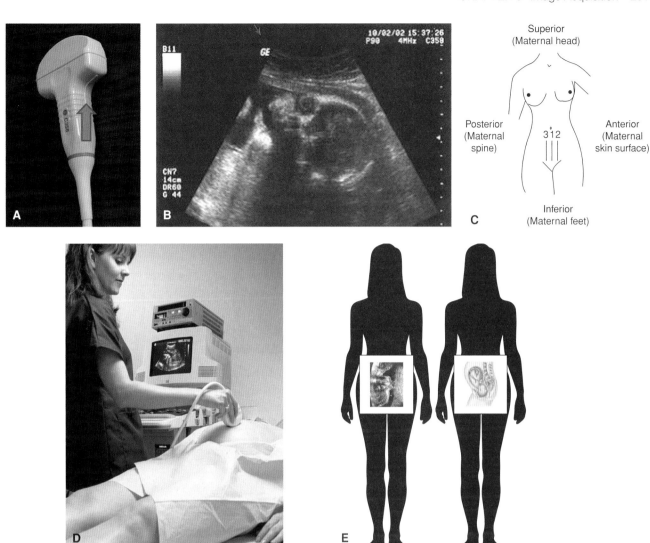

FIGURE 9–1. Visual progression as the transducer receives an image and it is transmitted to the operator. The notch on transducer **(A)** corresponds to the side and/or the top of the monitor displaying the company's logo **(B)** to differenti-ate right from left and superior from inferior. On schematic drawing **C,** again, the notch of the transducer is directed toward the woman's head (superior). So, on the corresponding image **(B)**, the top of the screen is toward the woman's head, the bottom of the screen is toward her feet, and the image is a mirror image of right/left (screen left is patient's right and vice versa). **D** shows the relationship of the transducer placement (longitudinal) on the woman's uterus producing the image on the monitor. **E** takes that image off of the screen and places it on the silhouettes to show the ultrasound image in comparison with the fetal anatomic image. This example demonstrates how the fetal presentation can be determined by initially placing the transducer longitudinally, beginning suprapubically and moving superior toward the maternal sterum. That which is under the transducer superpubically is the presenting part (vertex in the image above). (*continued*)

and the thickness of the transducer element. There are basically four different probe shapes used in obstetrical imaging: linear, sector, curved linear, and the intracavity or endovaginal transducer. These probes typically range in frequency from 2.5 MHz, which is 2.5 million cycles per second, to 10 MHz, which is 10 million cycles per second. Probe selection is based on imaging needs.

The display or shape of the screen varies depend-ing on the type of transducer used. The sector transducer produces more of a wedge-type format whereas linear transducers produce a rectangular format (Figure 9–2).

Transducers for transabdominal OB/GYN imag-ing generally range from 3 to 6 MHz, whereas endovaginal transducers use a higher frequency, to 5 to 10 MHz. Transducers are expensive, often in the $10,000 price range because of their specialized functions. The transducer is also the most often and most easily damaged component of the machine. If a transducer is dropped, the piezoelectric elements or "crystals" can be easily damaged.

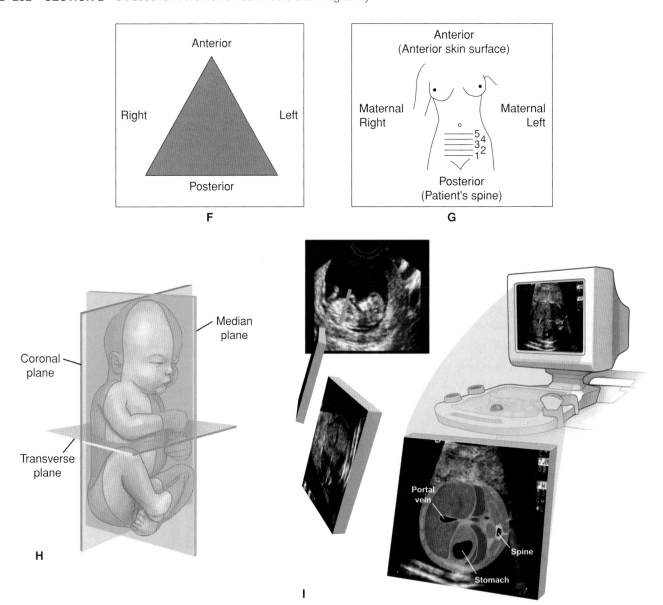

FIGURE 9–1. (*Continued*) **F** is a schematic representation of the monitor indicating direction and postion if the notch on the transducer is positioned toward the patient's right side, in the transverse plane (**G**). The top of the image corresponds to the patient's anterior, bottom of image is patient's posterior, and the right and left correspond directly with the patient. **H** demonstrates the coronal, medial, and transverse (sagittal) planes of the fetus. **I** shows the progression of imaging from the time the transducer is placed on the fetus: a "slice" of anatomic structure is visualized by the transducer. That "slice" is transmitted to the ultrasound monitor. In that process, the slice is "rotated" or "flipped" (similar to a slice of bread being removed from the loaf and "flipped" onto the monitor). Using this same type of demonstration, the fetal abdominal "slice" is taken and and rotated prior to being viewed on the monitor.

The difference in transducers is the resolution of the image it produces and the ability to delineate various tissue densities. For instance, a fluid-filled bladder or an area of fresh blood will have no or minimal echoes (anechoic or hypoechoic) returned to the transducer, so the image displayed is darker than the surrounding tissues or black. As blood begins to clot, more echoes will be returned to the transducer and will be displayed as different shades of gray. The denser the tissue or reflector, the whiter or brighter

(hyperechoic) the image will be. A combination of fluid and tissue will appear in varying degrees of black, gray, or white.

An important concept to remember when choosing the appropriate transducer is that the higher the frequency of the transducer, the greater the resolution but the shallower the penetration. Inversely, the lower the frequency, the lower the resolution, and the greater or deeper the penetration will be. The frequency of the transducer, the transducer diameter, and the distance/

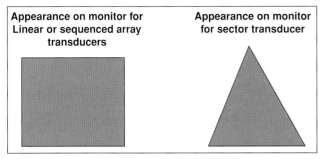

FIGURE 9–2. Monitor display formats for two types of ultrasound transducers.

depth of the structure being examined are pivotal in the production of the image quality. Other factors that influence which transducer to choose include the type of ultrasound exam to be performed. These include the approach (abdominal versus vaginal), fetal gestational age, amount of abdominal adipose tissue, and what types of transducers are available.

The development of the transvaginal (TV) or endovaginal (EV) ultrasound has produced the greatest impact on obstetric and gynecologic imaging in recent years, especially in the first trimester. Using the TV probe, fetal cardiac activity is identifiable as early as four weeks' postconception, and ectopic pregnancies are now more accurately diagnosed. In the gynecologic evaluation, endometrial thickness can be easily measured with the TV prove. For the woman undergoing advanced reproductive technologies, ovarian function and follicular response can be monitored and evaluated. Transvaginal imaging may even be implemented throughout pregnancy for those areas of interest that do not require deep penetration. These may include evaluation of the lower uterine segment, prior cesarean section scar evaluation, cervical length measurement, and placental evaluation in low-lying placentas or previa.

Transducer Maintenance

Endovaginal transducers need to be cleaned and disinfected after each patient. The American Institute of Ultrasound in Medicine (AIUM) provides detailed instructions in cleaning and disinfecting the TV probes. When performed properly, a reduction in microbes by 99% can be achieved.[2] With endocavity ultrasound probes, however, there is the potential for coming into contact with mucus membranes. Additionally, although the probe needs to be routinely protected by a single-use disposable probe cover, AIUM states that leakage rates of 0.9% to 2% for condoms and 8% to 81% for commercial probe covers have been observed in recent studies. Therefore, it is recommended that the probe be cleaned followed by high-level disinfection between each use and a probe cover or condom be used as an aid to keeping the probe clean.

SCAN PLANES

Orientation of the ultrasound image is paramount in the interpretation of the data. When referring to the scan plane, the terms most often used are *sagittal* (*longitudinal*), *transverse,* and *coronal* (Figure 9–3). The terms longitudinal and transverse refer to the placement and relationship of the transducer to the anatomy (Figures 9–4 and 9–5). The terms sagittal and coronal are used when referring to the view obtained by the probe.

The median plane is a vertical plane that divides the body into anterior and posterior segments through the midline of the body. The planes parallel to the midline are sagittal or longitudinal. At right angles to all of these planes are the coronal planes. The transverse plane divides the body into superior and inferior segments.

When the abdominal transducer is in the longitudinal plane, the "notch" indicator on the probe should be pointing to the patient's head so that the image on the screen should be maternal head to the left of the screen and maternal feet to the right of the screen. An easy way to check to see if the probe is being held correctly is by placing a finger under the transducer head and noting what side of the image on the screen is affected. Imaging in the transverse plane involves turning the transducer 90 degrees counterclockwise. In this plane, the patient's right is to the left of the

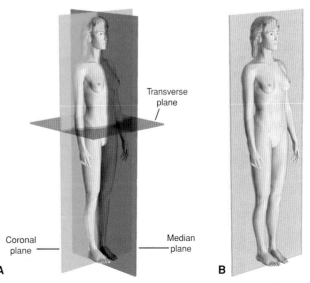

FIGURE 9–3. Anatomic planes: transverse, coronal [in both **A** (green) and **B** (blue)], and medial.

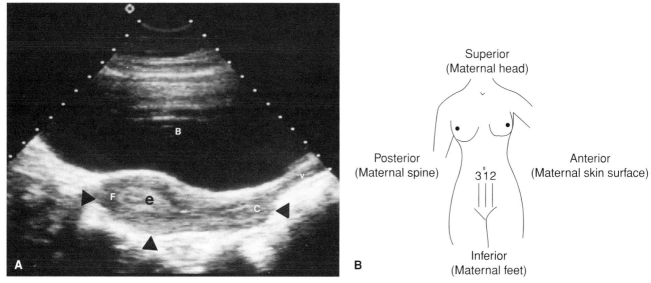

FIGURE 9–4. Transabdominal image **(A)** as seen on the display monitor with the longitudinal scan planes noted on the schematic **(B)**. The image demonstrates the maternal bladder (B) and the uterus (U) showing the relaxed detrusor muscle (DM) surrounding the inner mucosal layer (MU). In the longitudinal image, the body is divided into right and left, and the image is displayed as if you are looking in from the right side.

screen, and the maternal left is on the screen right. This mirrored-imaged approach is also used for x-ray, computed tomography (CT), and magnetic resonance imaging (MRI) imaging (Figure 9–1). The instruction manual specific to the machine being used will describe the proper technique needed to acquire the appropriate image direction. In gynecologic imaging, as in all imaging, it is extremely important not to confuse the patient's right and left sides.

Coronal views of the female pelvis are not typically acquired transabdominally; however, the coronal view will be discussed further when referring to transvaginal scanning. Coronal views divide the anatomy into front and back segments.

When determining fetal position transabdominally, begin with the probe in the longitudinal or transverse plane low in the pelvis or at the cervix and gradually move the transducer superiorly. The fetal part at the cervix is the presenting part. If the fetus is not in a cephalic presentation, follow the fetus's spine to the head. Next, find the stomach and the heart to ensure correct (left-sided) situs. This will determine the *fetal lie*. (For example, ask yourself: Is the head cephalic or breech? Is the spine toward the maternal left, right, anterior, or posterior? Given this, which side of the baby is up?)

Transvaginal orientation of the image requires a different perspective. The scan planes are no longer

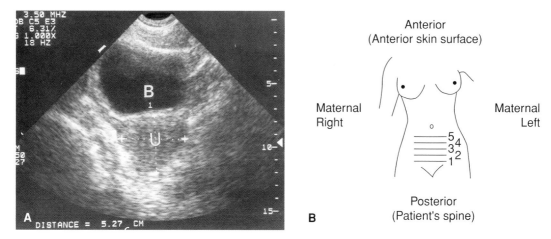

FIGURE 9–5. Transverse, transabdominal image **(A)** of a distended bladder superior to the uterus. Compare with scan planes in schematic **(B)**.

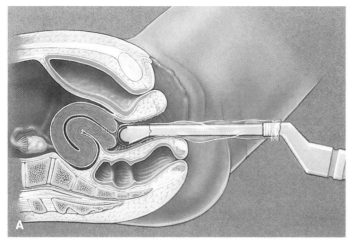

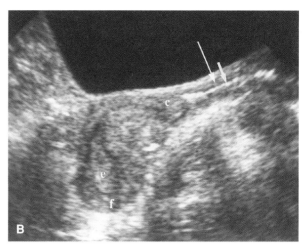

FIGURE 9–6. **(A)** diagram of transvaginal probe and retroflexed uterus. **(B)** Transvaginal sagittal image showing vagina at large arrow. Small arrow indicates the white strip, which is the endovaginal canal.

longitudinal and transverse but longitudinal and coronal. Transvaginal orientation does take practice. Remember, the top of the screen is where the probe is located, the bottom of the screen is toward the patient's head (Figures 9–6, 9–7, and 9–8).

ULTRASOUND BIOEFFECTS: THERMAL AND NONTHERMAL

When ultrasound waves propagate or move through tissue, there is the potential for damage to that tissue.

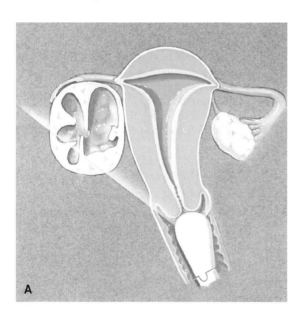

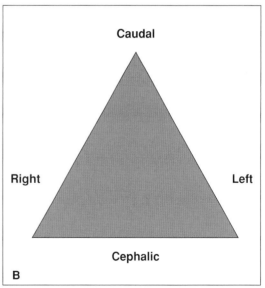

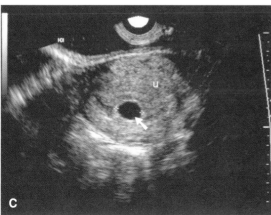

FIGURE 9–7. Transvaginal coronal view **(A)** with image and **(B)** schematic of image direction. The transducer tip **(A)** is at the cervix, and the transducer notch in this diagram is on the left. The cervix is closest to the transducer tip and therefore represents the top of the monitor (image **B**). The uterine fundus is farther from the tip of the transducer and is therefore at the bottom of the monitor screen **(C)**. The image is "inverted" in representation. Maternal right/left are the same as monitor right/left.

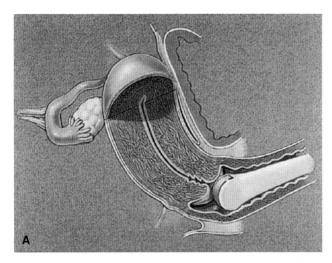

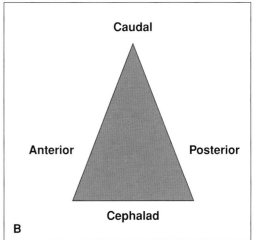

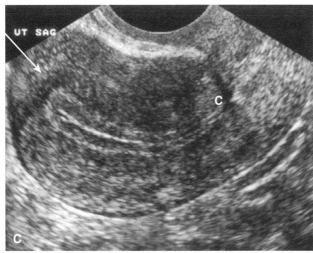

FIGURE 9–8. Transvaginal sagittal view. **(A)** Transvaginal probe tip at cervix. **(B)** Schematic of image direction when transducer is in this position. **(C)** The acquired image from this transducer placement. The transducer tip **(A)** is at the cervix, and the transducer notch in this diagram is up. The uterine fundus is on the left (arrow), and the cervix on the right in **C**.

There are two known mechanisms that can cause damage to the bone and tissue: thermal and nonthermal mechanisms.

Thermal Effects

With thermal effects, the tissue absorbs the ultrasound wave and heat builds. Bone has the highest absorption, and the temperature can rise rapidly. Adult bone absorbs nearly all of the ultrasound energy, whereas fetal bone heat absorption depends on the amount of calcification that has occurred. In soft tissue (i.e., organs), absorption is less than bone. Water or amniotic fluid, on the other hand, typically does not absorb ultrasonic energy and experience little temperature rise.

The first potential mechanism for causing thermal effect is in the volume of tissue exposed to the ultrasound beam. The greatest rise in temperature occurs in the area between where the ultrasound beam enters the tissue and the *focal zone*, which is where the resolution is the greatest. In addition, the volume of tissue exposed depends on the type of scanning technique: is the beam moving or being held stationary? It takes time for the temperature to rise; therefore, the longer the transducer remains in one place, the greater the possibility for the temperature to rise. Additionally, some ultrasound waves are transmitted in pulsed-wave form, meaning that there is a burst of energy and then a period during which no energy is transmitted. There can be a cumulative effect if the pulsed energy is used in a concentrated area over a prolonged period of time.

In scanned modes of ultrasound, such as B-mode and color flow Doppler, the energy is moving and being distributed over a large area. Therefore, the highest temperature is typically at the surface where the ultrasound beam enters the body, as is the case if the transducer is stationary and you are angling or heel-toeing the probe only.

In spectral Doppler, the power is concentrated along a single line, and energy is deposited along that stationary beam or *sample gate*. These are known as *unscanned modes*. The energy is being focused over a smaller volume of tissue than with the scanned modes, thus the highest temperature is found between the surface and the focus. In the obese woman, her adipose tissue can absorb much of the heat, but in the woman with a thin abdominal wall, the energy is transmitted to the fetus. It is similar to holding a hot iron over a piece of cloth for a prolonged period of time versus moving the iron over the entire piece of clothing. Similarly, it is also the difference between holding a hot iron over a folded towel on top of the cloth versus holding the iron directly on the cloth. On the other hand, M-mode utilizes grayscale or B-mode scanning and therefore does not increase the energy. For this reason, in the first trimester, only M-mode should be used to record fetal heart rate, not pulsed Doppler.

The person performing the ultrasound examination has the ability to minimize the temperature rise.[3] Temperature increases depend on intensity, the duration of exposure in one location, the transducer focal point size and location, and the absorption of the energy. The intensity of the sound wave depends on the equipment chosen for the exam and, therefore, is operator dependent. The duration of exposure is also controlled by the operator. The fixed-focused transducers have a focus that can't be changed, but the operator can change the focus on multielement array transducers. Understanding how the equipment works is of paramount importance in reducing thermal exposure to the patient. The goal is to obtain the necessary medical images using the lowest amount of energy and least amount of exposure time.

Nonthermal Effects

Nonthermal bioeffects are also referred to as *mechanical bioeffects* and are not understood as well as thermal effects. They seem to be caused by ultrasound pressure waves passing through or near areas with gas or air pockets, thus causing tissue motion. This is known as *cavitation.* Cavitation is defined as the generation, growth, vibration, and possible collapse of microbubbles within the tissue. It is possible for cavitation to occur in diagnostic ultrasound. However, there is no evidence thus far that diagnostic ultrasound exposure has caused cavitation in humans in the absence of gas bubbles. The concern for the creation of cavitation is when contrast agents are used. However, to minimize the risk of cavitation, always keep the output as low as possible and keep the ultrasound examination time as short as possible to obtain the imaging information needed.[3]

OUTPUT DISPLAY

The output display, which displays the indices that relate to the potential for bioeffects, is displayed on the image screen. These indices were established by the National Electrical Manufacturers Association, the U.S. Food and Drug Administration (FDA), the AIUM, and several other societies. The standard is called the Standard for Real-time Display of Thermal and Mechanical Acoustic Output Indices on Diagnostic Ultrasound Equipment, but it is more commonly called the Output Display Standard or ODS.

Two types of indices are displayed on the ODS. Thermal mechanisms are referred to as the thermal index (TI), and mechanical or nonthermal mechanisms are referred to as mechanical index (M1). The goal of users of diagnostic medical imaging equipment is to acquire the best quality images yet keep the T1 and MI as low reasonably possible.[4] An output display is not required if the equipment is not capable of exceeding an MI or a TI of 1. However, if the transducer and system are capable of exceeding a TI and/or MI of 1, then the display values must be displayed. Increments can be displayed as low as 0.4.

Keep in mind that the thermal indices are only a relative indicator of temperature rise, not an indication of actual temperature. TIs are categorized into three types based on the density of fetal tissue being scanned. The soft tissue index (TIS) informs us as to whether a change in the instrument setting will lead to an increase in temperature within soft homogeneous tissues. The TIC provides the same information for the cranial bone or any bone at or near the surface of the scanning plane. The bone TI (TIB) provides information on temperature changes in bone at or near the focus after the beam has traversed the soft tissue.

ULTRASOUND SAFETY: THE ALARA PRINCIPLE

The ALARA Principle simply stands for "as low as reasonably achievable." In ultrasound, exposure should be kept as low as possible while still acquiring diagnostic images and information.[5] To accomplish this, when using ultrasound for any type of examination, always follow these principles:

- Use the lowest power to acquire the image.
- Use the least amount of time to acquire necessary image.
- Use power or color Doppler only as necessary.

- Do not use pulsed Doppler unless necessary because it creates the greatest energy.
- TI should be ≤1.0.

IMAGE PROCESSING

Transmission controls on the keyboard of the ultrasound machine allow the operator to control the ultrasound output and improve the quality of the image. The controls that affect the intensity include:

- *The Application Selection control* allows the operator to select the type of ultrasound being done (i.e., fetal, ophthalmic, peripheral blood vessel). Different types of exams utilize different intensities. The maximum intensity for each type of exam is regulated by the FDA.
- *The Output Intensity control* (also called transmit, power, or output) is automatically determined once the application or preset is chosen. However, most equipment allows the operator to change intensity levels.
- *The Choice of Field for Exam control* (i.e., B-mode, M-mode, or Doppler) is based on whether the ultrasound beam is stationary or in motion, which affects the energy absorbed by the tissue. If the beam is stationary, the targeted exam area receives increased ultrasound energy.
- *The Pulse Repetition Frequency (PRF) control* determines the output. The higher the PRF, the higher the output.
- *Focusing* occurs when the beam is narrowed, which results in better lateral resolution. Improving lateral resolution means that the beam will be focused longer on one area. It is possible to set the transducer focus at the proper depth to improve the image of that structure without increasing the intensity.
- *Pulse Length* is the length of time the pulse is on. The longer it is on, the greater the likelihood of raising tissue temperature.
- *The Transducer Type* selects the frequency of the transducer. The higher the frequency of the transducer, the greater the output intensity needed to image at greater depths. Therefore, if greater depth is needed, it is recommended to switch to a lower frequency transducer to improve the quality of the image, thus avoiding increasing the intensity. Depth should always be adjusted to include the region of interest. For example, while performing a pregnancy scan, adjust the depth to include

the posterior uterus, but there is no need to image back to the maternal spine.

Manufacturers are required to provide a default setting for the output levels that conform to safe levels. The default levels are automatically set when the machine is turned on but can be adjusted by the operator. If the output levels are changed, careful observation of the TI and MI is imperative. Also, if preset default output levels are being used, there is still a possibility of increasing risk of harm if the exposure time is not minimized.

A second set of controls, referred to as *receiver controls,* affect the image display without having any effect on the output:

- *Receiver Gain controls* control the amplification of the returning signal or echo that is being reflected back by the tissue or fluid; these may be referred to as the *near gain* and *far gain* control. When attempting to image a structure that is deeper within the body cavity, increasing the far gain may improve the quality of the image. When imaging a structure closer to the surface, increasing the near gain control may improve visualization of those structures.
- *Time-Gain compensation (TGC) or overall gain compensation* is also known as the depth gain compensation (DGC). The TGC equalizes the differing intensity of received echoes that may initially be unequal due to differences in reflector depth. For example, for visualizing a fetal part that may be close to the anterior surface of the maternal abdomen and also be able to visualize the placenta, which may be on the posterior wall of the uterus, the TGC would be adjusted so that the sound waves reflected from the placenta, which need to travel farther, are amplified and the sound waves being received from more anterior structures are dampened. This will equalize all of the received signals.
- Many ultrasound machines come with an *automatic gain control* that will automatically adjust the gains to maximize the image quality.
- *Postprocessing of images* includes such functions as the *cine-loop.* Cine-loop allows the operator to move backward or forward through the stored images to locate the best image frame for a particular measurement or for documentation purposes. Most ultrasound machines store multiple images while scanning; this allows the operator to "rewind" or look back through prior images to find the best view of the area of interest.

BASIC CONTROLS AND SETTINGS

Overall gain does not change the frequency or the intensity of the transducer. It determines how much amplification is accomplished in the receiver of the transducer; it is similar to the volume control on a stereo system. Most of the work done by the transducer is done in the "listening" phase of the process. Less than 1% of the transducer's time is spent in transmitting sound waves into the body, leaving more than 99% of the time designated just for receiving the signals. This is called *duty cycle* or *duty factor*.

The time gain compensation (TGC) is also known as the depth gain compensation (DGC). The TGC equalizes the differing intensity of received echoes that may initially be unequal due to differences in reflector depth. For example, when visualizing the posterior uterus in an obese patient, more sound waves are absorbed. In this case, the TGC slope may be steeper than in a patient of normal habitus.

ARTIFACTS

Artifacts are distortions of the anatomic structures on the image. Proper adjustment of two operator-dependent variables—overall gain and TGC—along with appropriate transducer selection can eliminate many of the artifacts commonly seen in ultrasound imaging.

The application of coupling gel eliminates the most common imaging artifacts. Gel is a liquid medium, so that the ultrasound beam can be transmitted through the skin. Ultrasound gel is most commonly used, but substances such as mineral oil have also been used. Also, a good contact between the transducer and the skin or body surface will eliminate air artifacts.

Signal attenuation is another factor in the productions of artifact. Attenuation is a decrease in the amplitude and intensity of the ultrasound signal as the sound travels through a medium such as tissue. Attenuation may occur for any of three reasons: (1) conversion, in which sound is changed into heat; (2) reflection, in which some of the sound waves are returned from the boundary of a medium; and/or (3) scattering, which is the diffusion or redirection of sound in several directions.

Reflection, refraction, reverberation, and mirror imaging are some other types of ultrasound artifacts. For example, a reflection artifact occurs when a strong echo is returned to the transducer from a large acoustic interface (Figure 9–9). This echo

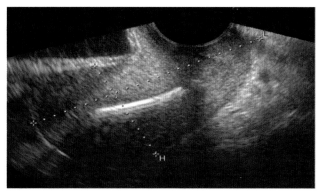

FIGURE 9–9. Reverberation of sound waves off of dense interuterine device (IUD; appearing hyperechoic as a "double line") making structure look "thickened."

bounces back to the same tissues, causing additional echoes parallel and equidistant to the first. Shadowing artifact occurs when the sound beam fails to pass through an object (e.g., a bone does not allow any sound to pass through it) and there is only a shadow seen behind it (Figure 9–10).

Ultrasound operators can often minimize artifact simply by manipulating the transducer. Artifacts are, however, essential for accurate diagnosis. For example, bone typically creates shadow. In a fetus with osteogenesis imperfecta, a strong shadow will not be present.

Artifact may also be the product of the machine itself. There may be a problem with the internal electronics of the machine, such as a broken crystal in the head of the transducer or air bubbles trapped beneath the surface of the transducer membrane. These issues must to be repaired by the manufacturer or someone qualified in ultrasound machine or transducer repair. Preventive maintenance and care of transducers add to the longevity of the equipment and help to maintain the quality of the image.

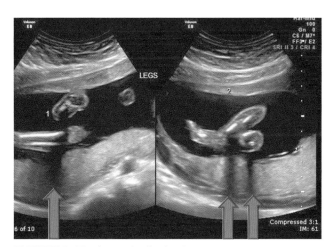

FIGURE 9–10. Acoustic shadowing, at arrows.

ACQUIRING THE BEST IMAGES

The movement of the transducer by the operator greatly influences the quality and accuracy of the image. Techniques that can be used to improve image acquisition include:

- Sliding the transducer across the abdomen to change the area of observation to a different slice or window.
- Using a window that minimizes the depth needed. This will increase resolution.
- Rocking the transducer to focus on an area of interest or to broaden the field of view while staying in the same plane.
- Rotating the transducer from the transverse to the sagittal to view the same structure but from a different angle.
- Compressing the transducer against the patient's skin to improve contact between the transducer and the structure being assessed. Caution must be used with compression because it can not only cause patient discomfort, but can also alter the appearance and measurement of a structure, thus creating inaccurate measurements.

- Scanning from the lateral approach, in obese patients, under the pannus or through the umbilicus to decrease the depth needed.

Proper adjustment of these two operator dependent variables (overall gain and TGC) along with appropriate transducer selection can minimize many of the artifacts commonly seen in ultrasound imaging.

REFERENCES

1. American Institute of Ultrasound in Medicine (AIUM). *Recommended Ultrasound Terminology*. 3rd ed. AIUM 2009.
2. American Institute of Ultrasound in Medicine (AIUM). AIUM Guidelines for Cleaning and Preparing Endocavitary Ultrasound Transducers Between Patients. 2003. Retrieved from: http://aium.org/officialStatements/27
3. American Institute of Ultrasound in Medicine (AIUM). *Medical Ultrasound Safety*. 2nd ed. AIUM; 2009.
4. American Institute of Ultrasound in Medicine (AIUM). Statement on Heat. 2009. Retrieved from: http://aium.org/officialStatements/17
5. American Institute of Ultrasound in Medicine (AIUM). *AIUM As Low As Reasonably Achievable (ALARA) Principle*. 2008. Retrieved from: http://aium.org/officialStatements/39

Point-of-Care Sonography in Gynecology and Reproductive Medicine

The three most common indications for point-of-care (POC) sonography in gynecology include the evaluation of the endometrial thickness, the measurement of follicles during ovarian stimulation with assisted reproductive technologies, and the localization of intrauterine devices (IUDs) pre- and postinsertion. In addition, POC sonography is utilized to measure retained residual urine following birth and in urogynecologic bladder assessments, among other indications.

However, prior to performing any gynecologic sonogram, it is essential to know the anatomy of the female pelvis. It is recommended to have a standard pelvic sonogram performed prior to performing any POC ultrasound. Following the performance of a complete pelvic sonogram, a "limited" or POC gynecologic ultrasound examination can be restricted to a specific organ or measurement.[1] The purpose of this chapter is to describe the anatomic structures and the measurement of these structures sonographically, as well as the documentation and communication of findings.

In the gynecologic or reproductive medicine specialty, a limited or POC sonogram may involve any one or all of the processes listed in Table 10–1. Although POC

TABLE 10–1 LIMITED PELVIC ULTRASOUND EXAMINATION

1. Identification of uterine position and ovaries (including uterine size, shape, and orientation; the endometrium; the myometrium; and the cervix)
2. Measurement of uterus/endometrial thickness
3. Location and measurement of ovarian follicles
4. Identification of an early intrauterine gestational sac (following reproductive medicine procedure)
5. Identification of the yolk sac
6. Identification of number of embryo (s), and measuring embryonic length; and/or
7. Identification of early fetal cardiac activity

Adapted from AWHONN,[12] AIUM,[7] and ASRM.[13]

sonograms following a successful assisted reproductive procedure may include sonographic confirmation of pregnancy, sonography in the first trimester of pregnancy is discussed in Chapter 11.

ULTRASOUND ANATOMY OF THE FEMALE PELVIS

The female pelvis can be imaged using the transabdominal (TA) or transvaginal (TV) approach. TA sonography (TAS) requires a full urinary bladder to displace air-filled bowel from the lower abdomen and to provide an acoustic window through which to visualize the pelvic organs (Figure 10–1). An acoustic window is a structure that has no acoustic impedance (no returning ultrasound signals) and is referred to as *anechoic*. This absence of returning sound waves imparts a black image on the monitor. This lack of impedance allows for passage of sound and enhanced visualization of deeper structures. In the TA approach, the depth of penetration into the body is much deeper, so more structures can be accessed, but it has inherently less resolution than the TV approach.

TVS requires an empty urinary bladder and is performed with high-frequency transducers. High frequency is better for resolution and visualization of the structures, but the depth of penetration of a high-resolution transducer, such as the vaginal probe, is shallower. For TV ultrasound, this penetration depth is accomplished by literally getting physically closer to the structures by way of the tip of the vaginal wand being in close proximity to the structure being imaged. In many circumstances, it is helpful to use both TAS and TVS to visualize the entire pelvis.

URINARY BLADDER

The urinary bladder is an important landmark in identifying pelvic anatomy. The bladder walls are

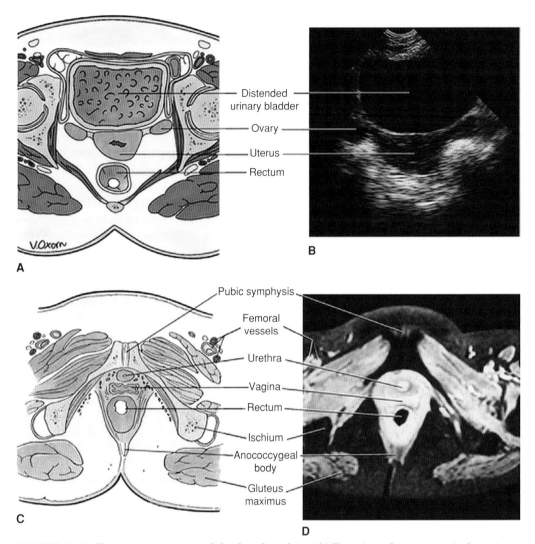

FIGURE 10–1. Transverse sections of the female pelvis. **(A)** Drawing of an anatomical section through the urinary bladder, uterus, and rectum. **(B)** Transverse ultrasound scan. **(C)** Drawing of an anatomical section through the urethra, vagina, and rectum. **(D)** Transverse magnetic resonance image (MRI).

composed of a thick (detrusor) muscle that is lined with a thin mucosa and covered externally by a serosal layer. Bladder distention causes a thinning and stretching of the bladder wall, which then appears as a thin echogenic line. With partial distention, the detrusor muscle is relaxed and appears as a hypoechoic layer around the inner mucosa (Figure 10–2). Ureters can be recognized when they are abnormally filled with fluid. They can be distinguished from the adjacent iliac vessels by their more echogenic walls, anatomical path, and by color Doppler. A urine jet can be seen in grayscale or color Doppler as the ureters enter into the posterior portion of the bladder.

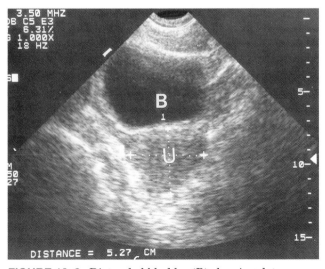

FIGURE 10–2. Distended bladder (B) showing detrusor muscle at arrow, and uterus (U).

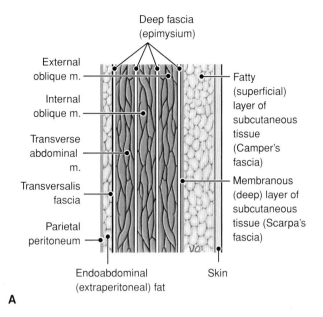

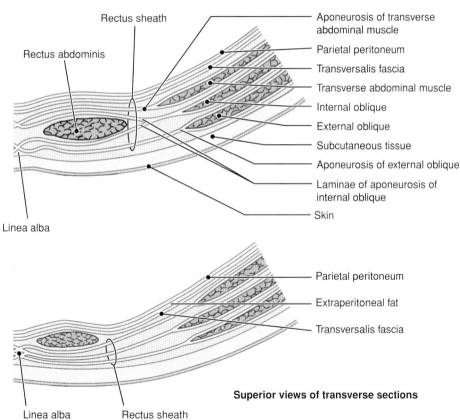

FIGURE 10–3. Diagram of longitudinal and transverse sections of the abdominal wall, showing the rectus abdominis muscle and the contributions of the lateral abdominal muscles to its sheath.

PELVIC MUSCULATURE

On ultrasound, muscles appear as hypoechoic bands of tissue, with low-level echoes and thin linear hyperechoic striations. The skeletal muscles of the false pelvis include the rectus and transverse abdominis and the iliopsoas muscles (Figures 10–3 and 10–4).

The muscles of the true pelvis include the obturator internus muscles, the piriformis muscles, and

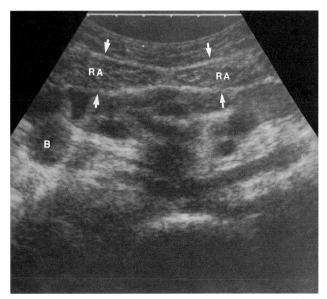

FIGURE 10–4. Transverse image of the anterior abdominal wall, showing the rectus abdominus muscle (RA), the anterior and posterior rectus sheath (arrows), and loops of bowel (B) in the abdominal cavity.

the muscles of the pelvic diaphragm. The latter are composed of three paired muscles: the coccygeus, the pubococcygeus, and the iliococcygeus, which form the floor of the true pelvis and support the pelvic organs (Figures 10–5 and 10–6).

The pubococcygeus and iliococcygeus muscles together form the levator ani muscles (Figure 10–7). The iliopsoas muscles can be identified in the sagittal (longitudinal) imaging as linear structures along the pelvic sidewall that are medial and slightly anterior to the iliacus muscles and as ovoid structures that

are anterior and lateral to the urinary bladder on transverse imaging (Figure 10–8).

The obturator internus muscles run parallel to the lateral walls of the bladder on transverse scans, but are more difficult to identify in the sagittal plane. The muscles of the pelvic diaphragm are seen best in the transverse plane at the level of the cervix.

Many pelvic muscles are difficult to evaluate sonographically. It is not unusual for normal muscles to be mistaken for free fluid, a mass, or other pathology; therefore, it is important to recognize the appearance of muscles, where they attach, and how each muscle is oriented.

PELVIC VASCULATURE

The common iliac arteries branch into the internal and external arteries. The internal and external iliac veins join to form the common iliac vein. The internal iliac vessels lie posterior and slightly lateral to the ovaries and are important landmarks to help identify and locate the ovaries (Figure 10–9), especially when the ovaries are small and lacking follicles.

The internal iliac arteries have a width of 5 to 7 mm and are pulsatile, whereas the veins are typically larger (1 cm), more medially located, and do not pulsate. The blood supply to the uterus and vagina

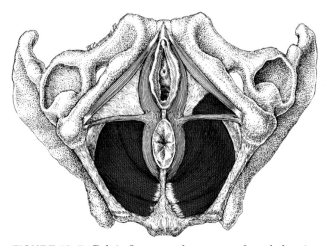

FIGURE 10–5. Pelvic floor muscles as seen from below in the supine female subject. The muscles of the pelvic diaphragm are dark red, and the associated pelvic muscles are light red.

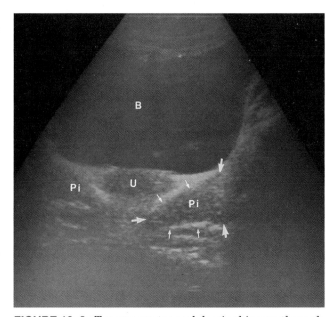

FIGURE 10–6. Transverse transabdominal image through a full bladder (B) showing the uterus (U) and the piriformis muscles (Pi) within the arrows, posterior to the cervix.

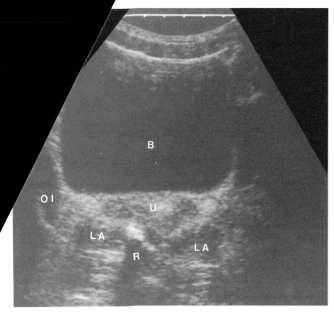

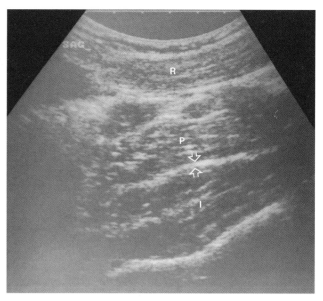

FIGURE 10–7. Transverse transabdominal image of levator ani (LA) muscles, the right obturator internus muscle (OI), bladder (B), and rectum (R), posterior to cervix.

FIGURE 10–8. Sagittal transabdominal image with transducer angled laterally to demonstrate the long axis of the psoas major (P), and the iliacus muscles (I), with interposed fascial plan (arrows).

is via the uterine artery, which is a branch of the internal iliac artery (Figure 10–10).

The uterine arteries give rise to the arcuate arteries, which encircle the uterus and branch into the radial arteries. The radial arteries pass through the myometrium, become the straight arteries at the level of the endometrium, and then branch to form spiral arteries. The blood supply to the endometrium

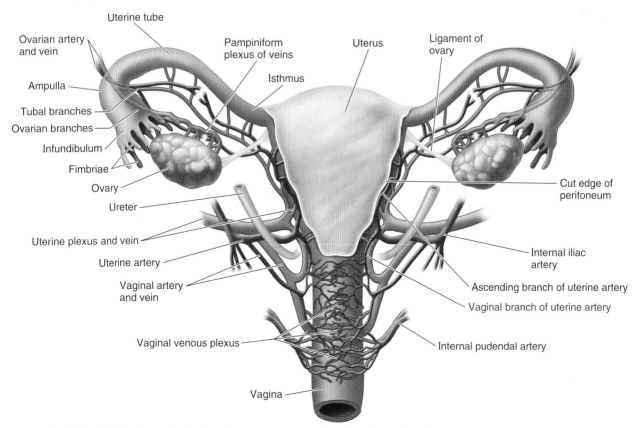

FIGURE 10–9. (A) Blood supply to the uterus, ovaries, and vagina. (*continued*)

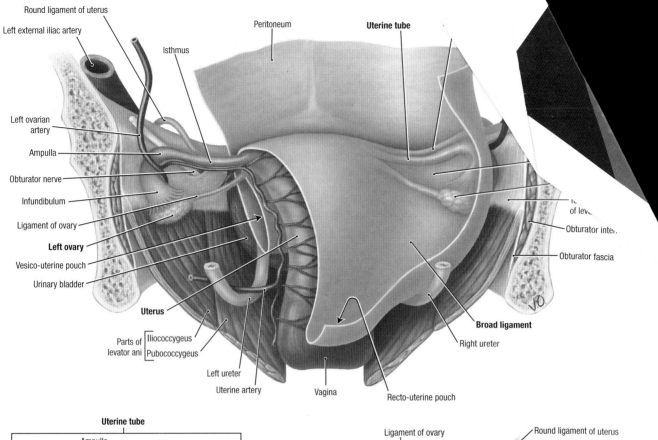

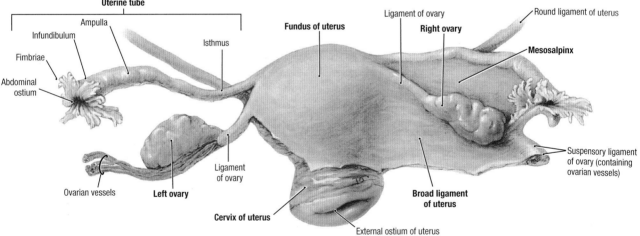

FIGURE 10–9. (*Continued*) **(B)** Broad ligaments.

is from the straight and spiral arteries, the latter being responsive to hormonal changes of the menstrual cycle. The ovarian blood supply is from both the ovarian and uterine artery and vein. The ovarian artery enters the ovarian hilum via the mesovarium, whereas the uterine artery reaches the ovarian hilum via the broad ligament.

UTERUS

The uterus is the most prominent landmark in the pelvis and can be visualized by both TA and TV ultra-sound (Figures 10–11 and 10–12). In the nonpregnant uterus, the cervix represents approximately one-third to one-half of the total uterine length and is approximately twice the diameter of the corpus. The adult uterus is approximately 6 to 8 cm in length and 3 to 5 cm wide.

The typical uterine position is anteverted, although a full bladder will displace an anteverted uterus into a more horizontal position (Figure 10–13). Variations include retroverted uterus, which is the posterior angulation of the uterus and cervix relative to the vagina; retroflexed uterus, which describes the posterior angulation

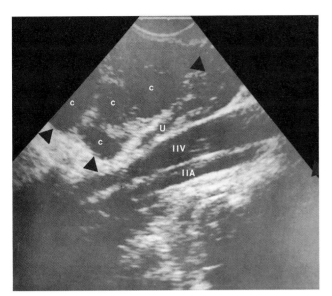

FIGURE 10–10. Sagittal transvaginal scan of left internal iliac artery (IIA) and vein (IIV) posterior to the ovary (arrowheads).

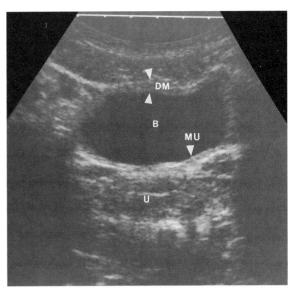

FIGURE 10–12. Transvaginal sagittal image of the uterus (within arrowheads) showing the uterine fundus and the proximal portion of the cervix. M, myometrium; E, endometrium.

of the uterine corpus relative to the cervix; and anteflexed, which is the anterior angulation of the uterine corpus relative to the cervix (Figures 10–14 and 10–15).

Myometrium

The myometrium, which exhibits medium to low-level homogeneous echoes, can be distinguished from the endometrium, which varies in thickness and echogenicity throughout the menstrual cycle. Uterine blood vessels can be imaged using both TA and TV sonography. When seen, arcuate arteries appear as anechoic tubular structures at the periphery of the myometrium. Calcifications may be seen within the arcuate arteries of elderly patients and appear as echogenic foci along the periphery of the uterus.

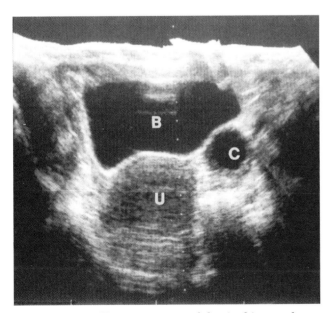

FIGURE 10–11. Transverse transabdominal image showing the anechoic distended bladder (B), uterus (U), and the smooth-walled anechoic corpus luteum cyst (C) in the left ovary. (From Ronald L. Eisenberg, *An Atlas of Differential Diagnosis,* 4th ed. Philadelphia: Lippincott Williams & Wilkins; 2003.)

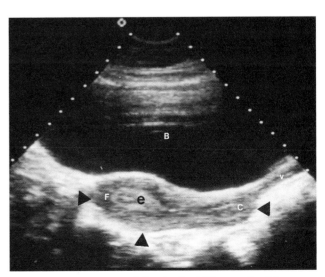

FIGURE 10–13. Transabdominal midline sagittal image of the uterus (within arrowheads), viewed through a distended anechoic urinary bladder (B). The endometrium (e) can be distinguished from the surrounding myometrium. F, fundus; C, cervix; V, vagina.

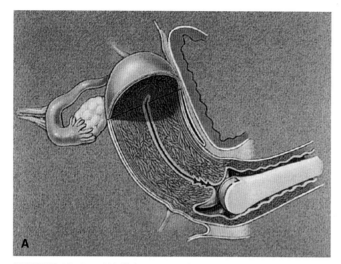
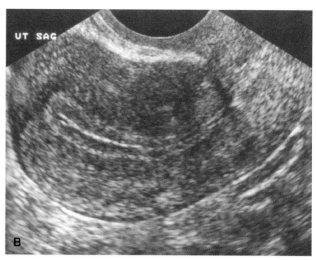

FIGURE 10–14. **(A)** Schematic of vaginal probe directed in the sagittal view of anteflexed uterus. **(B)** Transvaginal sagittal image of the anteflexed uterus in the panel A.

Endometrium

The endometrium is composed of a basal and a functional layer. Changes occur in the uterus in response to estradiol fluctuations and are reflected in overall uterine volume and in the thickness and echogenicity of the endometrium.

After menses, the endometrium appears as a thin echogenic stripe. During the follicular phase, there is a gradual increase, with an increase in endometrial thickness as the endometrium proliferates. The endometrium then appears as a triple line or trilaminar complex composed of the interfaces between the myometrium, endometrium, and the central midline stripe. After ovulation, the secretory endometrium appears thicker and more echogenic (Figure 10–16).

To measure the endometrial thickness, the endometrium should be sonographically viewed in the sagittal plane with a continuous view from the cervix to the fundus. The measurement should include both layers of the endometrium.[2] Place the calipers at the bright leading edge and measure to the bright far edge as noted in the above (Figure 10–16).

The incidence of malignancy in postmenopausal bleeding ranges from 1% to 14%. TV sonography should be the first diagnostic testing done because of the extremely high-negative predictive value of a thin echogenic endometrial stripe. Women with postmenopausal bleeding with an endometrial measurement of 4 mm or less have a risk of malignancy of 1/917, and this measurement reliably excludes endometrial

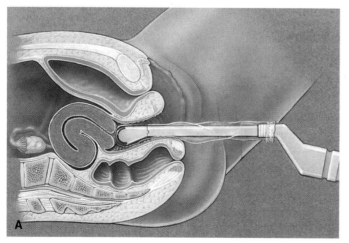
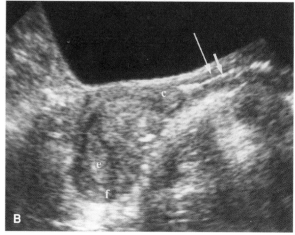

FIGURE 10–15. **(A)** Schematic of vaginal probe directed in sagittal view of retroflexed uterus. **(B)** Transvaginal sagittal image comparison with the schematic in A of retroflexed uterus. White arrows at vagina, which appears elongated secondary to a full bladder. Repeating the scan with an empty bladder would be recommended.

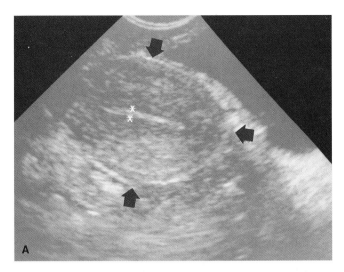

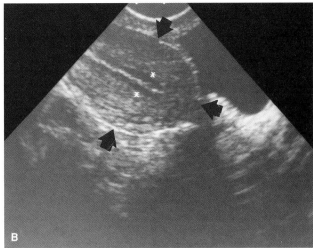

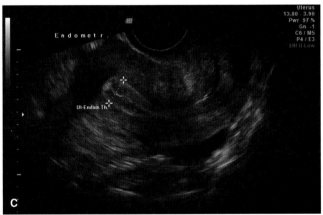

FIGURE 10–16. Changes in the endometrium during the menstrual cycle. **(A)** Early follicular phase after menses showing the uterus (arrows) and the endometrium (white "line" between stars). **(B)** Late proliferative phase, showing the typical triple-line of the endometrium (white line between stars) and the uterus (arrows). **(C)** Early secretory phase, showing the endometrium (between white [+] and the uterus [yellow stars]).

carcinoma. If the endometrial thickness is greater than 4 to 5 mm in a symptomatic postmenopausal woman, pathology cannot be ruled out.[3] In some women, visualization may not be adequate, and a sonohysterography with TV sonography may be needed to visualize the endometrial cavity (Figure 10–17).

CERVIX AND VAGINA

The cervix can be visualized with TV sonography. During TV scanning, the transducer should be placed at or near the external os. This allows for optimal visualization of the cervix as well as the uterus. If the vagina needs to be imaged, the transducer can be partially withdrawn. Mucus within the cervical canal appears echogenic, except during the periovulatory period, when it contains more fluid and appears hypoechoic (Figure 10–18). Small inclusion (nabothian) cysts are frequently seen within the muscle of the cervix at the region of the cervical canal. They appear as thin-walled hypoechoic structures usually less than 1 cm in size. Measurement of cervical length is discussed in Chapter 12.

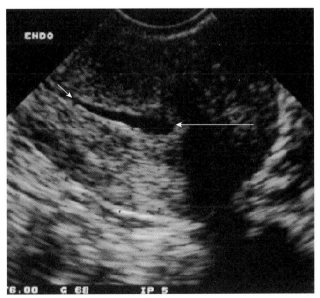

FIGURE 10–17. Sonohysterogram showing normal uterine cavity (anechoic area between arrows).

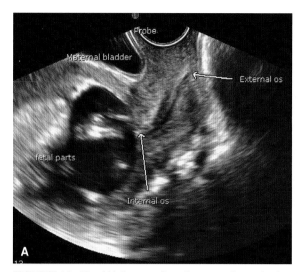
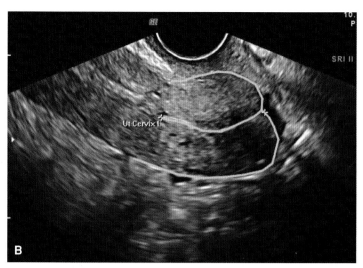

FIGURE 10–18. (**A**) Internal and external cervical os. (**B**) Cervical length with cervix outlined.

On TA examination, the vagina can be seen immediately posterior to the bladder neck. It appears as a collapsed tube exhibiting low-level echoes with a strong central echo from the apposed surfaces of the vaginal mucosa (Figure 10–19).

PELVIC ADNEXA

Bowel

The sonographic appearance of bowel depends on the amount of fluid, gas, and fecal material within its lumen (Figure 10–20). Loops of small bowel can be seen around the uterus and ovaries during TV scanning, often showing peristalsis.

Gas in the small intestine can sometimes obscure adequate visualization of the ovaries. The sigmoid colon and rectum frequently appear echogenic, with posterior wall shadowing from gas and fecal contents. The peristaltic activity demonstrated in small bowel is not seen in the sigmoid colon and rectum, but the peristalsis can sometimes help to discriminate a pelvic mass from other structures.

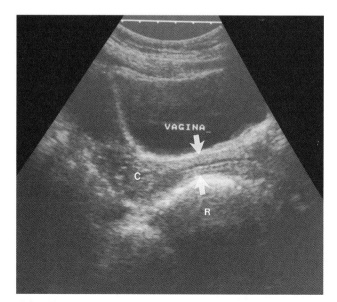

FIGURE 10–19. Midline sagittal transabdominal image of the vagina (between arrows) with the black stripe indicating cervical canal. The vagina is anterior to the rectum (R), posterior to the bladder, and inferior to the cervix (C).

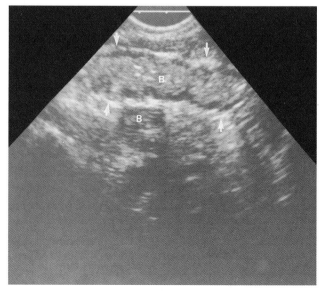

FIGURE 10–20. Transvaginal coronal image of a loop of small intestine among arrows, demonstrating submucosal folds and echogenic bowel (B) contents.

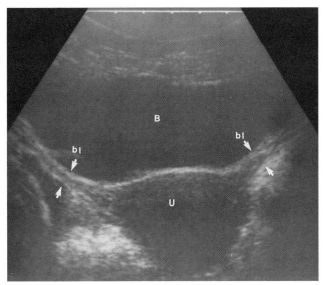

FIGURE 10–21. Transverse transabdominal image of the uterus at the level of the fundus (white arrow at echogenic "line"). The broad ligament (bl) is seen as a tubular structure extending laterally from the uterine corni (between arrows). Normal fallopian tubes are not routinely identified. The bladder (B) and uterus (U) are also identified.

Fallopian Tubes

Normal fallopian tubes, which measure approximately 10 cm in length, are not routinely identified. Since they are small and tortuous, they can be difficult to distinguish from the broad ligament, which appears as band of low-level echoes extending from the uterine cornu lateral to the ovaries (Figure 10–21).

Ovaries

The ovaries are usually located between the uterine fundus and the pelvic sidewall, medial to the

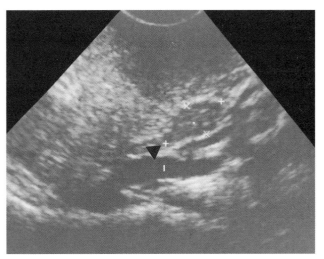

FIGURE 10–23. Transvaginal sagittal image of a postmenopausal ovary (between + marks). The iliac (i) vessels help to identify the ovary when it is small with few visible follicles (arrowhead).

iliopsoas muscles and external iliac vessels, and anterior to the internal iliac vessels. However, the precise location of the ovaries may vary, and they may be identified in the cul-de-sac or above the uterine fundus. Sonographically, ovaries appear as distinct ovoid structures, slightly less echogenic or isoechoic than the myometrium, and contain follicles in premenopausal women (Figure 10–22). The internal iliac vessels also serve as useful ovarian landmarks, especially after menopause, when ovaries are small and devoid of follicles (Figure 10–23).

When the TA approach is used, a full bladder is necessary to visualize the ovaries in the sagittal and transverse planes. Gentle pressure can be applied to the abdominal wall to displace bowel and optimize

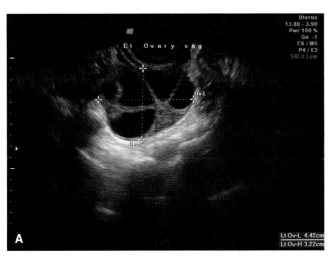
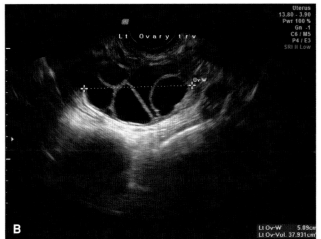

FIGURE 10–22. Transvaginal sagittal scans of left ovarian measurements with multiple developing follicles (anechoic "circles").

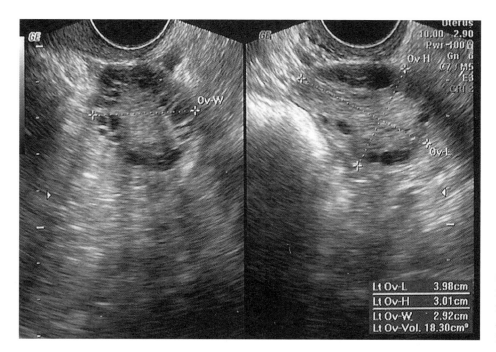

FIGURE 10–24. The measurements needed to obtain ovarian volume (between + signs). Also note more than 10 follicles present on each ovary.

visualization of each ovary. When the bladder is full, it can be used as an acoustic window to better evaluate the ovary. For example, when imaging the right ovary, slide the transducer toward the patient's left side and angle through the bladder to the right ovary. TV imaging of the ovary may be difficult if bowel shadowing is excessive, if the ovaries are displaced, or if they are small (as in postmenopausal women).

To identify the ovaries using TV scanning, begin in a coronal plane near the cornua of the uterus. Follow the broad ligament into the adnexa to the ovary. Scan the ovary in the coronal plane by angling the transducer anterior to posterior. In the sagittal plane, images are obtained by angling the transducer lateral (at the iliac vessels) to medial (back to the uterus). The entire adnexa should be evaluated for free fluid, masses, or cysts.

Ovarian size is expressed in terms of ovarian volume, which is calculated using the formula for a prolate ellipse (length × width × height × 0.523) (Figure 10–24). Ovarian size increases throughout childhood and puberty and fluctuates across the menstrual cycle in association with growth and ovulation of the dominant follicle. Ovarian volume decreases after menopause.

Ovarian volume and follicular number are essential ultrasound diagnostic criteria for polycystic ovary syndrome (PCOS). PCOS affects 6% to 10% of all women and often starts in adolescence. The Rotterdam Criteria defines ovaries as polycystic if there are 12 or more follicles measuring 2 to 9 mm (FNPS; follicle number per single cross-section of the ovary) and/or

ovarian volume (OV) of greater than 10 cm³.[4] Since 2003, there have been questions about these measurements because many normal women meet these criteria. A recent study done by Lujel et al. with Cornell University and Canadian researchers demonstrated a higher diagnostic sensitivity when the total number of follicles per ovary (FNPO) was more than two, as measured using multisector or three-dimensional (3D) scanning.[5] Although ovarian volume has been considered to be a hallmark diagnostic criteria, Atiomo et al.[6] found the following findings were more sensitive as diagnostic criteria for PCOS than ovarian volume: 10 or more follicles per ovary, peripheral distribution of follicles, and stromal brightness. PCOS is the most common cause of irregular menses and the most common cause of infertility in women, so ultrasound becomes a critical tool in providing early detection and management (Figure 10–25).[6]

ASSISTED REPRODUCTIVE PROCEDURES

When assisted reproductive technologies and ovarian-stimulating medications are being utilized, production of multiple follicles can occur. The follicular growth is followed by serial sonographic measurements. Because follicles are fluid-filled, they appear anechoic (Figure 10–26).

There is a close correlation between increasing levels of estradiol and the increasing size of the

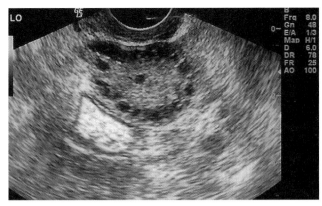

FIGURE 10–25. Multiple follicles are noted around the periphery of the ovary. Follicles appear numerous and are easily imaged.

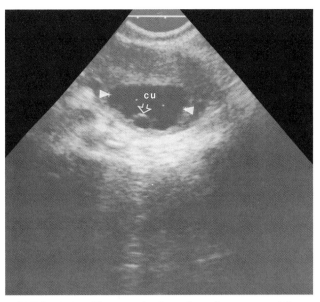

FIGURE 10–27. Transvaginal section of an ovary with a preovulatory follicle (arrowheads) of 28 mm. The cumulus oophorous (cu) can be seen projecting from the wall of the follicle into the follicular fluid (arrow).

dominant follicle, as estimated by measurements of mean follicle diameter or total surface area. There is also a close correlation between estimated follicular volume by ultrasound and those assessed at the time of laparoscopy. Although follicular growth and ovulation can be assessed with great accuracy, the use of follicle size alone as an absolute predictor of ovulation is limited because of variation in follicle size at rupture. Other sonographic findings may help to predict imminent ovulation more precisely. These include the "double contour" sign, which represents separation of the theca layer from the granulosa cell layer or visualization of the cumulus oophorus 12 to 24 hours prior to ovulation (Figure 10–27).

With assisted reproductive technologies, the follicular number and interval growth are followed closely with both hormone levels and sonographic imaging. Once the ovary is identified, the ovarian size (length, AP and transverse) is determined. All follicles, cysts, or masses should be noted. Follicles are measured in two dimensions at the largest diameter.[2,7] With in vitro fertilization, the goal is to induce multiple follicles in each ovary. During a normal or noninduced cycle, generally only a single follicle dominates and enlarges while the oocyte inside matures. A follicular measurement of more than 18 mm is considered to contain a mature egg. According to Rosen, Shen, Dobson, Rinaudo, McCulloch, and Cedars, the odds of a mature oocyte resulting from a 16 to 18 mm follicle size was 37% when compared to follicles measuring more than 18 mm. The odds decreased progressively with decreasing follicular size.[8] Any follicle greater than 10 mm should be measured and documented. If there are multiple follicles present, as in a stimulated in vitro fertilization cycle, the largest follicles should be measured and the total number of follicles documented according to established protocol.

After follicular collapse, the corpus luteum appears as a hypoechoic structure with irregular walls and internal echoes. Thereafter, the size and general appearance of the corpus luteum are variable. The structure may enlarge and fill with echogenic material corresponding to fresh hemorrhagic material. Over time, it can organize to produce a complex pattern of cystic areas and solid strands (Figure 10–28).

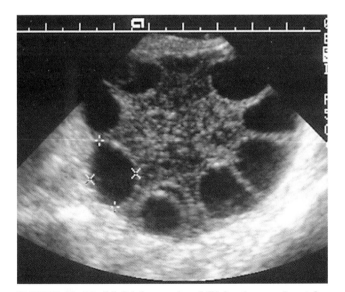

FIGURE 10–26. Multiple ovarian follicles (approximately nine) that have been induced by ovarian stimulation medication in assisted reproductive medicine, with measurement of one follicle at cursors.

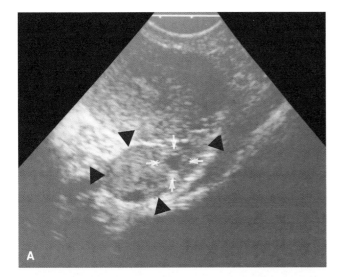

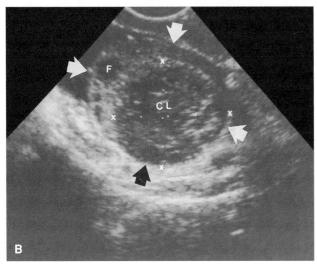

FIGURE 10–28. Sagittal section of the ovary after follicle rupture, showing variable appearances of the corpus luteum (CL). **(A)** Collapsed, thick-walled structure (arrowheads). **(B)** CL (arrows) contains echogenic hemorrhagic material and another follicle (F).

There is no relationship between the size and appearance of the corpus luteum and progesterone secretion. With color Doppler, a ring of color may be noted around a corpus luteum.

Sonography is also crucial in the retrieval of the oocytes in assisted reproduction. The reproductive medicine physician uses a TV ultrasound probe fitted with a retrieval needle. TA ultrasound guidance may be used as an adjunct to the retrieval. With the patient lightly sedated, the TV ultrasound transducer is used to identify each follicle. The retrieval needle is then advanced into each follicle and the fluid and oocyte are aspirated with gentle suction. The contents are collected in a small tube, and the process of oocyte identification and assessment begins.

With successful fertilization of the ovum or ova, sonography may also be used to assist with the guidance of embryo(s) transfer transcervically into the endometrial cavity. The catheter used for insertion of the embryo(s) is easily seen with a TA transducer.

USE OF COLOR DOPPLER

Color Doppler and pulsed-wave Doppler can be used to evaluate changes in pelvic blood flow across the ovulatory cycle. The Doppler classification is based on the presence and duration or absence of diastolic flow in the pelvic arteries.

Doppler ultrasound has also assumed a significant role in the evaluation of the ovaries in the perimenopausal as well as the menopausal woman. Superimposed color Doppler imaging of the ovaries allows possible detection of normal, suspicious, and pathologic blood flow characteristics in the blood vessels that helps distinguish between benign and malignant lesions.[9]

Additionally, Doppler can assist in the characterization of adnexal masses, such as tuboovarian abscess.[9] This can be beneficial when differentiating a tuboovarian abscess from a hydrosalpinx.

SONOGRAPHIC LOCALIZATION OF INTRAUTERINE DEVICE

Many providers use ultrasound to assist with the insertion of IUDs. TV assessment of uterine size and position may be done prior to insertion, as well as to verify or confirm IUD placement after insertion (Figures 10–29 and 10–30). If on subsequent examinations the IUD string is not palpable or cannot be

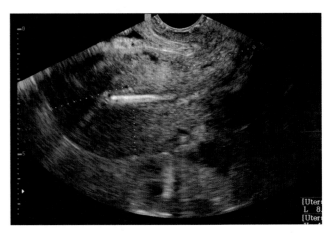

FIGURE 10–29. Sagittal image of uterine cavity with intrauterine device (IUD; hyperechoic area).

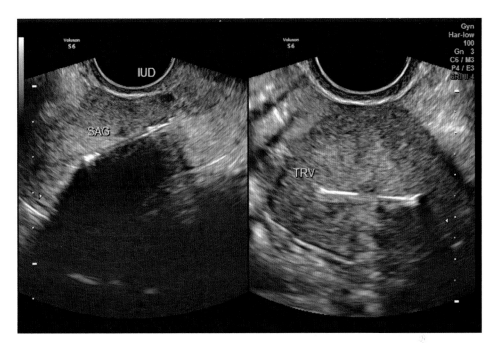

FIGURE 10–30. The intra-uterine device (IUD) is noted to be in the endometrial canal within the uterine cavity, and its hyperechoic bright white "line" (at arrowhead) is seen in the sagittal and transverse planes.

seen on speculum exam, the IUD location may be determined sonographically. For a number of reasons, ultrasound is the recommended initial imaging modality of choice in IUD localization: sonography equipment is generally readily available, has lower cost than other imaging modalities, lacks ionizing radiation along with radiation concerns, and is minimally invasive in nature. If the IUD cannot be seen with a POC TV scan, a standard (complete) pelvic ultrasound examination is warranted, often to include 3D volume assessments. 3D imaging can sometimes aid in identifying IUD malposition within the endometrium or myometrium. If the IUD has migrated outside the uterine cavity into the bowel, bowel cavity, or bladder, sonographic visualization of the IUD can be difficult due to bowel gas.[10] If the IUD cannot be identified sonographically, a plain film of the abdomen may be beneficial.

DOCUMENTATION AND SUBSEQUENT CARE

All findings from a POC sonogram should be documented in the medical record. Based on pelvic ultrasound guidelines, all POC sonograms performed in conjunction with reproductive medicine technologies and/or gynecologic assessment include specific information about each anatomic structures. Some structures, such as ovarian follicles or endometrial thickness, require measurements. All of the findings need to be documented.

Because a POC sonogram is neither a diagnostic nor a comprehensive pelvic ultrasound examination, recommendations also exist for the appropriate timing for comprehensive pelvic ultrasound. In reproductive medicine, it is advised that a comprehension pelvic ultrasound to assess for pelvic pathology be performed 4 to 6 months *prior* to the beginning of a stimulated cycle. Any POC sonogram performed for a specific gynecologic complaint may also warrant follow-up with a comprehensive scan.

Gynecologic and POC pelvic sonograms performed by nurses, midwives, or advanced practice nurses should be done with appropriate physician supervision.[11–13] The definition of "supervision" may vary depending on state laws and institutional policies. Nonetheless, a pre-established means for communicating findings and/or inconclusive results should be determined and clarified, along with establishing a line of contact for physician consultation and collaboration.

CONCLUSION

Nurses, midwives, advanced nurse practitioners, and physician assistants who have received the appropriate education and training may perform POC components of the pelvic ultrasound examination that are based on institutional policies and procedures, the scope of practice, and laws within the state. Each POC pelvic sonogram does have established guidelines that should be followed for each specific procedure, as well as a format for comprehensive documentation of findings.

REFERENCES

1. American Institute of Ultrasound in Medicine (AIUM). *Practice Guideline for the Performance of Ultrasound Examinations of the Female Pelvis.* Laurel, MD: AIUM; 2006.
2. American College of Obstetricians and Gynecologists (ACOG). The role of transvaginal ultrasonography in the evaluation of postmenopausal bleeding. Committee Opinion No. 440. Washington, DC: ACOG; 2009. http://www.aium.org/
3. Goldstein SR. Sonography in postmenopausal bleeding. *J Ultrasound Med.* 2012;31:333–336.
4. Kurjak A, Kupesic S, Simunic V. Ultrasonic assessment of the peri- and postmenopausal ovary. *Maturitas.* 2002;41(4):245–254.
5. Atiomo WU, Pearson S, Shaw S, et al. Ultrasound criteria in the diagnosis of polycystic ovary syndrome (PCOS). *Ultrasound Med Biol.* 2000 July;26(6):977–980.
6. Lujan ME, Jarrett BY, Brooks ED, et al. Updated ultrasound criteria for polycystic ovary syndrome: reliable thresholds for elevated follicle population and ovarian volume. *Hum Reprod.* 2013 May;28(5):1361–1368.
7. American Institute of Ultrasound in Medicine (AIUM). *Practice Guideline: Ultrasound of the Female Pelvis for Infertility and Reproductive Medicine.* Laurel, MD: AIUM; 2008.
8. Rosen M, Shen S, Dobson A, et al. A quantitative assessment of follicle size on oocyte developmental competence. *Fertil Steril.* 2008;90(3):684–690.
9. Zatel Y, Sorian D, Lipitz S, et al. Contribution of color Doppler flow to the ultrasonographic diagnosis of tubal abnormalities. *J Ultrasound Med.* 2000;19(9):645–649.
10. Nilsestuen L. IUD perforation to the urinary bladder: ultrasonographic diagnosis. *J Diagn Med Sonogr.* 2013;29(3):126–129.
11. American Society for Reproductive Medicine (ASRM). *Position Statement on Nurses Performing Focused Ultrasound Examinations in a Gynecology/Infertility Setting.* Birmingham, AL: ASRM; 2009.
12. Association of Women's Health, Obstetric and Neonatal Nurses (AWHONN). *Ultrasound Examinations Performed by Nurses in Obstetric, Gynecologic, and Reproductive Medicine Settings: Clinical Competencies and Education Guide.* 3rd ed. Washington, DC: AWHONN; 2010.
13. American Society of Reproductive Medicine (ASRM). Use of exogenous gonadotropins in anovulatory women (Practice Committee Technical Bulletin). *Fertil Steril.* 2008;90:S7–S12.

CHAPTER 11

Point-of-Care Sonography in the First Trimester

During the first trimester of pregnancy, clinical situations may warrant a limited or point-of-care (POC) ultrasound examination when a specific piece of information is needed to provide optimum bedside care in a timely fashion. Some of the more common clinical presentations leading to a POC ultrasound examination include vaginal spotting or bleeding, lower abdominal cramping or pain, or the inability of the clinician to auscultate fetal heart rate (FHR). However, a POC ultrasound is not intended to replace a standard first-trimester ultrasound. If a standard ultrasound study has not been performed prior to the POC imaging, it is recommended that, whenever reasonably possible, the POC scan be followed with a complete standard study.[1] But if critical information is needed when a standard ultrasound is not available, a POC ultrasound is a valuable tool for providing timely diagnostic assistance.

The intention of this chapter is to describe each of the components of the standard first-trimester ultrasound examination from which components may be used for the POC sonogram. For comparison purposes, some abnormal findings are presented to assist with distinctions from normal findings.

INDICATIONS FOR FIRST TRIMESTER STANDARD SONOGRAM

In 1984, The National Institutes of Health convened a task force to determine if routine sonography was appropriate for all pregnancies. Their conclusion was that not all pregnant women would benefit from a routine ultrasound, and therefore a list of appropriate indications was generated for sonography for all trimesters of pregnancy.[2] That basic premise still exists today; however, the indications for a first-trimester ultrasound examination have been updated in recent years[1,3] and are shown in Box 11–1. It should be noted that many of the individual indications identified are also indications for a POC ultrasound examination under certain clinical situations.

DISCRIMINATORY ZONE IN FIRST TRIMESTER EVALUATION

Serum screening for quantitative beta human chorionic gonadotropin (β-hCG) has been the "gold standard" for many years in assessing the stable patient for an abnormal pregnancy. Although it is not diagnostic, it still may be used in conjunction with sonographic evaluation. However, the best approach for patient management will depend on both the availability of the testing procedure, the skills of the clinician performing the sonogram, and the interpretation of the results of each.

In the past, certain ranges or cutoffs of β-hCG levels (known as the "discriminatory zone") were used in conjunction with specific first-trimester ultrasound findings to differentiate between viable and nonviable pregnancies. Research has shown many drawbacks to that system, and its use is no longer recommended. Doublet and Benson[4] determined that there are potential errors in image interpretation that can lead to errors in management when utilizing this approach: (1) the failure to conclude there is a definite or probable viable pregnancy in conflict with ultrasound images showing such a finding, and

 BOX 11–1 | **Indications for First-Trimester Ultrasound Examination**

Confirm the presence of an intrauterine pregnancy
Evaluate a suspected ectopic pregnancy
Define the cause of vaginal bleeding
Evaluate pelvic pain
Estimate gestation age
Diagnose or evaluate multiple gestations
Confirm cardiac activity
Localize and remove an intrauterine device
Assess for certain fetal anomalies
Evaluate maternal pelvic masses or uterine abnormalities
As an adjunct to chorionic villus sampling, embryo transfer
Measure nuchal translucency as part of aneuploidy screening
Evaluate a suspected hydatidiform mole

Adapted from AIUM[1] and ACOG.[3]

(2) the failure to conclude that there is sonographic confirmation or likelihood of the presence of an ectopic pregnancy despite ultrasound images supporting that finding.

The first potential error may come from failing to see a "double sac sign (DSS)" or the "intradecidual sign (IDS)," interpreting the findings as a nonviable pregnancy, and moving forward with medical or surgical intervention. The double sac sign is thought to represent the two layers of decidua surrounding the intrauterine fluid collection and does occur in most, but not all, normal pregnancies. There is no data to support that the absence of this finding is consistent with an abnormal pregnancy.

The second problem is the misdiagnosis of a pseudogestational sac, which refers to fluid in the uterine cavity that is occasionally seen in women with an ectopic pregnancy. Fluid in the endometrium is more likely to be a gestational sac than a pseudogestational sac. When nonspecific intrauterine fluid collection is seen, the odds of a gestational sac over a pseudogestational sac are approximately 245:1.

If no intrauterine sac is seen and the patient's quantitative β-hCG is well above a discriminatory level where one expects to see an intrauterine pregnancy (IUP), there should be concern for an ectopic pregnancy. If a sonogram shows a definite extrauterine pregnancy (embryo with cardiac activity), then the presence or absence of a pseudogestational sac is clinically irrelevant.[3]

Doublet and Benson[5] also investigated the interobserver agreement, frequency of occurrence, and the prognostic importance of the DSS, the IDS, and other sonographic findings in early pregnancies. As for the occurrence of these signs, the interobserver agreement was poor because the sonographic images frequently did not demonstrate either sign. The presence of a DSS or IDS was also unrelated to β-hCG levels, first-trimester outcome, presence of an inner echogenic ring, or decidual presence. The conclusion was that the sonographic appearance of an early gestational sac, before visualization of a yolk sac or embryo, is highly variable. Therefore, it is advised that if a round or oval intrauterine fluid collection is sonographically visualized in a woman with a positive β-hCG, it should be treated as a gestational sac until proven otherwise, regardless of whether it demonstrates a DSS or an IDS. Performing medical and surgical interventions has the potential to damage an IUP, and these procedures should be avoided unless a viable pregnancy

is definitely excluded by follow-up β-hCG values or sonograms.[5]

TRANSVAGINAL SONOGRAPHY IN THE FIRST TRIMESTER

One of the most important prognostic indicators in the first trimester is the crown–rump length (CRL) of the fetus. It is the most accurate biometric measurement for the prediction of gestational age, as well as having predictive value in determining survivability of a pregnancy.[6] The development of the vaginal sonography, along with improved resolution, has led to improved accuracy. Transvaginal sonography (TVS) uses higher frequency transducers, which provides a 40% to 50% improvement in lateral and axial resolution over transabdominal sonography (TAS). Although the American Institute of Ultrasound in Medicine (AIUM)[1] states that first-trimester ultrasound may be performed by the TA approach only, most sonographers employ both TV and TA transducers during the standard first-trimester scan. Initially, patient acceptance in the use of the vaginal probe was a concern, but when women presented with early pregnancy issues, the TV probe was acceptable.[7]

THE STANDARD SONOGRAPHIC EXAM IN THE FIRST TRIMESTER OF PREGNANCY

Membranes, Yolk Sac, and Umbilical Cord

With a normally developing pregnancy, certain parameters are expected to be visible by TVS at specific gestational ages. The identifiable gestational sac is typically present at 5 weeks' gestation. The yolk sac, located within the chorioamniotic space, becomes visible at 5.5 weeks. A small fetal pole containing an active fetal heart can be seen by 6 to 6.5 weeks, with the beat occurring around the same time. The thin and wispy amniotic membrane is sonographically visualized at 7 weeks. The chorioamniotic space obliterates as the amniotic cavity grows to the size of the chorion. By 14 to 16 weeks' gestation, the amnion fuses with the chorion, making the two sonographically indistinguishable. Further details are described below.

Gestational Sac

Endometrial implantation of the blastocyst occurs approximately 9.5 days after conception. Prior to

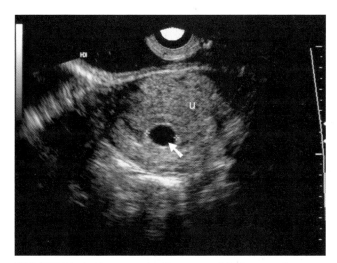

FIGURE 11–1. Transvaginal sonographic image of a normal 6.5-week gestational sac (arrow) showing the sac within the uterus (U).

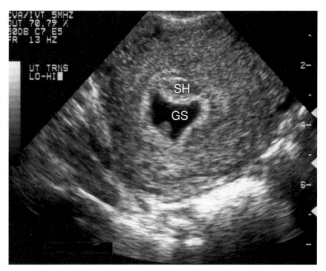

FIGURE 11–3. An irregular gestational sac, as seen in this transvaginal image, has been associated with an abnormal pregnancy. GS, gestational sac; SH, subchorionic hemorrhage.

the identification of a normal gestational sac, the endometrium appears secretory. Sonographically, a double-echogenic ring or decidual reaction is produced by the decidual capsularis and the decidua parietalis.

The normal gestational sac can be seen as early as 4 to 5 weeks of gestation or when the sac is 2 to 5 mm in size.[6,8] The gestational sac size has been used to predict gestational age before the identification of the embryo. The normal gestational sac typically appears ellipsoid or circular in shape. Sonographically, the sac appears as a hypoechoic or anechoic area in or near the midline of the uterus

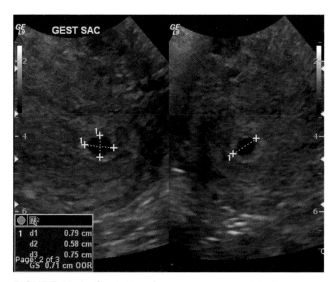

FIGURE 11–2. Gestational sac measurement in two coronal views. The sac is the anechoic area within the uterine cavity, which is hyperechoic.

(Figure 11–1). The gestational sac size is obtained by measuring the gestational sac in all three dimensions at the chorionic margin (Figure 11–2). One of these planes should be made at the largest diameter of the sac. These measurements are then averaged together.

A mean sac diameter of 25 mm or greater with no visible embryo is diagnostic of a failed pregnancy. An abnormal shape to the gestational sac may suggest an abnormal pregnancy (Figure 11–3).[9] Additionally, the gestational sac should increase in size by 1 to 1.2 mm/day. Any abnormal growth of the gestational sac is a poor prognostic sign.[10]

The yolk sac is the next structure that becomes visible, typically between 5 and 6 weeks of gestation. It is located outside the amnion and appears as an echogenic ring with an anechoic center (Figures 11–4 and 11–5). Recent studies suggest that an irregular yolk sac shape is unrelated to an increased risk of spontaneous abortion.[11]

The yolk sac, fetal pole, and fetal heart can be seen earlier by TV ultrasound than by the TA approach (Table 11–1). Therefore, if the scan has been performed transabdominally without evidence of any of the identifiable fetal anatomy or landmarks, a TV approach should be used.

The Embryo/Fetus

An embryo can first be identified with a TV transducer at approximately 5 to 6 weeks' gestation. Cardiac motion should be observed when the embryo is 2 mm

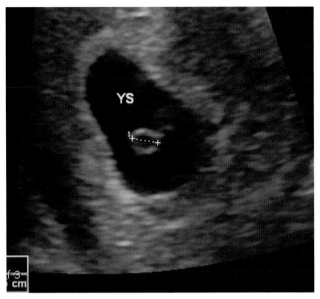

FIGURE 11–4. Gestational sac with presence of yolk sac, measured (YS).

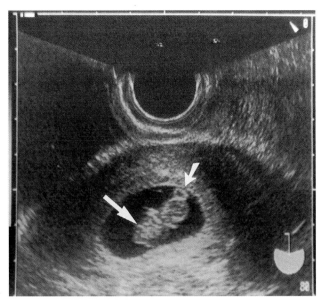

FIGURE 11–5. Yolk sac (at top, smaller arrow) and fetal pole.

or greater in length. If cardiac activity is not observed when the embryo is greater than 7 mm in length, a subsequent scan 1 week later is recommended to confirm a viable versus a nonviable pregnancy. This should be performed prior to any medical or surgical interventions.[1,3] The fetal number should be confidently identified beginning at approximately 8 weeks' gestation.

Crown–Rump Length Measurement

Even with extraordinary advances in high-resolution technology, the most accurate method for determining gestational age remains the fetal CRL (Figure 11–6). In spite of radical improvements in imaging and the ability to date pregnancy accurately (especially with assisted reproductive technologies), there has been minimal improvement in the accuracy of CRL. Accuracy of this early pregnancy ultrasound is measured in terms of a low margin of error, which remains at plus or minus 3 days of the calculated date.[3] Advanced biometry in the first trimester, such as measurement of the biparietal diameter, head circumference, and abdominal circumference has been studied, and growth charts have been created for the first trimester.[12] After about 11 or 12 weeks, the fetal posture may vary between flexion and extension leading to more variance in the estimated gestational age. The CRL, however, continues to be the most accurate predictor of gestational age. As pregnancy advances, this margin of error becomes greater; it will never be as low (or accurate) as it is in the early weeks.

Sonographic Finding at Earliest Gestation	Visualized via Transvaginal Scan by:	Visualized via Transabdominal Scan by:
Intrauterine Sac	4.5–5 weeks' measuring 2–4 mm	5.5 weeks'
Cardiac activity	5 weeks'	6 weeks'
Yolk sac	5 weeks' measuring 3–5 mm	5.5–6 weeks

TABLE 11–1 TRANSVAGINAL (TV) VERSUS TRANSABDOMINAL (TA) ULTRASOUND: EARLIEST VISUALIZED SONOGRAPHIC FINDINGS

Adapted from AIUM,[1] ACOG,[3] and Campion.[25]

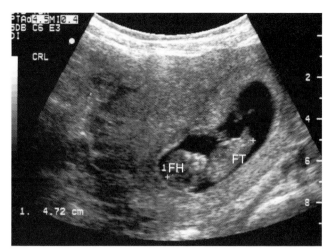

FIGURE 11–6. Transabdominal image of an 11-week, 2-day fetus showing a typical crown-rump length measurement (between cursors). FH, fetal head; FT, fetal torso.

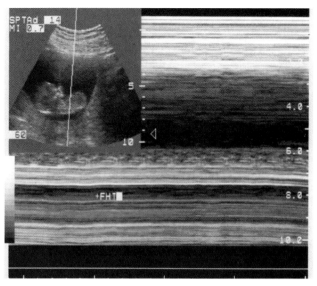

FIGURE 11–7. M-mode ultrasound is useful in documenting fetal heart motion. M-mode records one-line sonographic information and displays it over time, so that structures that move within that line show a "wavy" pattern on the display.

The CRL measures 8 to 14 mm in the sixth week of pregnancy, 14 to 20 mm in the seventh week, and 21 to 30 mm in the eighth week. The early embryo grows approximately 2 mm/day during the first trimester.

With few exceptions, the CRL in the normal pregnancy is thought to be biologically stable and thus reproducible and reliable. It usually is not influenced by intrinsic variables such as racial variation or extrinsic variables such as altitude. Two exceptions to this observation have been demonstrated in one recent study: (1) female embryos showed slightly smaller CRL than male embryos, and (2) embryos of diabetic mothers had slightly smaller CRLs than did embryos of nondiabetic mothers. Female fetuses grow considerably more slowly than male fetuses, and these differences are observed from early gestation. However, the female fetus is not merely a smaller version of the male fetus; rather, there is a sex-specific growth pattern for each of the individual fetal biometric indices. These findings provide support for the use of sex-specific sonographic models for fetal weight estimation, as well as the use of sex-specific reference growth charts.[13]

Fetal Heart Motion

Fetal heart motion can be seen with TV ultrasonography at approximately 5 weeks (CRL of 2–4 mm) in 80% of cases and by 7 weeks in 100% of cases (Figure 11–7).[14] Cardiac motion is usually seen when the embryo is at least 5 mm in length.

The presence or absence of cardiac activity should be documented with a video clip or M-mode imaging, avoiding use of color or spectral Doppler.[1] When attempting to obtain the FHR with a diagnostic ultrasound system, the AIUM recommends using M-mode first because of its lower acoustic intensity. Spectral Doppler has higher acoustic intensity and should not be used. This restriction does not apply to traditional handheld Doppler devices without imaging capabilities that are used to auscultate FHR.[15]

Heart rate may prove to be a useful method of assessing gestational age and in the prediction of impending fetal loss. Fetal loss has been associated not only with the ultrasound finding of a small gestational sac, but also fetal bradycardia (<90–100 bpm).[16]

Fetal Structural Abnormalities

Many fetal structural abnormalities have been identified in the first trimester (Figure 11–8). A limited anatomic survey can be accomplished as early as 12 weeks' gestation, but not all anomalies can be identified this early.[17,18] Anomalies can occur as either isolated findings or as part of a syndrome. Although a variety of defects have been identified in early pregnancy, an abnormal nuchal translucency (NT) is the most reliable.

Nuchal Translucency

The "prominent nuchal membrane" was first described in 1990 by Szabo and Gellen[19] and is now referred to

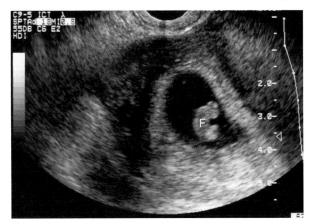

FIGURE 11–8. This fetus (F) was found to be anomalous at the time of this 9-week ultrasound examination. Although a heartbeat could be seen, no normal fetal anatomy could be visualized.

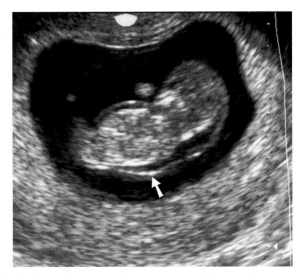

FIGURE 11–10. In addition to the nuchal translucency (NT), this fetus has diffuse anasarca (widespread edema) pushing skin away from torso (arrow). Chorionic villus sampling showed this fetus to have monosomy X (Turner's syndrome).

as *nuchal translucency*.[18] Nuchal translucency is an abnormal collection of fluid in the posterior cervical (nuchal) area of the fetus that can be detected as early as 9 weeks. These fluid accumulations have been described as localized or diffuse, thick or septated, transient or permanent collections of fluid (Figures 11–9 and 11–10).

Normal nuchal thickening (as opposed to "translucency") increases with gestational age. Therefore, it is recommended that the NT measurement be performed between 10 and 13 weeks' gestation, with a cutoff measurement typically of less than 3 mm and dependent on CRL. With a measurement of more than 3 mm there is a 10% increase in major

congenital anomalies. With a measurement of 6 mm, the risk of anomaly increases to 90%.[7] An extended fetal neck can result in a falsely increased measurement. Additionally, careful attention needs to be given to the placement of the calipers when obtaining the measurement so as to avoid mistaking the amnion, a spinal defect, or encephalocele for nuchal thickening.[20,21]

If possible, the nuchal region should be assessed during the first-trimester sonogram. The measurement should be used in conjunction with biochemical markers to determine the risk for aneuploidy and/or other abnormalities. The measurements must be done at a precise level by an experienced practitioner to ensure the accuracy of the result.[1]

Adnexa and Uterus

The complete first-trimester sonographic examination should include an assessment of the myometrium and the adnexa.[3] Evaluation of the adnexa can include a TA as well as a TV ultrasound examination. The depth of penetration of the TV sound beam is restricted due to its high frequency and can restrict visualization of the deep adnexa. As a result, large masses such as those extending from the uterine fundus, can missed. In these situations, a TA ultrasound examination should also be performed.

The uterus and the adnexa should also be evaluated for masses and evidence of an extrauterine

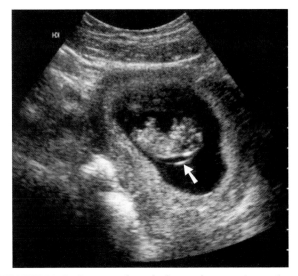

FIGURE 11–9. Increased nuchal translucency (arrow) was seen during ultrasound examination of this 11-week fetus with trisomy 21.

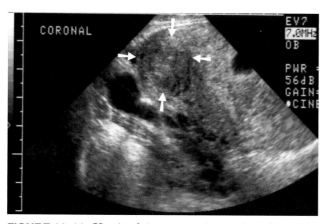

FIGURE 11–11. Uterine leiomyomas (arrows), such as this one seen on a transabdominal sonographic image, are common and often are observed during routine examination.

BOX 11–2	Imaging Parameters for the Standard First-Trimester Ultrasound Examination

Evaluation and documentation of the uterus, cervix, adnexal structures, and cul-de-sac

Evaluation and documentation of gestational sac and location

Document the presence/absence of a yolk sac and/or embryo

Crown–rump length measurement obtained and documented

Presence or absence of cardiac activity documented with 2-dimensional video clip or M-mode

Fetal number documented

Embryonic/fetal anatomy appropriate for first trimester assessed and documented

Nuchal region imaged and documented

Adapted from AIUM[1] and ACOG.[3]

gestation. The cul-de-sac should be evaluated for the presence or absence of fluid.[1,3]

The normal myometrium should have a uniformly homogenous, echogenic appearance. The peritoneum (perimetrium) and endometrium are stronger reflectors and appear more echogenic by ultrasound. Uterine masses, such as leiomyomata, may present as discrete entities in the myometrial substance, or they may appear as diffuse thickening of the myometrium. Commonly, the diffuse thickening is adenomyosis rather than a fibroid, with true fibroids having definitive borders. Submucosal leiomyomata or polyps in the endometrial cavity may distort the usual linear appearance of the endometrial echo (Figure 11–11). Pedunculated leiomyomata that extend into the adnexa can mimic solid or complex adnexal masses.

Both ovaries should also be investigated during the first-trimester standard scan. A corpus luteal cyst of pregnancy is a common adnexal finding in the first trimester. It is usually unilateral and can appear anechoic or complex. It may become hemorrhagic, resulting in echo-filled appearing texture, or it may develop thick walls. The corpus luteal cyst typically resolves by 16 weeks' gestation. Rarely, the corpus luteal cyst can grossly enlarge, becoming symptomatic and measuring more than 10 cm.

The standard first-trimester obstetric sonogram is summarized in Box 11–2.

SONOGRAPHY IN EARLY PREGNANCY FAILURE: DIFFERENTIAL DIAGNOSIS

Threatened Abortion

The two most common indications for a first-trimester sonogram are vaginal bleeding or spotting and abdominal or pelvic pain, both of which may be indicative of a threatened abortion. When used appropriately, POC sonography can be used confidently to distinguish the normal IUP from such pathologic conditions as missed and spontaneous abortion, ectopic pregnancy, or hydatidiform mole.

As mentioned, the identification of various sonographic landmarks, such as detection of heart motion or a yolk sac, has served to predict successful pregnancy continuation. In addition, much effort has been applied to finding biochemical and sonographic parameters with prognostic capabilities in cases of threatened abortion. More recently, another ultrasound prognostic sign, subchorionic bleeding, has been described. This finding is characterized by a hypoechoic collection of fluid outside the gestational sac. It has been associated with miscarriage and/or preterm labor, but in most cases it is an insignificant finding.[22–24]

Anembryonic Gestation or Nonliving Embryo/Fetus

An anembryonic pregnancy usually represents an early IUP failure with subsequent embryonic disintegration. This gives the appearance of an "empty sac." The anembryonic (blighted ovum) pregnancy can be diagnosed confidently when the mean gestational sac size is greater than 25 mm with no embryo identified.[8,25] TVS has allowed for an earlier confident diagnosis. Once a mean gestational sac diameter of 10 mm is achieved, a yolk sac should be identifiable. If a yolk sac cannot be seen at this time,

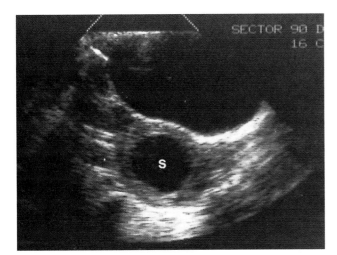

FIGURE 11–12. Sagittal transabdominal image showing an anembryonic (blighted ovum) gestational sac (S).

an anembryonic pregnancy may be diagnosed (Figure 11–12).

Missed Abortion

The missed abortion has been defined as an intrauterine embryo with a CRL of greater than 15 mm without fetal cardiac motion. Sonographically, these fetuses can be hydropic with diffuse edema.[10,11]

PREGNANCY OF UNKNOWN LOCATION (PUL)

If during either a POC sonogram or a standard first-trimester ultrasound examination the location of the pregnancy cannot be definitively determined, the diagnosis may be a pregnancy of unknown location (PUL). Bernhardt and associates propose a consensus statement with definitions of population, target disease, and final outcome.[26] The following categorization suggested by Bernhardt and associates includes:

1. *Definite extrauterine pregnancy (EP):* Extrauterine gestational sac with yolk sac and/or embryo (with or without cardiac activity)
2. *Probable EP:* Homogeneous adnexal mass or extrauterine sac-like structure
3. *PUL:* No signs of either EP or IUP
4. *Probable IUP:* Intrauterine echogenic sac-like structure
5. *Definite IUP:* Intrauterine gestational sac with yolk sac and/or embryo (with or without cardiac activity)

Ectopic Pregnancy

In addition to tools such as serum quantitative β-hCG levels and physical examination, sonography plays a pivotal role in the diagnosis and management of the ectopic pregnancy. The most widely accepted diagnostic application of sonography in the suspected ectopic pregnancy is the lack of identification of an IUP in the presence of sufficiently high serum quantitative β-hCG levels that would normally be seen with an IUP.

Conversely, the presence of an IUP or yolk sac virtually excludes the possibility of an ectopic pregnancy, except for the risk of a heterotopic pregnancy (one twin intrauterine and one twin extrauterine). The risk of heterotopic pregnancy is 1/30,000 for spontaneous conceptions and 1/6,000 in assisted reproduction conceptions.[27]

Ultrasound findings of an ectopic pregnancy may include an empty uterus with or without a thickened endometrium, a pseudogestational sac in the uterus, a concurrent intrauterine (heterotopic) pregnancy, or the absence of a gestational sac at 6 weeks' gestation (Figures 11–13 and 11–14). In approximately 10% to 20% of ectopic pregnancies, a gestational sac can be seen outside the endometrial cavity with an identifiable embryonic/fetal pole and an active heartbeat. This provides convincing evidence of an ectopic pregnancy. More commonly, findings of a noncystic adnexal mass and/or fluid (simple or complex) in the posterior cul-de-sac are observed with the ectopic pregnancy.

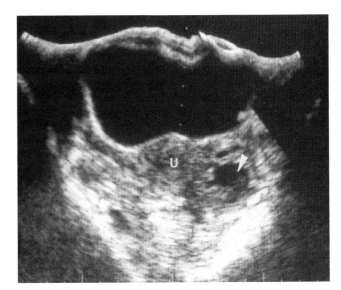

FIGURE 11–13. Transverse image of ectopic pregnancy (arrowhead) and uterus (U).

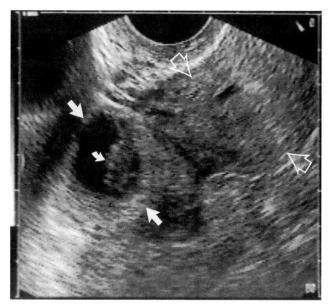

FIGURE 11–14. Transvaginal image of a right adnexal ectopic pregnancy with a gestational sac (large arrows) and fetal pole (small arrow). The uterus is seen (hollow arrows) with a small amount of endometrial fluid.

TROPHOBLASTIC DISEASE

Trophoblastic disease is a rare complication of pregnancy that may present as vaginal bleeding; it is also known as a *molar pregnancy*. It results from a degeneration of placental tissue and occurs in 1 in 3,000 pregnancies in Caucasian women but in as many as 1 in 250 pregnancies in Asian women. There are basically two types: a complete mole, in which there is no embryonic tissue (Figure 11–15), and an incomplete

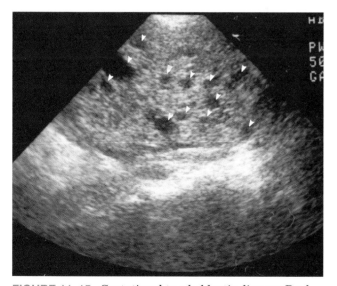

FIGURE 11–15. Gestational trophoblastic disease: Real-time image of the uterus reveals a soft-tissue mass with multiple cystic areas (arrowheads) of varying sizes, often described as a grape-like pattern.

mole, in which the embryo develops in the presence of a hydropic placenta.[10]

CONCLUSION

Advances in reproductive technologies and medical therapies have contributed to higher pregnancy rates and, thus, higher rates of complications in the first trimester. Physical, biochemical, and sonographic assessments are intimately interwoven in the evaluation of patients with early pregnancy complications. Several clinically relevant and realistic goals of sonography in the first trimester are (1) visualization and localization of the gestational sac and the exclusion of an ectopic pregnancy, (2) early identification of nonviable pregnancies, (3) determination of the number of embryos, (4) estimation of gestational age, and (5) early diagnosis of fetal abnormalities. Additionally, high-resolution vaginal ultrasound has greatly enhanced the clinician's ability to assess the pregnancy.

Additionally, in the stable woman with an inconclusive sonogram, subsequent repeat sonogram(s) may improve accuracy of diagnosis. A completely empty uterus, even without evidence of endometrial fluid collection, with a β-hCG level of greater than 2,000 does not exclude the development of a normal IUP.[28]

POC ultrasound in the first trimester offers many advantages in patient care. It can eliminate delay in diagnosis, management, and treatment. By doing so, it also improves patient safety and satisfaction. However, performing a more limited ultrasound examination instead of a standard sonogram carries some inherent risks. A general rule of thumb is that if something is not visualized when it is expected to be seen, or if the pregnancy is not clearly identified in the uterus, a standard ultrasound examination is indicated.

REFERENCES

1. American Institute of Ultrasound in Medicine (AIUM). *AIUM Practice Guidelines: Obstetric Ultrasound.* Laurel, MD: AIUM; 2013.
2. National Institutes of Health. *Diagnostic Ultrasound in Pregnancy.* NIH Publication No. 84-667. Bethesda, MD: U.S. Department of Health and Human Services/NIH; 1984.
3. American College of Obstetricians and Gynecologists (ACOG). *Ultrasonography in Pregnancy.* Technical Bulletin No. 101. Washington, DC: ACOG; 2009.
4. Doublet PM, Benson CB. First, do no harm . . . to early pregnancies. *J Ultrasound Med.* 2010;29:685–689.

5. Doubilet PM, Benson CB. Double sac sign and intra-decidual sign in early pregnancy. *J Ultrasound Med.* 2013;32:1207–1214.

6. Dutta RL, Economides DL. Patient acceptance of trans-vaginal sonography in the early pregnancy unit setting. *Ultrasound Obstet Gynecol.* 2003;22(5):503–507.

7. Smith NC, Smith PM. *Obstetric Ultrasound Made Easy.* Edinburgh: Churchill Livingstone; 2003.

8. Laing FC, Frates MC. Ultrasound Evaluation During the First Trimester. In: PW Callen, ed., *Ultrasonography in Obstetrics and Gynecology,* 4th ed. Philadelphia: Saunders; 2000:105–145.

9. Nyberg DA, Laing FC, Filly RA. Threatened abortion: Sonographic distinction of normal and abnormal gestation sacs. *Radiology.* 1986;158:397.

10. Jaffe R, Abramowicz J. *Manual of Obstetric and Gynecologic Ultrasound.* Philadelphia: Lippincott-Raven; 1997.

11. Tan S, Pektas MK, Arslan H. Sonographic evaluation of the yolk sac. *J Ultrasound Med.* 2012;31:87–95.

12. Salomon LJ, Bernard JP, Duyme M, et al. Revisiting first-trimester biometry. *Ultrasound Obstet Gynecol.* 2003;22(1):63–66.

13. Melamed N, Meisner I, Mashiach R, et al. Fetal sex and intrauterine growth patterns. *J Ultrasound Med.* 2013;32:35–43.

14. Smith N, Smith, P. *Obstetric Ultrasound Made Easy.* Sapin, Philadelphia, PA: Elsevier Science; 2002.

15. American Institute of Ultrasound in Medicine (AIUM). *AIUM Statement on Measurement of Fetal Heart Rate.* Laurel, MD: AIUM; 2011.

16. Makrydimas G, Sebire NJ, Lolis D, et al. Fetal loss following ultrasound diagnosis of a live fetus at 6–10 weeks gestation. *Ultrasound Obstet Gynecol.* 2003;22(4):368–372.

17. Monteagudo A, Timor-Tritsch IE. First trimester anatomy scan: pushing the limits. What can we see now? *Curr Opin Obstet Gynecol.* 2003;15(2):131–141.

18. Benacerraf B. Ultrasound Evaluation of Chromosomal Abnormalities. In: PW Callen, ed., *Ultrasonography in Obstetrics and Gynecology.* 4th ed. Philadelphia: Saunders; 2000:38–67.

19. Taipale P, Ammala M, Salonen R, Hiilesmaa V. Learning curve in ultrasonographic screening for selected fetal structural anomalies in early pregnancy. *Obstet Gynecol.* 2003;101(2):273–278.

20. Szabo J, Gellen I. Nuchal fluid accumulation in trisomy 21 detected by vaginosonography in first trimester (letter). *Lancet.* 1990;336:1133.

21. Stephenson SR. Sonographic signs of fetal neural tube and central nervous system defects. *JDMS.* 2003;19:347–357.

22. Harris RD, Alexander RD. Ultrasound of the Placenta and Umbilical Cord. In: PW Callen, ed., *Ultrasonography in Obstetrics and Gynecology,* 4th ed. Philadelphia: Saunders; 2000:597–625.

23. Deutchman M, Tubay AT, Turok D. First trimester bleeding. *Am Fam Physician.* 2009 June 1;79(11):985–992.

24. Yamada T, Atsuki Y, Wakasaya A, et al. Characteristics of patients with subchorionic hematomas in the second trimester. *J Obstet Gynaecol Res.* 2012 Jan;38(1):180–184.

25. Champion E, Doubilet P, Benson C, Blaivas M. Current concepts: Diagnostic criteria for nonviable pregnancy early in the first trimester. *N Engl J Med.* 2013 Oct 10;369:1443–1451.

26. Barnhart K, van Mello NM, Bourne T, et al. Pregnancy of unknown location: a consensus statement of nomenclature, definitions, and outcome. *Fertil Steril.* 2011 March 1;95(3):857–866.

27. Hill J. Assisted reproduction and the multiple pregnancy: Increasing the risks for heterotopic pregnancy. *JDMS.* 2003;19:28–260.

28. Doubilet P, Benson C. Further evidence against the reliability of the human chorionic gonadotropin discriminatory level. *J Ultrasound Med.* 2011;30:1637–1642.

CHAPTER 12

Point-of-Care Sonography in the Second and Third Trimesters

Assessment of symptoms and complaints by pregnant women in the second and third trimesters can be expedited and decision making improved by utilizing sonography in the evaluation of both maternal and fetal conditions. Some of the common maternal symptoms include bleeding and pain, both of which warrant the use of point-of-care (POC) ultrasound at the bedside because timely results are needed.

Another situation in which a POC ultrasound exam is indicated is when a woman who has not had prenatal care presents with signs and symptoms of active labor. Under those circumstances, it may be imperative to determine fetal gestational age and weight, should the delivery be imminent and/or transfer to another facility indicated. Knowing approximate sonographic fetal gestational age may also assist in determining the need for tocolytics, steroid administration, and neonatal interventions and thus may impact long-term outcome.

In all clinical situations warranting a POC sonogram that do not result in birth, a standard sonogram should be performed as follow-up. This is particularly important if one has never been performed during the pregnancy.

STANDARD SECOND- AND THIRD-TRIMESTER EXAMINATION

The standard ultrasound performed in the second and third trimesters entails a complete survey, which includes taking fetal measurements, evaluating specific fetal anatomy, identifying the presence or absence of fetal cardiac activity, identifying the fetal number (i.e., twins), determining fetal presentation, identifying placental localization, and assessing the amniotic fluid. Additionally, when technically feasible, the maternal cervix and adnexa should be examined based on clinical indicators (Table 12–1).[1–3] Some measurements are used more frequently than others. This chapter focuses on the methods currently used in practice in estimating fetal age and weight.

FETAL BIOMETRY

Fetal biometry is the sonographic method of obtaining fetal measurements and comparing these findings to already-established fetal growth tables and growth curves. The individual anatomic measurement or combinations of anatomic measurements will correspond to ranges of fetal weights and gestational age. The most common measurements used in the second and third trimester of pregnancy include (1) fetal head biparietal diameter (BPD), (2) fetal head circumference (HC), (3) fetal femur length (FL), and (4) fetal abdominal circumference (AC).[4–7]

The gestational age of a pregnancy should never be assigned a new due date based on a second- or

TABLE 12–1	INDICATIONS FOR SECOND- AND THIRD-TRIMESTER STANDARD ULTRASOUND EXAMINATION
Estimation of Gestational Age and Weight	Suspected Ectopic Pregnancy
Evaluation of Fetal Growth	Rule out Fetal Demise
Evaluation of Fetal Well Being	Suspected Uterine Anomaly
Assessment of Amniotic Fluid	Suspected Placental Abruption
Vaginal Bleeding	Adjunct to External Cephalic Version
Cervical Insufficiency	Premature Rupture of Membranes (PROM)
Adjunct to Cerclage Placement	Abnormal Biochemical Markers
Determination of Presenting Part	Follow-up Evaluation of Fetal Anomaly
Fetal Number	Follow-up of Placental Location
Adjunct to Amniocentesis or Other Procedure	History of Prior Infant with Anomaly
Size/Dates Discrepancy	Assess for Indicators for Risk of Aneuploidy
Pelvic Mass	Screening for Fetal Anomalies
Suspected Hydatidiform Mole	Abdominal or Pelvic Pain

Adapted from AIUM.[1]

third-trimester sonogram *if* a first trimester dating ultrasound has already been performed.[1] Recalculating the gestational age of a pregnancy at this late point increases the risk of missing a fetal growth disorder. For example, if the third-trimester fetal growth scan indicates a gestational age of 3 weeks less than the gestational age determined by sonogram in the first trimester, that discrepancy in "dating" may actually indicate a growth-restricted fetus.

Fetal Biparietal Diameter

The BPD measurement is one of the four most common measurements used to determine fetal age. The BPD can be accurately measured after week 12 of the pregnancy. The proper sonographic image is obtained in a transverse view of the head. The correct level is identified when the thalami and the cavum septum pellucidi are visualized and the cerebellar hemispheres are not visible.[1]

The measurement is obtained by placing a caliper on the proximal or outside edge of the skull nearest the transducer and the second caliper on the inside of the distal skull. This is referred to as the outer-to-inner skull measurement or leading edge-to-leading edge (Figure 12–1). The inside distal edge of the skull is used because the farther the sound waves travel, the greater the likelihood of creating artifact or a thicker appearing skull. If the outer edge of the distal skull is used, the BPD (and thus the gestational age) will erroneously be determined to be larger with an incorrectly advanced gestational age and higher weight.

The BPD measurement is then compared to the BPD table, and the menstrual age in weeks will be determined. Modern ultrasound equipment contains software tables that automatically calculate fetal age and weight. These measurements and estimations of gestational age are based on the fetal head being more oval in shape. Other less common head shapes include a rounder appearance, known as brachycephalic, or an elongated shape, known as dolichocephalic, which may cause the BPD measurement to be misleading.[1]

Head Circumference

Due to the variations in head shape, measurement of the HC is utilized. The HC is considered more precise in determining fetal age because the measurement is not shape dependent.[1] As with the BPD, the HC can be measured after 12 weeks. The HC is obtained in the same view as the BPD, and an ellipse is used to encircle the head (Figures 12-1B and 12–2).

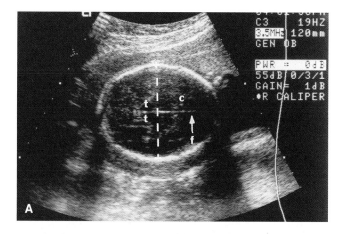

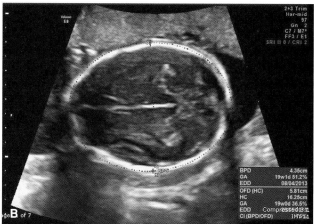

FIGURE 12–1. (A) Biparietal diameter (BPD). T, on each side of the thalami; c, over the cavum septi pellucidi; f, at the arrow is the falx cerebri, an echogenic line from anterior to posterior in the cranium. The first caliper is placed on the proximal or outside edge of the skull nearest the transducer and the second caliper on the inside of the distal skull. **(B)** Biparietal diameter on vertical axis. Note caliper placement. Ellipse indicates HC.

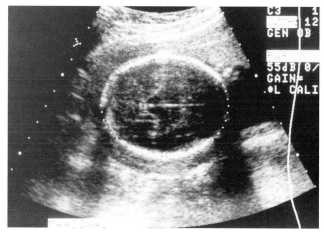

FIGURE 12–2. Head circumference (ellipse encircling skull at level of biparietal diameter [BPD]).

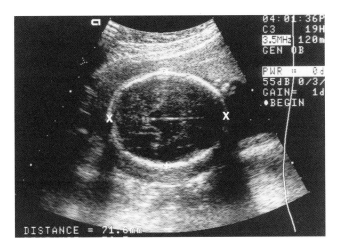

FIGURE 12-3. Cephalic index. Biparietal diameter (BPD; measured from + to +) multiplied by occipital frontal diameter (from × to ×).

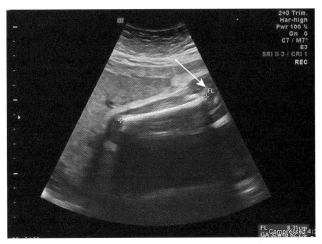

FIGURE 12-5. Hyperechoic femur at arrow, with correct placement of cursors (at each end) for measuring femur length. The epiphyses (arrow) are excluded from the measurement.

The calipers can also be placed on the lateral skull. A method used less frequently is the cephalic index (CI). The CI equals the BPD divided by the occipital-frontal diameter multiplied by 100 (Figure 12–3). The CI is an indicator of head shape that is used in the sonographic literature.

When measuring the BPD and HC, the cerebellum should not be visible. If it is, the scanning plane is too low (Figure 12–4).

Fetal Femur Length

The FL measurement is used in assessing fetal growth. This measurement is optimal at 15 weeks and remains accurate until approximately 32 weeks'. The femur is measured in a longitudinal position. The proper view is obtained when the longest measurement of femur is visualized. The diaphysis of the femur is echogenic and can display posterior shadowing depending on gestational age.

The measurement is done by placing a caliper at each end of the diaphysis (excluding the epiphysis). The epiphysis is hypoechoic, becoming hyperechoic after 32 weeks' gestation (Figure 12–5). For the best resolution, the femur closest to the transducer should be measured. After 32 weeks' or if the posterior (deep) femur is being measured, the femur can appear bowed.[2] Abnormal bowing may also be seen in fetuses with skeletal abnormalities such as hypomineralization or osteogenesis imperfecta, which can lead to bone fractures (Figure 12–6).

The femur length measurement is calculated by the ultrasound system. To evaluate proper growth, various ratios are used in determining intrauterine growth restriction (IUGR). A common ratio used to estimate proportional growth is femur length to abdominal circumference.

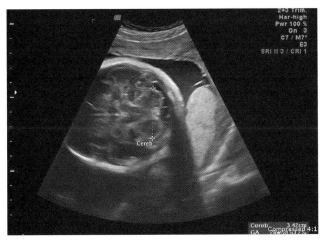

FIGURE 12-4. Measurement of the cerebellum.

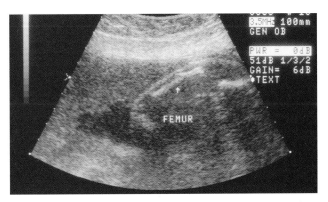

FIGURE 12-6. Femur with hypomineralization. Note the break in the femur at the arrow.

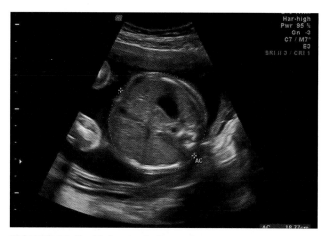

FIGURE 12–7. Abdominal circumference.

Fetal Abdominal Circumference

The AC is used to evaluate fetal growth and fetal age. This measurement is made by obtaining a transverse image of the fetal abdomen at the level of the stomach and the umbilical vein joining the portal vein, which forms a "J" shape (Figures 12–7 and 12–8).[1]

To obtain this level, image the fetus in a longitudinal axis, turn the transducer into a transverse position at the level of the stomach, and move the transducer superior and inferior until the correct fetal parts are seen. If the fetal kidneys are visualized, then the level is too low in the fetal abdomen. Then place one caliper on the outside of the anterior skin edge of the abdomen and the other caliper on the outside skin edge of the posterior spine. The ellipse is then opened and expanded to cover the outer portion of the abdomen. The skin line needs to be included. The resulting value is calculated by the ultrasound system.

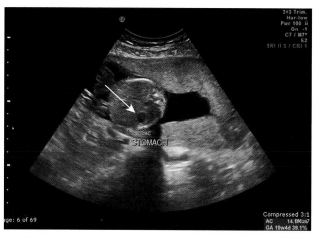

FIGURE 12–8. Transverse image of level for abdominal circumference. AC, abdominal circumference. Note the anechoic stomach bubble.

ESTIMATED FETAL WEIGHT

The estimated fetal weight (EFW) is achieved by utilizing combinations of fetal anatomic measurements, such as by using the AC and BPD measurements. These measurements are then plotted on a growth chart displaying EFW. A second method utilizes the AC and the FL. These growth charts were created in the 1970s and 1980s, but still hold true at present.[8] However, in most cases, instead of the clinician needing to plot the measurements on a graph, the software in the ultrasound machine performs the calculations and then displays the result on the report page along with the estimated gestational age and estimated date of delivery.

Newer formulas that use three measurements such as HC, AC, and FL to calculate EFW are available in some software packages that come with the newer ultrasound machines. In some cases, they have proved to be more accurate. However, the Hadlock is generally recognized as most accurate over the full range of fetal weights from 500 to 5,000 g.[8]

If a fetus is being evaluated for a growth concern, the comparative scans should be performed every 2 to 4 weeks[1] and plotted on growth charts (Appendix D). A growth scan performed sooner can yield erroneous results. Fetal weight predictions may have an error rate as high as +/–15%. A study by Ben-Haroush et al.[9] showed that EFW by sonogram had a high correlation with actual birth weight, except in preterm premature rupture of the membranes (PPROM) and larger for gestational age (LGA) fetuses. In the PPROM cases, an underestimated EFW occurred, and in the LGA cases, an overestimation occurred. In a second study, the authors stated that "the true value of ultrasonography in the management of fetal macrosomia may be its ability to rule out the diagnosis."[10]

Gender is an additional consideration for estimating gestational age as well as estimating fetal weight. Gender-specific growth charts (Appendix D) may be used to optimize the prediction of EFW.[11,12] This was further substantiated by Melmed et al. in 2013,[13] whose study showed that female fetuses grow considerably slower than male fetuses from an early gestation onward. In this study, the female fetus appeared not to be merely a smaller version of the male fetus, but rather they observed a sex-specific growth pattern for each of the individual fetal biometric indices. These findings provide further support for the use of sex-specific sonographic models for fetal weight estimation, as well as the use of sex-specific reference growth charts.

The accuracy of sonographic formulas (Hadlock and Shepard) for estimating weight in singleton gestations was recently studied in twin pregnancies. All widely used EFW formulas performed equally well in estimating birth weight in twin gestations. However, most women delivered between 33 and 36 weeks' gestation, thus limiting the studies to gestations of under 36 weeks.[14]

THE FETAL ANATOMIC SURVEY

A standard sonogram performed after 18 weeks' gestation includes minimal elements of a fetal anatomic screen (Table 12–2).

Deviations from Normal Fetal Anatomy

Evaluation of fetal anatomy is not a part of a POC sonogram. However, to obtain anatomic landmarks for estimating fetal age and weight, knowing normal fetal anatomy is important. One method for learning normal anatomy is to compare it with abnormal anatomic features. A few significant anatomic abnormalities will be described and images presented in the following section to compare normal and abnormal anatomy.

Fetal Head

The fetal cranium normally appears as a hyperechoic oval. Anencephaly is identified by sonography when the fetal cranium cannot be visualized. The com-

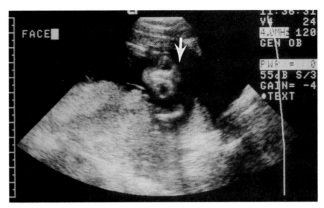

FIGURE 12–9. Anencephalic. Note that the cranium is not over the eyes (at arrows). Eyes appear hypoechoic.

mon appearance is noted by the absence of cranium from the forehead up, along with bulging orbits (Figure 12–9), which are hypoechoic on sonography.

Lateral Ventricles

At the superior level of the head are the lateral ventricles. The choroid plexus are located within the ventricles and produce cerebral spinal fluid (CSF). The ventricles carry CSF through the brain. The lateral ventricles are divided into various portions: the frontal, the body, and the occipital. They are located anteriorly, midportion, and posteriorly, respectively.

It is recommended that the lateral ventricular measurement be taken at the level of the atria to evaluate for hydrocephalus and other anomalies such as Dandy-Walker malformation (Figure 12–10). This measurement can be routinely obtained after 12 weeks' gestation. The normal measurement should not be greater than 10 mm.

TABLE 12–2 MINIMAL ELEMENTS OF A STANDARD EXAMINATION OF FETAL ANATOMY

Head, Face, Neck	Cerebellum Choroid Plexus Cisterna Magna Lateral Cerebral Ventricles Midline Falx Cavum Septi Pellucidi Upper Lip	**Spine**	Cervical, Thoracic, Lumbar, and Sacral Spine
Chest	Four-Chamber View Left ventricular outflow tract Right ventricular outflow tract	**Extremities**	Presence/absence of legs and arms
Abdomen	Stomach (presence, size, and situs) Kidneys Urinary Bladder Umbilical Cord Insertion Side into Fetal Abdomen Umbilical cord vessel number	**Sex**	Multiple Gestations and when Medically Indicated

Adapted from AIUM.[1]

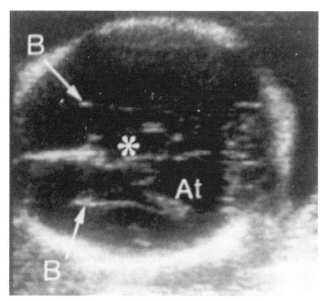

FIGURE 12–10. Axial scan through the lateral ventricles showing typical enlargement of the atria (At) and widely separated bodies (B) with the upward displacement of the third ventricle (*).

The choroid plexus is hyperechoic, homogeneous tissue and should be evaluated for simple cysts. Single cysts or multiple cysts creating a mottled appearance to the choroid plexus can be seen before 22 weeks but should resolve after that gestation.

Cerebellum

The cerebellum is located in the posterior-inferior portion of the brain. The image is obtained by placing the transducer in a coronal position at the frontal bone and angling posterior to the base of the skull (Figure 12–11). The transducer may also be angled inferior to the BPD/HC measurement level.

Measuring the cerebellum is helpful in determining gestational age.

The cerebellum is responsible for the coordination of muscular movements. The shape of the cerebellum is also important. The normal cerebellum is dumbbell-shaped, similar to Figure 12–8. If, however, the cerebellum is "banana-shaped," it can be indicative of a neural tube defect. This shape has been designated the "banana sign." This abnormality, along with dilated lateral ventricles, is known as a Chiari malformation (previously named Arnold Chiari) and is associated with spinal defects.

Cerebellar measurements can also be used in cases of suspected symmetric growth restriction to differentiate IUGR from a small for gestational age (SGA) fetus. The cerebellum is often the last to be compromised in the setting of IUGR.

Cisterna Magna

Posterior to the cerebellum is the cisternal magna, normally measuring 2 to 10 mm (Figure 12–12). This measurement may also be helpful in evaluating for Dandy-Walker malformation. Also, the cisterna magna will be obliterated in the setting of Chiari malformations and many neural tube defects.

Spine

The spine is divided into five segments: cervical, thoracic, lumbar, sacral, and coccyx. The spine can be evaluated in longitudinal, transverse, and/or coronal views. The spine is typically ossified after 15 weeks and, depending on fetal position, can be visualized at this age. To evaluate for spinal closure, a careful scan of each vertebrae, as well as the skin line,

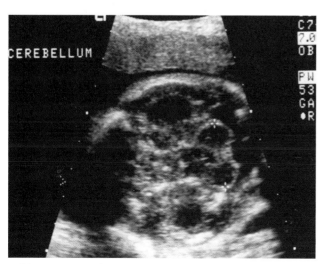

FIGURE 12–11. Cerebellum, between "+" signs.

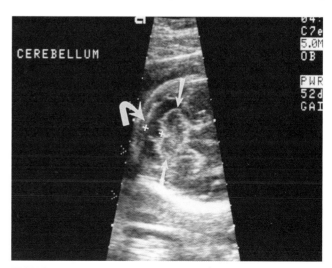

FIGURE 12–12. Cisterna magna (curved arrow) with the measurement between the "+" signs. The cerebellum is between the straight arrows.

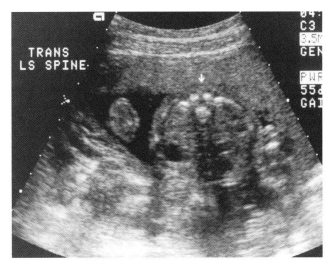

FIGURE 12–13. Transverse view of the spine. The arrow indicates the ossification centers, which in this image are normal.

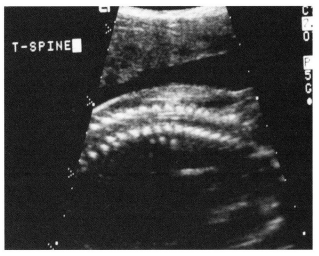

FIGURE 12–15. Thoracic spine in longitudinal view.

is imaged in the transverse position. This position permits visualization of the three ossification centers (Figure 12–13). Any splaying of the ossification centers will indicate an abnormality. The longitudinal plane is helpful for imaging and evaluating a complete skin line, as well as the normal spinal curvatures (Figures 12–14, 12–15, and 12–16).

Abnormalities such as cystic hygroma and encephalocele can be identified at the level of the cervical spine. The most common location for spina bifida and myelomeningocele are the lumbar and sacral spine, although they can occur at any level. Sacrococcygeal teratomas occur at the sacrum and coccyx. Due to these abnormalities, skin closure over the vertebrae is important to image and observe (Figure 12–17).

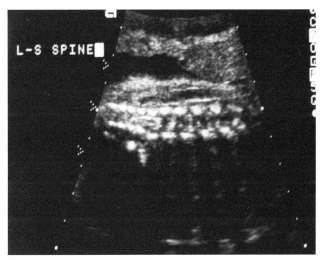

FIGURE 12–16. Lumbar-sacral spine in longitudinal view.

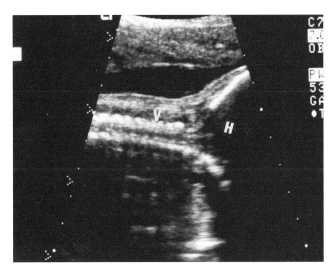

FIGURE 12–14. Longitudinal view of cervical spine. H, head; V, vertebrae.

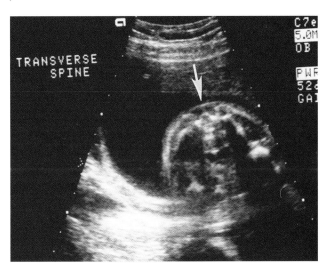

FIGURE 12–17. Transverse view of the lumbar-sacral spine. Note the intact skin closure (arrow).

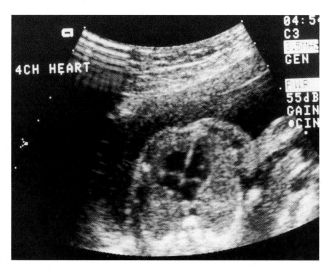

FIGURE 12–18. Axial view of four-chamber fetal heart.

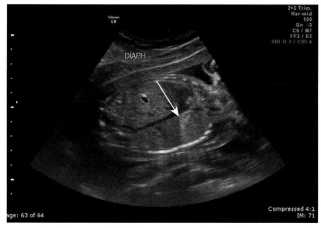

FIGURE 12–20. Longitudinal view of the fetal chest and abdomen. Note the diaphragm (arrow) separating abdominal contents from chest contents.

Chest/Heart

The heart is imaged in an axial approach allowing visualization of the four chambers (Figure 12–18). The heart should comprise one-third of the fetal chest. Fetal heart motion is confirmed using M-mode sonography, and this view then archived (Figure 12–19).

Abdomen

The structures in the fetal abdomen that need to be identified during the sonographic evaluation are the stomach, three-vessel umbilical cord, bowel, liver, and gallbladder. One important landmark is the fetal diaphragm (Figure 12–20), which divides the contents of the abdomen from the chest. The diaphragm is also a useful landmark in the

observation of fetal breathing movements during a biophysical profile (see Chapter 13). Since the stomach is fluid-filled, sonographically it will appear anechoic (Figure 12–8). It remains this way until term, when the fetus may swallow amniotic fluid containing meconium and/or vernix, which will then appear as hyperechoic debris within the stomach. A left-sided stomach needs to be confirmed at each sonogram.

The three-vessel umbilical cord is identified in the transverse view. It contains one larger vessel that is the umbilical vein and two smaller vessels that are the umbilical arteries (Figure 12–21). A two-vessel cord would be considered an abnormality and requires further investigation of all other systems.

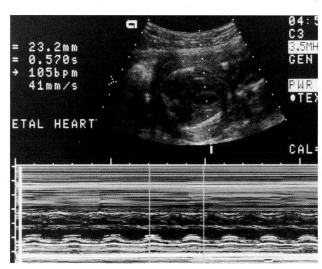

FIGURE 12–19. M-mode tracing of fetal heart verifying cardiac motion.

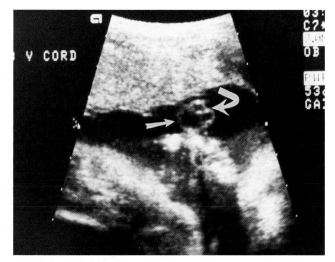

FIGURE 12–21. Transverse view of three-vessel umbilical cord. Large arrow points at the large hypoechoic umbilical vein; curved arrow indicates the two smaller hypoechoic arteries.

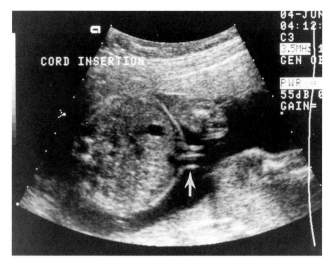

FIGURE 12–22. Cord insertion into fetal abdomen (arrow).

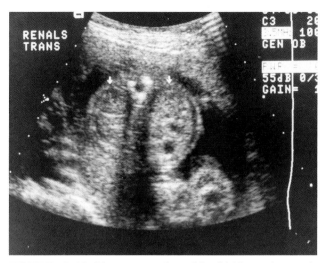

FIGURE 12–23. Transverse view of fetal kidneys (arrows).

The umbilical vein enters the abdomen and joins the portal vein in the liver. The umbilical arteries originate at the fetal iliac arteries, extend along each side of the fetal bladder to the anterior abdominal wall, and return to the placenta. The cord insertion site is at the level where the arteries and vein are viewed entering the abdomen (Figure 12–22). This is a vital image, necessary to assess for any type of abdominal wall defects such as gastroschisis and omphalocele.

The fetal gallbladder appears as an ovoid, fluid-filled, tear-drop shaped structure to the right and inferior to the intrahepatic section of the umbilical vein. It can also be visualized and may be confused with the umbilical vein due to their proximity. Nonetheless, the gallbladder should be imaged.

Kidneys

Beginning at approximately 16 weeks' gestation, the fetal kidneys may be visualized and evaluated transabdominally. They are located inferior to the level of the stomach. The kidneys are viewed in a transverse approach and are located on either side of the spine (Figure 12–23). Both the right and left kidney should be visualized. The kidneys are evaluated for hydronephrosis and cystic or solid masses. A longitudinal or coronal view of the kidneys will assist in differentiating the kidneys from the adrenal glands, which are located cephalad to the kidneys.

Bladder

The fetal bladder is identified as an anechoic structure located between the iliac crests (Figure 12–24). The

bladder will change in volume during the course of the sonogram. This filling and emptying of the bladder will verify that the bladder is free of urethral obstruction.

Other Views and Measurements

The aorta and iliac arteries may be visualized to assess fetal circulation (Figure 12–25).

Gender can be difficult to determine in a breech position. Determination of the gender can be done by viewing between both femurs (Figure 12–26). However, it is possible to misidentify the umbilical cord as a penis (Figure 12–27).

The nose and lips are very important views in determining facial defects, such as cleft lip and palate. Evaluation of the hands consists of counting digits and identifying normal hand position (Figure 12–28). The feet can also be evaluated for evidence of clubbing.

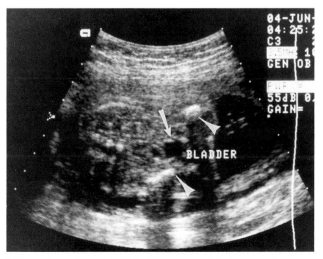

FIGURE 12–24. Fetal bladder (arrow) between iliac crests (arrowheads).

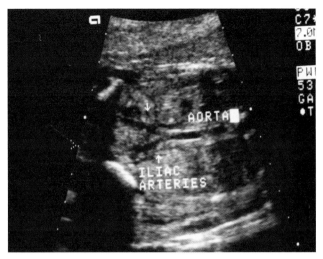

FIGURE 12–25. Fetal aorta (anechoic tubular structure) and iliac arteries branching from it.

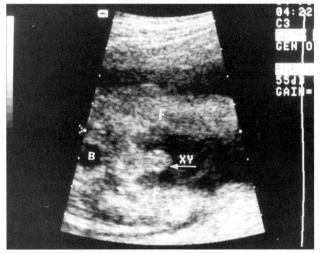

FIGURE 12–26. Male fetus. The penis is identified between the femur bones of each leg. F, femur; bones, xy, penis; B, bladder.

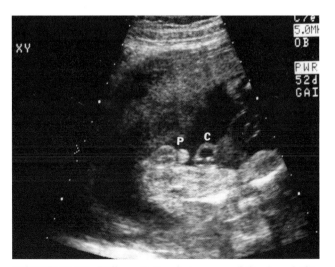

FIGURE 12–27. Differentiation between umbilical cord (C), which can be between the legs, and penis (P).

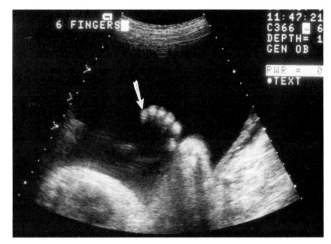

FIGURE 12–28. Fetal hand digits. Arrow indicates polydactyly (six fingers).

SONOGRAPHIC ASSESSMENT OF AMNIOTIC FLUID

Amniotic fluid assessment is part of the standard obstetric ultrasound exam and may be performed subjectively and described with such terms as increased, normal, or decreased. When objective fluid assessments are done during the standard second- and third-trimester sonograms or during a biophysical profile (BPP), the maximum vertical pocket measurement, 2 cm "deepest" pocket or the amniotic fluid index may be used (see Chapter 13).[1]

THE PLACENTA

Placental localization is part of the standard second- and third-trimester obstetrical sonograms. The placental appearance and location in relationship to the cervical os should be documented.[1] Sonographic appearance of placental tissue begins as echogenic focal thickening of the wall of the gestational sac early in pregnancy to a more homogenous appearance toward the end of the first trimester that continues throughout the duration of the pregnancy. Hyperechoic lines of calcification may be seen outlining the cotyledons as the placenta matures.

POC ultrasound of the placenta is indicated when a woman presents in the second or third trimester with the chief complaint of vaginal bleeding. Differential diagnosis of bleeding in pregnancy includes such etiologies as placental abruption and placenta previa, but can also be caused by cervical erosion, preterm labor, term labor, and lacerations, to name a few. Diagnosis of placental-related bleeding issues has significantly improved since the introduction of ultrasound into obstetric care.[1,2,15] Therefore, this section focuses on placental abruption, placenta previa, and other placental deviations that carry the risk for adverse maternal and fetal conditions.

Placenta Previa

Placenta previa refers to placental tissue that covers or partially covers the internal cervical os. The patient classically presents with painless vaginal bleeding. The incidence of placenta previa is 1 in 200 to 250 births. Of those, approximately 20% are complete and 80% are marginal or partial. However, in recent years, there has been an increase incidence of placenta previa directly related to the increased incidence of cesarean births. Potential complications from placenta previa include premature delivery and hemorrhage.

To avoid errors in sonographic interpretation, both the lower edge of the placenta and the internal cervical os must be visualized. In a study by Rosati and Guariglia,[16] transvaginal sonography (TVS) was used as the primary method for evaluating placental location in 10- to 16-week gestations. Although there was a high false-positive rate (placenta previa diagnosed by the early scan but not present later in pregnancy), the transvaginal (TV) approach can be effective in high-risk patients. TVS permits specific measurements from the lower margin of the placenta to the internal os. However, care must be taken not to apply the pressure of the transducer to the cervix or lower uterine segment because it could potentially cause bleeding or cause error in measurement. The transperineal approach may be a safer option. When a previa is diagnosed early in pregnancy, follow-up scans are imperative.[16] Care must be taken not to misinterpret an echogenic subchorionic hematoma overlying the cervix for placental tissue.

Sonographically, placenta previa appears as placental tissue covering all or part of the internal cervical os. This tissue may be normal echogenic placental tissue or hypoechoic venous lakes or vessels of the placenta. There may be displacement of the presenting fetal part from the internal os. Placenta previa can be excluded if one of the following can be demonstrated: (1) direct sonographic visualization of both the lower edge of the placenta and the internal cervical os, with the lower edge of the placenta seen separate from the cervix; (2) amniotic fluid between the presenting part and the cervix without interposed placental tissue; or (3) the presenting part immediately overlying the cervix without space for intervening placental tissue.

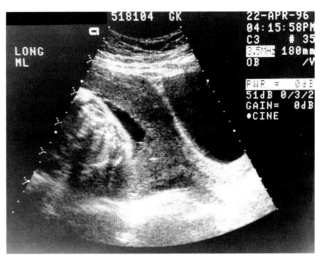

FIGURE 12–29. Complete placenta previa. Internal cervical os (small arrow), and placenta (*).

Distinguishing an asymmetric complete placenta previa from a partial placenta previa or a very low-lying placenta may be difficult.

Placenta previa is divided into the following categories based on the placental proximity to the cervical os: complete or total, partial, marginal, and low-lying. Total placental previa occurs when the placenta completely covers the cervical os. The placenta may be predominately on the anterior, posterior, or lateral uterine wall extending over the cervix, but often is not symmetrically located over the cervical os (Figure 12–29). When the placenta is concentrically implanted about the cervical os, the term *central placenta previa* is frequently used.

A partial placenta previa occurs when the placental edge covers a portion of the internal cervical os. A marginal placenta previa abuts the edge of the cervix but does not cover the cervical os. A low-lying placenta occurs when the placental edge is implanted on the lower uterine segment but does not encroach on the internal cervical os. If the placenta is less than 3 to 5 cm from the cervical os, it is considered a marginal previa.[17]

TVS has also shown to be very effective in the diagnosis of placenta previa. TVS permits specific measurements from the lower margin of the placenta to the internal os. Care must be taken not to apply the pressure of the transducer to the cervix or lower uterine segment because it could potentially cause bleeding or cause error in measurement.

A partial or marginal placenta previa that is seen during the second trimester should be sonographically reevaluated in the third trimester of pregnancy. Many times, the uterus has grown in such a manner that the placenta is no longer as close to or covering the internal cervical os. This movement of the placenta is sometimes referred to as *placental migration*. The apparent movement or motion appears to be a result of differential growth rates between the lower uterine segment and the placenta, with relatively rapid growth of the myometrium just above the level of the cervix.

Technical factors that can mimic placenta previa are focal uterine contractions or an overly distended bladder. A focal uterine contraction can be suspected if the myometrial wall is focally thickened (>1.5 cm). The placenta is usually more echogenic than the contracted uterine wall. Rescanning after 30 to 60 minutes generally allows sufficient time for the contraction to dissipate and to restore normal anatomic relationships.

During a transabdominal scan, an overly distended bladder may press against the lower uterine segment, bringing the anterior wall against the posterior wall and causing an artificially elongated cervix. If the cervix measures greater than 3 to 4 cm, then the bladder is probably overdistended. If this occurs, the woman can partially void, and the sonogram is repeated. If the placental location in relationship to the cervix still cannot be determined, have the patient void completely and repeat the sonogram.

Use of gentle transabdominal traction on the fetal head may allow visualization of the internal cervical os despite low position of the fetal head. If the cervical os cannot be adequately identified using the transabdominal ultrasound technique, TV and/or transperineal techniques may be used.

An alternate method of evaluating the internal cervical os is the transperineal or translabial approach. It requires no specialized equipment, vaginal penetration, or manipulation of the fetus. The bladder is emptied, and the woman is placed in the lithotomy position. A sector (abdominal) transducer covered with a condom or glove is placed in the sagittal orientation directly over or between the labia minora. The transducer is angled medially and laterally to image the entire internal surface of the cervix. The orientation of the image will be the same as with the TV transducer: the vagina is at the apex of the image (top of the screen), and the cervix is in a horizontal plane.

Vasa Previa

Vasa previa occurs in about 1 in 3,000 births. It is the result of the velamentous insertion of the umbilical cord in the lower uterine segment so that the unsupported cord vessels traverse through membranes and the internal cervical os (Figure 12–30). Vasa previa is associated with higher fetal mortality rates.

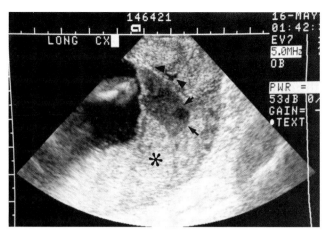

FIGURE 12–30. Variation of vasa previa. Transvaginal sonography demonstrates large area of vascularity by the internal cervical os. Vasa previa (arrows), internal cervical os (arrows), internal cervical os (arrowheads), placenta (*).

These unsupported vessels are prone to tearing when the membranes rupture, resulting in fetal exsanguination and death in at least 75% of the cases. There also may be compression of vessels by a presenting part, which compromises feto-placental circulation. There is a highly significant association between a second-trimester placenta previa and vasa previa at birth,[18] which further supports the need for follow-up sonographic evaluation of early scans.

O'Brien and Sheehan[19] believe that the location of the cord insertion is an integral part of all obstetric sonographic studies. Color Doppler ultrasound is extremely helpful in making the diagnosis of both vasa previa and velamentous insertion of the cord because of its ability to determine the cord insertion. If an abnormal cord insertion or any placental abnormality is noted, such as an extra lobe, a TV scan should be performed to further evaluate for any abnormality.[19]

Placenta Accreta

Placenta accreta is an abnormal attachment of the placenta in which the chorionic villi have grown directly into the myometrium. This is called a *placenta accreta vera*. It is attributed to complete or partial absence of the decidua basalis and imperfect development of the fibrin layer. If the villi have penetrated deeper into the myometrium, it is called *placenta increta*. If the uterine serosa has been penetrated, the villi pass through the uterus and often attach into the bladder or rectum.[20] This is referred to as *placenta percreta*. The term *placenta accreta* is generally used to refer to all three types (Figures 12–31 and 12–32).

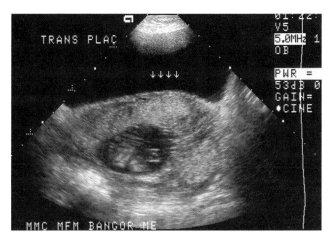

FIGURE 12–31. Transverse transabdominal image of placenta accreta (arrows pointing to invasion).

The most common predisposing factor for developing a placenta accreta is uterine scar from previous cesarean birth. Placenta accreta can cause antepartum bleeding, but in the majority of cases the bleeding is a consequence of coexisting placenta previa. The greatest risk of placenta accreta is during the third stage of labor when the placenta fails to separate and deliver, resulting in persistent postpartum bleeding and maternal hemorrhage. Severe hemorrhage, uterine perforation, and infection resulting from attempts at manual removal contribute to maternal morbidity and mortality. If manual extraction is unsuccessful, a surgical intervention may be necessary to control bleeding.

At times, placenta accreta may be visualized by ultrasound by analyzing the retroplacental complex. The retroplacental complex is a 1 to 2 cm hypoechoic band. In accreta, this band is either absent or less than 2 mm thick. Additionally, there is a loss of the normal decidual interface between the placenta and myometrium. The placenta can also have a "Swiss cheese" appearance and marked vasculature on color Doppler. If the placenta is posterior, a TV ultrasound with Doppler or magnetic resonance imaging (MRI) should be utilized.[20,21]

Other sonographic markers include:

- Absence or severe thinning of the hypoechoic myometrium between the placenta and uterine serosa-bladder wall
- Thinning, irregularity, or disruption of the linear hypoechoic uterine serosa-bladder wall complex
- Extension of tissue of placental echogenicity beyond the uterine serosa

Placental Abruption

Placenta abruption is also referred to as *placenta abruption, abruptio placentae, ablatio placentae,* and *premature separation* or *abnormally implanted placenta.* Sonographic examination is not as sensitive for the detection of abruption as it is for placenta previa. However, if a positive finding is noted, such as visualization of a hematoma, then the likelihood of an abruption is increased.[22]

The sonographic appearance of an abruption depends on its age. An acute hematoma may range from hyperechoic to isoechoic relative to the placenta. A resolving hematoma generally becomes hypoechoic or will have mixed echoes within a week of the onset of symptoms. This depends on the degree of organization. Within 2 weeks, the resolving hematoma will be anechoic (Figures 12–33 and 12–34). Color Doppler

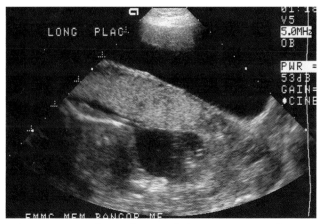

FIGURE 12–32. Sagittal view of placenta accreta also seen in Figure 12–31.

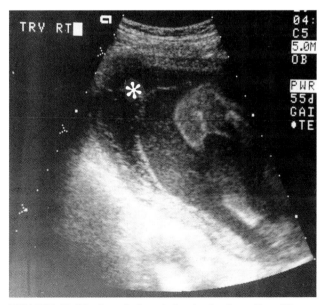

FIGURE 12–33. Isoechoic subchorionic abruption (*).

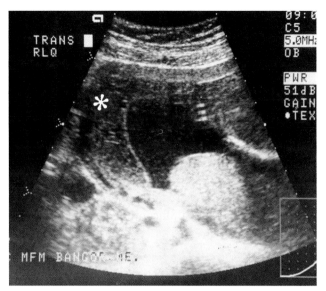

FIGURE 12–34. The same patient as in Figure 12–33, 18 days later. Note the mixed echogenicity of the abruption (*).

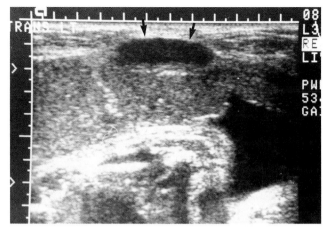

FIGURE 12–35. Retroplacental abruption demonstrating bleeding with the separation of the placenta from the uterine wall (arrows).

may be useful to determine a suspected abruption. The color Doppler box is positioned over the anatomic area of interest. The color filter is adjusted to the most sensitive low-flow setting, and the Doppler velocity scale to the low- or slow-flow setting. The presence of color flow in the suspected area will rule out abruption.

The color Doppler settings should be readjusted and the area of interest reimaged if no flow is demonstrated. Color amplitude power mapping, when available, is also helpful in visualizing flow. The probability of an abruption is greatly increased if flow is not demonstrated using these techniques.

Abruption may be categorized as retroplacental, subchorionic and marginal, or preplacental. Retroplacental abruption occurs when there is a separation of the placenta from the myometrial wall (Figure 12–35). Evidence suggests that retroplacental abruption usually results from the rupture of the decidual spiral arteries, with hemorrhage into the decidua basalis producing "high-pressure" bleeds. Most small retroplacental hematomas are asymptomatic, whereas large hematomas may have devastating consequences. Retroplacental hematomas are often linear or biconcave with well–defined margins (Figure 12–36). Large hematomas may deform the overlying placenta and produce bulging of the chorionic plate.

Acute retroplacental hematomas may be difficult to recognize because they dissect into the placenta and/or myometrium and are isoechoic to the adjacent placenta. In these cases, sonography may demonstrate

a thickened, heterogenous-appearing placenta that may measure up to 9 cm thick compared to a normal thickness of 4 to 5 cm.

With the finding of a thickened, heterogenous-appearing placenta, the differential diagnosis includes (1) normal retroplacental myometrium with prominent basal veins, (2) retroplacental myoma, (3) myometrial contraction, and (4) placental maturation along the basal plate. When an abruption is

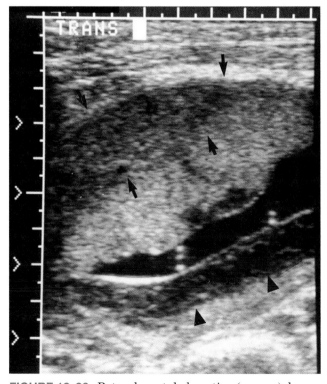

FIGURE 12–36. Retroplacental abruption (arrows) demonstrating a biconcave appearance. Subchorionic bleeding is noted (arrowheads).

diagnosed by ultrasound, follow-up sonograms are recommended to ensure that the placental abruption decreases in size and that fetal growth is appropriate for gestational age. Other fetal testing may be indicated.

Marginal Placental Abruption

A marginal placental abruption is seen at the periphery of the placenta and can result from tears of marginal veins, producing "low-pressure" bleeds. This most likely occurs because the placental membrane separates easier from the myometrium than the more firmly attached placenta.

The placental edge is elevated slightly, but marginal abruption is associated with little placental detachment and clinical symptoms are mild. The hematoma may extend away from the placenta to the subchorionic area.

In some situations, the subchorionic hematoma may be seen in a site remote from the placenta and is presumed to have originated from bleeding at the placental margin (Figure 12–37). Nearly all subchorionic hematomas arise from marginal abruptions, but in only one-half of the cases is placental detachment demonstrated by ultrasound. As the hematoma resolves, the detached placental membrane may be the only evidence of prior subchorionic hematoma.

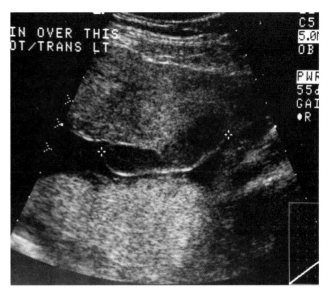

FIGURE 12–38. Preplacental bleeding with blood between the placenta and chorion anechoic area between **.

Marginal placental abruption is strongly associated with maternal smoking. The sonographic differential diagnosis includes (1) succenturiate lobe, (2) chorioangioma, (3) placenta previa, or (4) coexisting molar pregnancy.

Preplacental Abruption

Preplacental abruption occurs when there is a collection of blood between the placenta and the chorion or between the amnion and chorion, although the distinction between the two usually cannot be made by ultrasound (Figure 12–38). Large preplacental hematomas may produce clinical symptoms similar to placental abruption; however, placental detachment does not occur from preplacental hematomas.

Differentiating Placental Tissue from Other Structures

Unusual shapes or configurations of the placenta will impact the sonographic appearance of the structure and may impact birth outcome. A succenturiate or bilobed placenta (Figure 12–39) has an accessory lobe connected by either blood vessels within a membrane or by chorionic tissue to the main placental mass. Risks associated with this include retained placental tissue, as well as fetal hemorrhage. A circumvallate placenta is defined as placental implantation that extends beyond the limits of the chorionic plate. Other deviations from normal include amniotic bands, as well as abnormal placental size as seen in fetal hydrops.

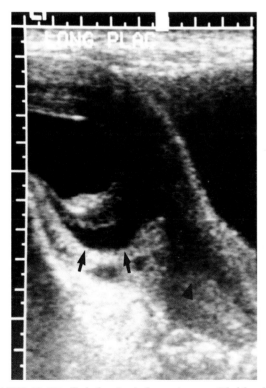

FIGURE 12–37. Subchorionic hematoma with blood (arrows) at internal os (arrowhead).

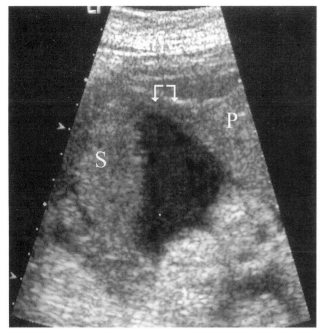

FIGURE 12–39. Succenturiate lobe. The succenturiate lobe (S) is connected to the placenta (P) by the bridge of tissue and vessels.

Placental tissue must also be differentiated from leiomyomas (fibroids) (Figure 12–40) and uterine contraction. Fibroids often distort the wall of the uterus and alter the contour. Uterine contractions can be determined either by palpation of the maternal abdomen or by continued sonographic observation until the contraction ends and the "mass" disappears.

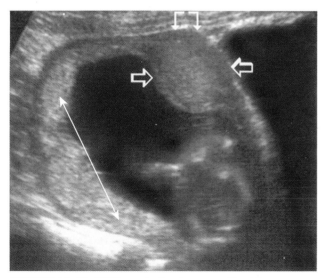

FIGURE 12–40. Differentiation between fibroid (between arrowheads) and placental tissue along right lateral uterine wall with double arrow indicating placental tissue. Note differences in types of echoes, with the fibroid appearing more isoechoic.

Placental Calcifications

As the placenta matures, some degree of calcification occurs, sonographically appearing as hyperechoic "patches." This formed the basis of placental grading that was once used as one parameter in the biophysical profile (see Chapter 13).

Placental Lakes

On examination of the placenta, hypoechoic areas within the placental tissue may be seen. These are called venous or placental lakes. Placental lakes are more likely to be found with a thick placenta (>3 cm at 20 weeks' gestation) and do not appear to be associated with any uteroplacental complication or adverse pregnancy outcome.[17,23]

Retained Placenta

When clinical suspicions point to possible retained placental products during the postpartum period, a sonogram may be ordered prior to surgical interventions. The sonographic findings are often nonspecific because blood clots and retained products show considerable overlap in their sonographic appearances. The most common finding of retained placental tissue is an endometrial mass (Figure 12–41).[24,25] The use of color Doppler, however, can further clarify a clot versus retained products. Clot within the endometrium typically does not display color flow. On the other hand, retained products often have a "stalk-like" or diffuse flow within the mass or endometrium.

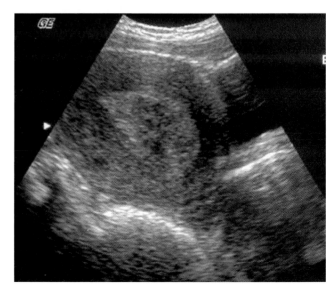

FIGURE 12–41. Retained placental tissue.

MATERNAL CERVICAL LENGTH MEASUREMENT: Betty Kay Taylor

Measuring cervical length has become a relatively common POC sonogram performed in response to a complaint of uterine activity or cramping. Until recently, the research pertaining to the association between cervical length and preterm birth has focused on the high-risk population, particularly women with a history of preterm birth. The benefit of the routine cervical length measurement was clearly established as a predictor for preterm birth in women with a history of prior preterm birth. However, since approximately 50% of preterm births occur in primigravidas, the need for a screening exam in this group was needed. Crane and Hutchens[26] showed that cervical length measurement done with TVU in asymptomatic high-risk women predicted spontaneous preterm birth at less than 35 weeks of gestation. Multiple studies have shown that a short cervix measured by ultrasound is a powerful predictor for preterm birth. As recommended by the American College of Obstetrics and Gynecology (ACOG), in high-risk pregnancies, treatment with injectable progesterone has proven successful in reducing the preterm birth rate.[27]

In 2010, a study by Cahill et al.[28] was undertaken to estimate a strategy that would be cost-effective for the treatment of preterm birth when a short cervix was diagnosed by ultrasound. The study focused on using ultrasound cervical length measurements as a screening in all pregnant women rather than scanning only those determined to be at risk based on history. Their conclusion was that universal screening for cervical length followed by treatment with progesterone gel of those determined to have a short cervical length was cost effective. They also showed that it resulted in a statistically significant reduction of preterm birth at less than 34 weeks' gestation.

The Cahill study was followed by a study by Hassan et al.[29] in 2011 specifically testing the efficacy of progesterone gel in reducing the rate of preterm birth in those women with an ultrasound-diagnosed short cervix between 19 and 23 weeks' gestation. This study was a prospective, randomized, double-blinded study and included 44 medical centers in 10 countries. A short cervix was defined as being between 10 and 20 mm in asymptomatic women. The results showed a substantial reduction in the rate of preterm delivery at less than 33 weeks' gestation and a significant decrease in the rate of respiratory distress syndrome (RDS). Based

on these studies, the current belief of many health care providers is that there is convincing evidence supporting routine cervical length measurements in all pregnant women in the second trimester of pregnancy.[30]

TV cervical ultrasound has been shown to be a reliable and reproducible method for assessing cervical length in the second trimester of pregnancy.[31] Transabdominal (TA) cervical length measurements performed with an empty bladder has shown a close correlation with TV ultrasound in some studies and may be the first step in cervical assessment.[32]

The ACOG recommends that the use of cervical length measurement may be helpful in determining which patients may do *not* need tocolysis. Cervical length ultrasound has a good negative predictive value in showing that those with a normal cervical length will not need tocolysis.[31]

Errors in scanning technique that can distort the appearance of the cervix or alter cervical measurements include putting too much pressure against the cervix with the vaginal probe or fundal pressure. An overly distended maternal bladder can also exert enough pressure to artificially elongate the cervix.

How to Measure Cervical Length

The distal portion of the uterus, the uterine cervix, consists primarily of cartilaginous connective tissue that serves to close the passageway from the uterus to the vagina. It softens with pregnancy, and prior to labor it begins to efface or thin. This process starts from the inner os of the cervix, the uterine end of the canal, and progresses toward the external os at the vaginal end[33,34] (Figures 12–42, 12–43, and 12–44). This internal effacement can be seen by ultrasound, but it cannot be felt by an examining

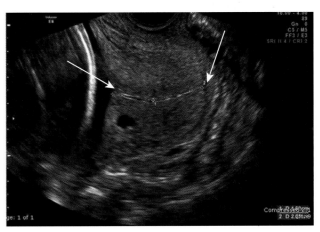

FIGURE 12–42. Cervical length, between arrows.

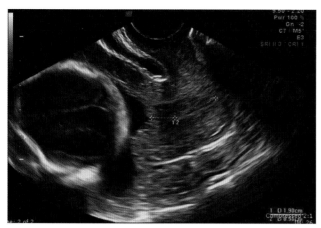

FIGURE 12–43. Cervical length noted between **. Note that because the cervix is curved, two lengths are determined and then added together.

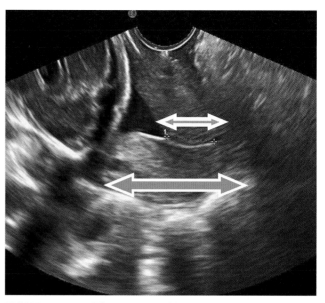

FIGURE 12–45. This cervix will feel longer (blue arrows) than its functional length (red).

finger[35,36] (Figures 12–45 and 12–46). The uneffaced, closed portion of the cervix can be measured by ultrasound.

Ultrasound measurement of cervical length is useful in several clinical situations:

- To evaluate the risk of preterm labor in symptomatic and asymptomatic women.
- To confirm or refute the suspicion of an incompetent cervix.
- To help determine whether a woman with symptoms of labor is likely to deliver in the near future, especially if she is preterm.

Ultrasound measurement of the cervix is a screening test that will not detect all women at risk for preterm labor. Also, many women deemed to be at risk will not deliver preterm even without treatment. However, cervical measurement can be helpful in determining when to transfer to a tertiary facility or initiate therapies such as treatment with progesterone or cervical cerclage. Importantly, it can help avoid costly and potentially risky treatments for women who are not likely to benefit from those treatments (prolonged hospitalization or prolonged home bed rest). The majority of women with symptoms suspicious for preterm labor will not proceed to delivery. Measuring cervical length has been shown to decrease the number of days of hospitalization and decrease the use of medication without increasing the number of preterm births.[37,38]

Cervical length measurements can also:

- Help predict the likelihood of a successful induction of labor (Crane, 2008)

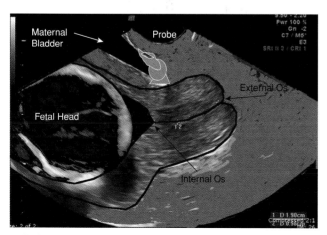

FIGURE 12–44. The same image as in Figure 12–43, but with the lower uterine segment, cervix, and cervical canal outlined for comparison.

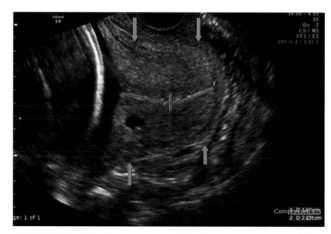

FIGURE 12–46. This cervix will feel shorter (between the blue arrows) than its functional length (measured in red).

- Evaluate the chance of a pregnancy continuing post term
- Evaluate the risk of cesarean birth[39]
- Help determine the timing of a maternal transport in women who need to deliver at a distance from their home due to complications of pregnancy or need for immediate neonatal care that is not available locally

Expertise in evaluating the anatomy of the lower uterine segment and cervix can be of value when assessing placental position relative to the cervix. Cervical length can be reliably measured once the lower uterine segment and the cervix can be differentiated. This occurs at around 14 weeks' gestation. Prior to this gestation, measuring cervical length is generally not recommended.[40]

Cervical sonogram is done with a high-frequency vaginal transducer (3 to 9 MHz). Measurement using the abdominal approach has generally not been found to be accurate.[41] Although transperineal or translabial methods can be successful, the technique is more difficult to master and may not always be successful even for the experienced sonographer.[42]

For the examiner performing digital exams, it may be helpful to begin with palpation of the cervix. This will help to locate the cervix and, if it is found to be more than 2 cm dilated, the measurement of cervical length by ultrasound can be abandoned as the patient is at risk for delivery.[42]

The pregnant woman should be reassured that a vaginal ultrasound is no more uncomfortable than a digital exam of the cervix. The woman should have an empty bladder, both for comfort and to prevent elongating the lower uterine segment and causing the cervix to appear longer. The woman can be placed in a supine position with her knees flexed as she would for a digital examination of the cervix. It may be helpful to elevate her buttocks with a folded blanket or have her put her fists under her buttocks. Alternately, she can be placed in lithotomy position with her feet in stirrups as if for a speculum examination.

The proper probe and frequency should be selected. The transducer should be covered with a probe cover or the finger of an exam glove. A generous amount of gel is applied on the inside and the outside of the probe cover, being careful to avoid air bubbles that will prevent the transmission of the sound waves and obscure the image.

The examiner will place his or her thumb on the directional guide on the probe (a notch or groove). The transducer should remain in the 12 o'clock position.

This position will result in a sagittal section or a slice parallel to the maternal long axis. The probe should be inserted gently and slowly while watching for the appropriate landmarks as they appear on the monitor. The corner of the maternal bladder and amniotic fluid should be visible. The internal os, the cervical canal, and the anterior and posterior lip of the cervix at the external os should be identifiable.[1] The left side of the screen will be cephalad. The right side will be caudal, extending into the vagina. The internal cervical os will be on the left and the external os on the right. With minimal gentle rocking, tilting, or rotation of the transducer, it should be possible to elongate the entire cervical canal (Figure 12–47).

Once an adequate view is obtained, the probe should be withdrawn so that the thickness of the anterior and posterior cervical tissue is similar. If the probe is pushing directly on the cervix, it can cause it to elongate, exaggerating its length.[43] A measurement is then taken from the external to the internal os of the cervix. The cervical canal is frequently curved, especially when the cervix is long. It may then be necessary to measure it in two or more separate pieces, adding the measurements together (Figure 12–48). Tracing the canal has been found to be less accurate than summing two straight measurements. If the cervix is short, it will often be straight.

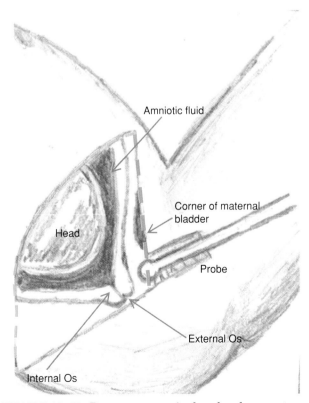

FIGURE 12–47. Proper transvaginal probe placement.

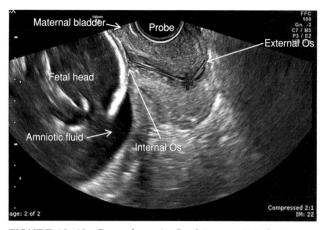

FIGURE 12–48. Curved cervix. In this case, it is better to measure in straight segments and add them together than it is to draw one straight line. A straight line will incorrectly show a shorter length.

At least three measurements should be taken, and the shortest of the three measurements used so as to err on the side of caution. The length of the cervix may be noted to change during the examination if there is a uterine contraction. This occasionally may be a dramatic change. The shortest measurement is most predictive of preterm birth.[44] Average cervical length prior to 22 weeks is 40 mm. From 22 to 32 weeks, the average length is 35 mm, and the cervix will continue to shorten until term. Between 22 and 30 weeks the 10th percentile for cervical length is 25 mm. A length less than this was shown to be statistically significant in association with preterm delivery, with the risk increasing as cervical length decreases.[45,46] Treatment with progesterone has been shown to be most effective when the cervical length is between 10 and 20 mm.[47]

Because the cervix effaces from the internal os to the external os, it precedes dilation and cannot be palpated by an examining finger. This process creates a characteristic funnel shape or "beaking" appearance that has been described as progressing from a "T" shape where the amniotic fluid meets the cervical canal, to a "Y" shape, to a "V," and finally to a "U" when membranes are bulging into the cervical canal (although the membranes may not yet be palpable in the vagina) (Figures 12–49, 12–50, 12–51, and 12–52). Although funneling is associated with a short cervix and preterm labor, the critical factor in predicting preterm birth is the closed length of the cervix, not the amount of funneling.[35,48]

When measuring cervical length by ultrasound:

- Do not perform before 14 to 15 weeks' gestation.
- Measure vaginally and not abdominally, when possible.
- Use plenty of gel and avoid air pockets under the probe cover.
- Do not measure with a full maternal bladder.
- Do not apply pressure to the cervix.
- Anterior width of the cervix should equal the posterior width.
- Both the internal os and external os should be viewed.
- The entire length of the cervical canal should be viewed.
- Do not rush. Allow time for a contraction to occur or subside.
- You do not need to measure the length if the cervix is more than 2 cm dilated by digital exam.
- Observe the image on the monitor in real time as the probe is inserted.

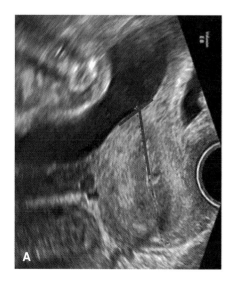

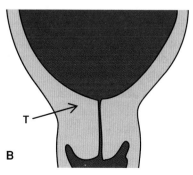

FIGURE 12–49. (A) Image of a long and closed cervix, with the internal cervical os closed at the level of the amniotic fluid (the top of the "T" running along this straight edge and the tail of the "T" running through the long cervix). **(B)** Schematic diagram illustrates this normal finding.

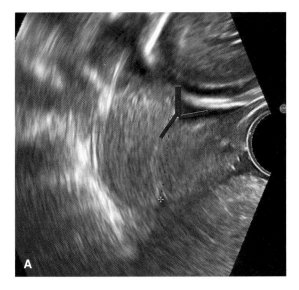

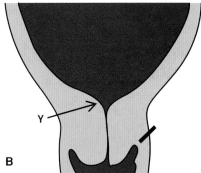

FIGURE 12–50. (A, B) The internal os is slightly open, changing the "T" more to a "Y."

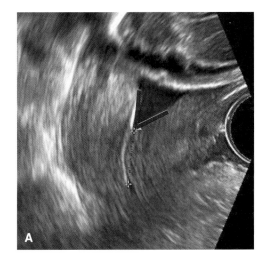

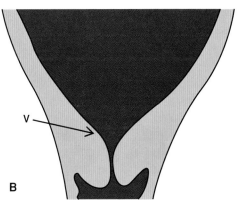

FIGURE 12–51. (A, B) As the cervix further effaces, the internal os opens and changes from a "U" shape to a "V" shape. The image shows the anechoic amniotic fluid dipping into the internal os.

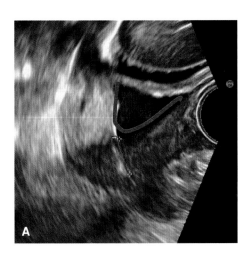

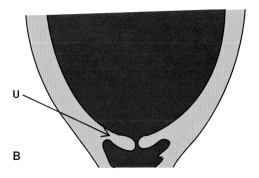

FIGURE 12–52. (A, B) As the internal os continues to shorten, the amniotic fluid fills the space and forms a "U" appearance, as shown in both the image and diagram. The arrow is pointing at the uterus.

- The risk assessment is based on closed cervical length, not the amount of funneling.

In summary, ultrasound measurement of cervical length can be of value in several clinical situations. It is better at predicting who will *not* deliver preterm than who will. POC bedside ultrasound can be a valuable tool for a rapid, painless assessment of the cervix.

CONCLUSION

POC sonography has multiple applications and indications during the second and third trimesters of pregnancy. These range from the diagnosis and management of possible preterm labor[49] to the clinical decision making in the woman presenting with no prenatal care and unknown pregnancy dating. Careful POC sonographic scanning with attention to the placenta and its borders is critical in making an accurate diagnosis when vaginal bleeding occurs in the second and third trimesters. Examination of the placenta and documentation of results need to include placental location, changes in echogenicity, placental thickness, and fluid collections. If the borders of the placenta are not clear in its relationship to the cervical os, consultation and collaboration is indicated. Finally, measurement of cervical length has become an integral part of the second- and third-trimester sonographic exam. And, of course, paramount to applying POC ultrasound skill to clinical practice is obtaining education and clinical competency. Regardless of the indication for POC sonography, there is no doubt that bedside ultrasound saves time and money, and promotes patient safety.

REFERENCES

1. American Institute of Ultrasound in Medicine (AIUM). *Practice Guideline: Obstetric Ultrasound.* Laurel, MD: Author; 2013.
2. American College of Radiology. ACR Practice Guidelines for the Performance Of Obstetrical Ultrasound. In: *ACR Practice Guidelines and Technical Standards,* 2007. Reston, VA: Author; 2007:1025–1033.
3. American College of Obstetricians and Gynecologists (ACOG). *Ultrasonography in Pregnancy* (Technical Bulletin No. 101). Washington, DC: Author; 2009.
4. Hadlock FP, Deter RL. Fetal biparietal diameter: A critical reevaluation of the relation to menstrual age by means of real-time ultrasound. *J Ultrasound Med.* 1982;1:(3):97–104.
5. Hadlock FP, Deter RL, Harrist RB, Park SK. Fetal head circumference: relation to menstrual age. *AJR.* 1982;138(4):649–653.
6. Hadlock FP, Deter DL, Harrist RB, Park SK. Fetal abdominal circumference as a predictor of menstrual age. *AJR.* 1982;139(2):367–370.
7. Hadlock FP, Harrist RB, Deter RL, Park SK. Femur length as a predictor of menstrual age: sonographically measured. *AJR.* 1982;138(5):875–878.
8. Kurmananvicius J, Burkhardt T, Wisser J, Huch R. Ultrasonographic fetal weight estimation: accuracy of formulas and accuracy of examiners by birth weight from 500–5,000 g. *J Perinatal Med.* 2004;32(2):155–161.
9. Ben-Haroush A, Yogev Y, Bar J, et al. Accuracy of sonographically estimated fetal weight in 840 women with different pregnancy complications prior to induction of labor. *Ultrasound Obstet Gynecol.* 2004;23(2):172–176.
10. Ben-Haroush A, Yogev Y, Hod M. Fetal weight estimation in diabetic pregnancies and suspected fetal macrosomia. *J Perinat Med.* 2003;32(2):113–121.
11. Schild RL, Sachs C, Fimmers R, et al. Sex-specific fetal weight prediction by ultrasound. *Ultrasound Obstet Gynecol.* 2004;23(1):30–35.
12. Schwarzler P, Bland JM, Holden D, et al. Sex-specific antenatal reference growth charts for uncomplicated singleton pregnancies at 15–40 weeks of gestation. *Ultrasound Obstet Gynecol.* 2004;23(1):23–29.
13. Melamed N, Meisner I, Mashiach R, et al. Fetal sex and intrauterine growth patterns. *J Ultrasound Med.* 2013;32:35–43.
14. Harper LM, Roehl KA, Tuuli MG, et al. Sonographic accuracy of estimated fetal weight in twins. *J Ultrasound Med.* 2013;32:625–630.
15. Williams PL, Laifer-Narin SL, Ragavendra N. US of abnormal uterine bleeding. *Radiographics.* 2003;23(3):703–718.
16. Rosati P, Guariglia L. Clinical significance of placenta previa detected at early routine transvaginal scan. *J Ultrasound Med.* 2000;19:581–585.
17. Smith NC, Smith PM. *Obstetric Ultrasound Made Easy.* Edinburgh: Churchill Livingstone; 2003.
18. Francois K, Mayer S, Harris C, Perlow JH. Association of vasa previa at delivery with a history of second-trimester placenta previa. *J Repro Med.* 2003;48(10);771–774.
19. O'Brien J, Sheehan K. Prenatal diagnosis of a velamentous cord insertion associated with vasa previa. *JDMS.* 2001;17:94–98.
20. Moore Lisa E, Gonzalez Ileana. Placenta percreta with bladder invasion diagnosed with sonography: images and clinical correlation. *J Diagn Med Sonogr.* 2008;24:238–241.
21. Harris RD, Alexander RD. Ultrasound of the placenta and umbilical cord. In: PW Callen, ed. *Ultrasonography in Obstetrics and Gynecology.* 4th ed. Philadelphia: W.B. Saunders; 2000:597–614.
22. Glantz C, Purnell L. Clinical utility of sonography in the diagnosis and treatment of placental abruption. *J Ultrasound Med.* 2002;21(8):837–840.
23. Thompson MO, Vines SK, Aquilina J, et al. Are placental lakes of any clinical significance? *Placenta.* 2002;23(8–9):685–690.
24. Durfee SM, Frates M, Luong A, Benson CB. The sonographic and color Doppler features of retained products of conception. *J Ultrasound Med.* 2005;24:1181–1186.

25. Kamaya A, Petrovitch I, Chen B, et al. Retained products of conception. Spectrum of color Doppler findings. *J Ultrasound Med.* 2009;28:1031–1041.

26. Crane JM, Hutchens D. Transvaginal sonographic measurement of cervical length to predict preterm birth in asymptomatic women at increased risk, a systemic review. *Ultrasound Obstet Gynecol.* 2008 May; 31(5):579–587.

27. American College of Obstetricians and Gynecologists (ACOG). *Use of Progesterone to Reduce Preterm Birth.* ACOG Committee Opinion No. 419. Washington, DC: Author; 2008.

28. Cahill A, Obido A, Caughey A, et al. Universal cervical length screening and treatment with vaginal progesterone to prevent preterm birth: A decision and economic analysis. *Am J Obstet Gynecol.* 2010;202(6).

29. Hassan S, Romero R, Vidyadhari D et al. Vaginal progesterone reduces the rate of preterm birth in women with a sonographic short cervix: A multicenter, randomized, double-blind, placebo-controlled trial. *Ultrasound Obstet Gynecol.* 2011;38:18–31.

30. Campbell S. Universal cervical-length and vaginal progesterone prevents early preterm births, reduces neonatal morbidity and is cost saving: Doing nothing is no longer an option. *Ultrasound Obstet Gynecol.* 2011; 38:1–9.

31. American College of Obstetricians and Gynecologists (ACOG). *Prediction and Prevention of Preterm Birth.* Technical Bulletin No. 130. Washington, DC: Author; 2012.

32. Saul L, Kurtzman T, Hagemann C, Ghamsary M, Wing D. Is transabdominal sonography of the cervix after voiding a reliable method of cervical length assessment? *J Ultrasound Med.* 27:1305–1311.

33. Gramellini D, Fieni S, Molina E, et al. Transvaginal sonographic cervical length changes during normal pregnancy. *J Ultrasound Med.* 2002;21(3):227–232.

34. Romero R, Nien JK, Chaiworapongsa T, et al. Does the presence of a funnel increase the risk of adverse perinatal outcome in a patient with a short cervix? *Am J Obstet Gynecol.* 2005;192(4):1060–1066.

35. Berghella V, Tolosa JE, Kuhlman KA, et al. Cervical ultrasonography compared to manual examination as a predictor of preterm delivery. *Am J Obstet Gynecol.* 1997;177:723–730.

36. Debbs RH, Chen J. Contemporary use of cerclage in pregnancy. *Clin Obstet Gynecol.* 2009;52:597–610.

37. Ness A, Visintine J, Ricci E, Berghella V. Does knowledge of cervical length and fetal fiibronectin affect management of women with threatened preterm labor? A randomized trial. *Am J Obstet Gynecol.* 2007 Oct; 197(4):426.e1–7.

38. Sanin-Blair J, Palacia M, Delgado J, et al. Impact of ultrasound cervical length assessment on duration of hospital stay in the clinical management of threatened preterm labor. *Ultrasound Obstet Gynecol.* 2004;24(7):756–760.

39. Smith GC, Celik E, To M, et al. Cervical length at midpregnancy and the risk of primary cesarean delivery. *N Engl J Med.* 2008;27;358(13):1346–1353.

40. Berghella V, Talucci M, Desai A. Does transvaginal sonographic measurement of cervical length before 14 weeks predict preterm delivery in high-risk pregnancies? *Ultrasound Obstet Gynecol.* 2003;21(2):140–144.

41. Berghella V, Bega B. Ultrasound Evaluation of the Cervix in Ultrasonography in Obstetrics and Gynecology. In: PW Callen, ed. *Ultrasonography in Obstetrics and Gynecology.* 5th ed. Philadelphia: Saunders; 2000:698–720.

42. Cicero S, Skentou C, Souka A, et al. Cervical length at 22–24 weeks of gestation: Comparison of transvaginal and transperineal-translabial ultrasonography. *Ultrasound Obstet Gynecol.* 2001;17(4):335–340.

43. Yost NP, Bloom SL, Twickler DM, Leveno KJ. Pitfalls in ultrasonic cervical length measurement for predicting preterm birth. *Obstet Gynecol.* 1999;93(4):510–516.

44. Rust OA, Atlas RO, Kimmel S, et al. Does the presence of a funnel increase the risk of adverse perinatal outcome in a patient with a short cervix? *Am J Obstet Gynecol.* 2005 Apr;192(4):1060–1066.

45. Goldenberg RL, Iams JD, Mercer BM, et al.; National Institute of Child Health and Human Development Maternal-Fetal Medicine Units Network. What we have learned about the predictors of preterm birth. *Semin Perinatol.* 2003 Jun;27(3):185–193.

46. Mercer BM, Goldenberg RL, Das A, et al. The preterm prediction study: a clinical risk assessment system. *Am J Obstet Gynecol.* 1996 Jun;174(6):1885–1893.

47. Berghella V. Novel developments on cervical length screening and progesterone for preventing preterm birth. *Br J Obstet Gynecol* 2009;116(2):182–187.

48. https://www.perinatalquality.org/CLEAR/default.aspx

49. Taylor BK. Sonographic assessment of cervical length and the risk of preterm birth. *J Obstet Gynecol Neonat Nurs.* 2011;40(5):617–631.

CHAPTER 13

Point-of-Care Sonographic Evaluation of Fetal Well-Being

One of the most utilized point-of-care sonograms to assess fetal well-being is the biophysical profile (BPP). The BPP is generally performed following a nonreactive nonstress test (NST); although, in some cases, it is the first line of antepartum testing employed in either its full application or with its modified use (the modified BPP). The purpose of this chapter is to describe each component of the sonographic portion of the BPP, along with further description of amniotic fluid assessment.

HISTORY OF THE BIOPHYSICAL PROFILE

The BPP was developed in 1980 by Manning and Associates[1] and utilizes traditional electronic fetal monitoring (EFM) in combination with a sonographic fetal evaluation. Manning viewed this technique as "undertaking an intrauterine physical examination, analogous to Apgar scoring."

As the fetal central nervous system (CNS) matures with advancing gestational age, fetal behavior develops in a specific order. Fetal tone (FT) begins to be evident by ultrasound around 7.5 to 8 weeks of gestation, followed by fetal movement (FM) beginning around 9 weeks' gestation. Fetal breathing becomes regular at 20 to 21 weeks, followed by development of fetal heart rate (FHR) control (the ability to accelerate and decelerate) at the end of the second or beginning of the third trimester.

With an insidious or chronic loss of fetal oxygenation, the fetus begins to lose these same behaviors, but in the *opposite* order in which they developed. So, in the event of chronic oxygen deprivation, initially there will be the loss of fetal heart reactivity followed by a decrease or loss of fetal breathing movements (FBM). If the oxygen deprivation continues, a decrease in amniotic fluid will occur. Ultimately, there will be a loss of FM with, finally, the loss of FT.[1] Although factors other than deoxygenation may cause a change in some or all of these behaviors, these are the parameters that, when present, were determined to be predictive of fetal oxygenation, and thus they are used as the basis of the BPP.

FHR reactivity, tone, movement, and breathing are CNS activities that respond to acute hypoxic changes. Additionally, decreased amniotic fluid volume (AFV), in the absence of ruptured membranes or fetal renal abnormalities, may be an indicator of chronic fetal compromise as oxygenated blood is shunted from the fetal kidneys to the vital organs. Knowledge of the five parameters, their progressive emergence throughout gestational age, and pattern of decline with increasing hypoxia can provide invaluable information regarding the oxygenation status of the fetus.

The five parameters assessed in the Manning BPP are:

1. Fetal heart reactivity (the nonstress test)
2. Fetal tone
3. Fetal movement
4. Fetal breathing activity
5. Amniotic fluid volume

The BPP has a very low false-negative rate, meaning that a score of 8/10 or 10/10 is highly predictive of adequate fetal oxygenation and the absence of fetal metabolic acidemia. However, each single BPP parameter has a high false-positive rate, meaning, for example, that absence of fetal breathing alone may be the result of sleep cycles, medication affects, or some unknown cause other than deoxygenation. The false-positive rate can be greatly reduced when the parameters are combined. The specific criterion for each parameter was defined by Manning with a scoring system of 2 points if the parameter is present and 0 if it is absent (Table 13–1).[1,2] There is no partial score.

In 1983, Vintzileos et al.[3] proposed a modification to Manning's scoring system. In addition to Manning's five parameters, Vintzileos introduced a sixth parameter: placental grading based on the degree of maturation of the placenta. A mature placenta is given the highest score, and the immature

TABLE 13-1 MANNING BIOPHYSICAL PROFILE SCORING SYSTEM

Criterion	Score 2	Score 0
Fetal tone	One episode of flexion/extension of fetal spine, limbs, or hand	Extremities in extension
Fetal movement	Three gross body movements including rolling	Two or fewer episodes of fetal movement
Fetal breathing	30 seconds of continuous breathing	Absence of respiratory effort
Nonstress test (NST)	Two accelerations 15 bpm × 15 seconds within 20 minutes	Nonreactive NST
Amniotic fluid volume	Largest fluid pocket >2 cm vertically or AFI >5 cm	Oligohydramnios

Adapted from Manning et al.[1]

placenta a low score. Additionally, the change to the scoring system for each parameter included adding a middle point value option, a score of 1, that accounted for the observation of partial fetal behaviors, borderline amniotic fluid levels, and/or the inability to grade the placenta (Table 13–2).[3]

Both forms of BPPs have similar neonatal outcome predictive value. Whichever BPP point system is chosen to be used in a particular health care setting should be clarified and established in a protocol. Potentially, clinical management could be adversely impacted if only a raw score is reported. For instance, a loss of 2 points for oligohydramnios and 2 points for absence of FM would give a score of 8 (out of 12) on the Vintzileos scale and a 6 (out of 10) on Manning's. In this example, the raw score of eight on the Vintzileos scale would be falsely reassuring if it is believed to be based on the Manning criteria. It is imperative to express the score with both the numerator and denominator (8/12 or 8/10) so that the test may be interpreted correctly. For the purposes of this chapter, the BPP parameters

TABLE 13-2 VINTZILEOS BIOPHYSICAL SCORING SYSTEM

Criterion	Score 2	Score 1	Score 0
Fetal tone	One episode of flexion/extension of extremity AND one episode of spine extension/flexion	One episode of flexion/extension of extremity OR one episode of spine extension/flexion	Extremities in extension
Fetal movement	At least three episodes of gross body movements within 30 minutes	One or two gross body movements within 30 minutes	Absence of gross body movements within 30 minutes
Fetal breathing	At least one episode of fetal breathing sustained for minimum of 60 seconds during 30 minutes	At least one episode of fetal breathing sustained for 30–60 seconds during 30 minutes	No fetal breathing or breathing lasting less than 30 seconds
Nonstress Test (NST)	At least ≥5 15 bpm × 15 seconds accelerations associated with fetal movement in 20 minute time frame	2–4 15 × 15 accelerations associated with fetal movement in 20 minute time frame	≤1 15 × 15 accelerations associated with fetal movement in 20 minute time frame
Amniotic fluid volume	>2 cm vertical pocket	A vertical pocket that measures <2 cm but >1 cm	Crowding of fetal small parts with <1 cm vertical fluid pocket
Placental grading	Score 0, 1, or 2	Placenta posterior and difficult to grade	Score 3

Adapted from Vintzileos et al.[3]

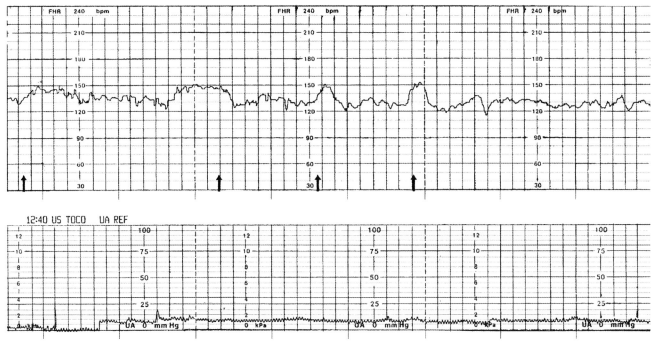

FIGURE 13–1. Reactive nonstress test (NST).

and scoring system presented will be based on the Manning 10-point criteria.

BIOPHYSICAL PROFILE (BPP) PARAMETERS

Fetal Heart Reactivity

Fetal heart reactivity is determined by performing an NST that is interpreted as reactive or nonreactive (see Chapter 4: Antepartum Assessment). Although the criteria for a reactive pattern may vary among institutions, the most commonly accepted criteria for a reactive NST is the presence of two accelerations within 20 minutes of testing. Each acceleration must last for 15 seconds, with a peak amplitude of 15 beats per minute (bpm) above the baseline FHR (Figure 13–1). The NST is considered nonreactive when it fails to meet the stated criteria for a reactive NST (i.e., fails to demonstrate adequate fetal heart rate accelerations; see Figure 13–2). An additional 20 minutes can be used to evaluate reactivity since it has been well-established that fetal sleep–wake cycles may be up to 40 minutes in length.[3,4]

A reactive NST is considered one of the best predictors of fetal well-being and the absence of fetal metabolic acidemia. However, a nonreactive NST has a false positive rate of 40% to 80%, meaning that the cause of the nonreactivity may be something other than

hypoxia. Therefore, a nonreactive NST needs to be followed by another form of fetal evaluation in order to differentiate the hypoxic from the nonhypoxic fetus. The BPP is the most commonly used follow-up test.[4,5]

Fetal Tone

FT is the first of the five parameters to develop during fetal CNS maturation. It is defined as the observer witnessing at least one of the following fetal activities: limb extension with return to flexion, flexion/extension of the spine, or the opening and closing of the hand.

Fetal Movement

FM is defined as the observation of flexion and extension of extremities and/or rolling motions of the fetal trunk. Three distinct episodes of FM are required to achieve a full score. Simultaneous movement of more than one body part is counted as a single movement, just as are isolated limb movements.

Fetal Breathing Movements

FBM increase in frequency and duration with advancing gestational age. Ultrasound observation reveals the presence of diaphragmatic and chest wall excursion often best visualized at the level of the diaphragm (Figure 13–3A,B). A minimum of 30 seconds of *continuous* fetal breathing is required. The presence

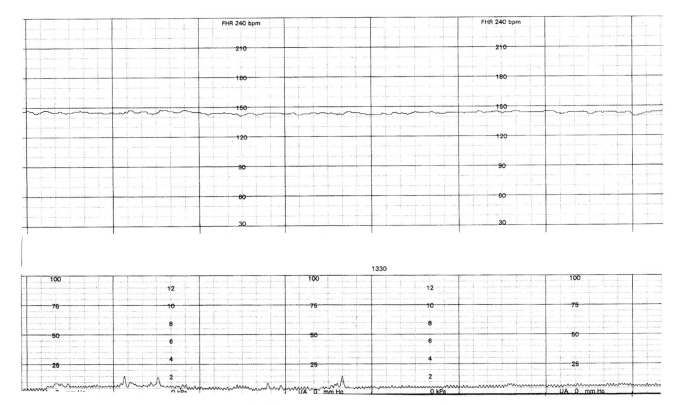

FIGURE 13–2. Nonreactive nonstress test (NST).

or absence of fetal breathing as a reliable indicator of well-being must be evaluated carefully. It is known that breathing movements are sporadic, vary with gestational age, exhibit diurnal variations, and are often absent in the presence of labor. FBMs are known to be reduced in women who have been fasting[6] and following glucocorticosteroid administration.[7]

Amniotic Fluid Volume

Amniotic fluid is measured either by the deepest pocket method or by the amniotic fluid index (AFI). The fluid measured should be free of fetal parts or umbilical cord. AFVs are stable between 26 and 38 weeks, after which a normal gradual decline may be observed. A normal AFI at term is considered an aggregate number of the sum of four fluid quadrants of more than 5 cm. Reduced amniotic fluid may be the result of normal decline or an indicator of chronic fetal compromise leading to reduced fetal renal profusion and reduced urinary output.[8] Regardless of the cause, a significantly reduced AFV is a risk factor because it may contribute to cord compression, poor perinatal outcome, and possibly fetal death. The current data show, however, that regardless of the method used to identify oligohydramnios (subjective, AFI, or deepest pocket), overdiagnosis of oligohydramnios is occurring. Overdiagnosis often leads to unnecessary

inductions and may contribute to the increase in neonatal morbidity and mortality without demonstrating improvement in perinatal outcomes.[8–10]

SONOGRAPHIC TECHNIQUES FOR AMNIOTIC FLUID ASSESSMENT

Two primary methods of fluid volume assessment are commonly used: the single-pocket AFV and the AFI. Using the single-pocket method, at least one pocket of amniotic fluid that is 2 cm or greater in vertical dimension is identified. Areas with umbilical cord visible should not be measured. Measuring up to the edge of the cord is acceptable (Figure 13–3A–C). An AFV of more than 2 cm receives two points on the Manning BPP scoring system and is considered normal fluid volume (Figure 13–3D).

The second method of fluid assessment is the AFI, which was developed by Phelan and his group.[9] The AFI is obtained by measuring the largest pocket of fluid in each of the four quadrants of the uterus (Figure 13–4). The sum of the four-quadrant measurements is the AFI. Serial AFI evaluations provide the clinician with a semiquantitative volume of fluid and the ability to assess overall changes with time and patient status. An AFI of 5 to 18 cm is considered normal at term. AFIs at or below 5 cm have been

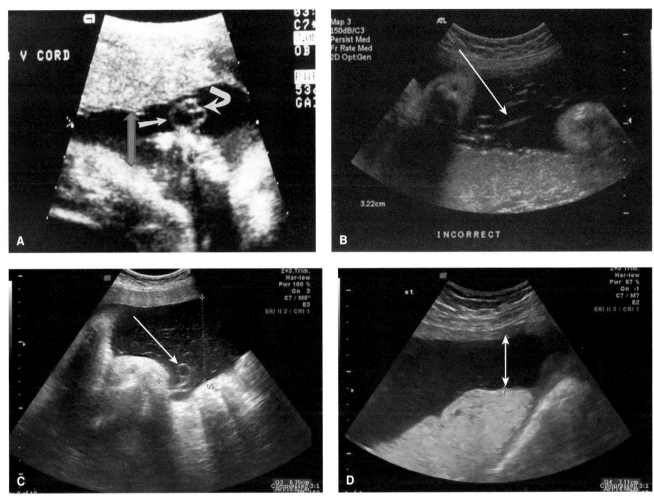

FIGURE 13–3. (A) Single-pocket fluid measurement at deepest pocket (colored arrow) excluding umbilical cord (between white arrows). (B) Single-pocket fluid measurement performed *incorrectly* (between cursors) because measurement includes areas of umbilical cord at arrow. (C) Single-pocket fluid measurement performed correctly by omitting area of umbilical cord at arrow. (D) Correct measurement of single fluid pocket, between arrow points.

diagnostic of oligohydramnios (Figure 13–5) and have been associated with nonreactive NSTs, variable decelerations, meconium staining, and 5-minute Apgar scores of less than 7,[9] as well as with an increase in operative delivery for fetal distress.

However, the association between an AFI of less than 5 cm measured within 7 days of birth has not been associated with decreasing umbilical artery pH or increasing base excess.[11,12] It has been postulated that this occurs because assessment of fluid volume is more accurate for identifying normal volume than for identifying oligohydramnios (Figures 13–4 and 13–5).[12–14]

There is also no clear consensus as to which method of assessing amniotic fluid is better, the AFV or AFI. Review of the literature is conflicting; however, the single deepest vertical pocket measurement seems to be a better choice at this point in time. The use of the AFI appears to increase the rate of induction without demonstrating improvement in perinatal outcome.[11,13]

Shanks and his group assessed the definition of oligohydramnios with adverse neonatal outcome. Their results showed that amniotic fluid indices vary with gestational age, and, when oligohydramnios is defined by percentile rather than a single measurement, it more accurately predicts fetuses at risk for NICU admission. An AFI of less than the fifth percentile was more predictive than an AFI of less than 5 cm (Figure 13–5).[14]

When oligohydramnios is diagnosed based on an AFI of less than 5 cm, medical intervention often follows as an induction of labor or surgical intervention. Amniotic fluid can increase with hydration and rest. In one study, women with *normal* amounts of amniotic fluid (AFI of 6 to 24 cm) were divided into two groups: (1) maternal rest in the left lateral decubitus position with oral hydration and (2) women positioned in the left lateral decubitus position alone. The results showed that the two groups had similar

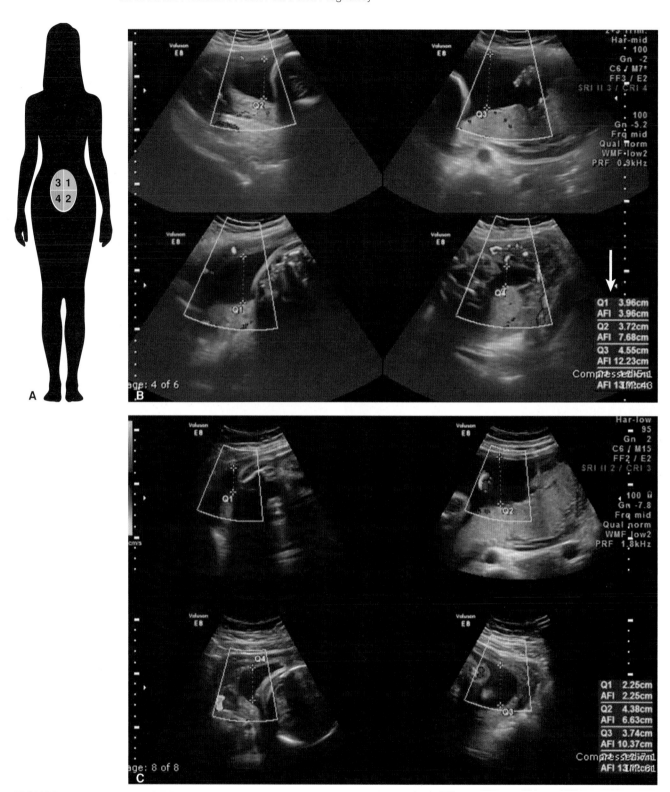

FIGURE 13–4. (A) Dividing the maternal abdomen into four quadrants for measuring the amniotic fluid index (AFI). **(B)** AFI with color flow Doppler identification of umbilical cord in pocket. Individual four-quadrant measurement of amniotic fluid between "+" signs. Note each quadrant measurement at large arrow that has been generated by the ultrasound machine, along with the total of the four quadrants. The total AFI is in the bottom right corner (arrow). **(C)** AFI with color flow Doppler of umbilical cord ensuring it is not included in the measurement.

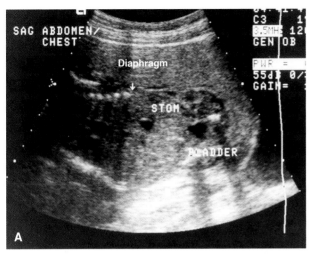
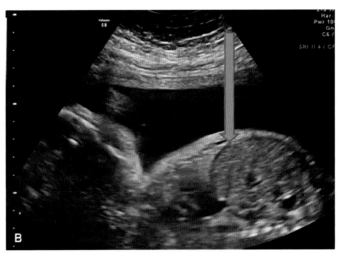

FIGURE 13–5. **(A)** Oligohydramnios with no measurable fluid observed, with confirmation of urine in the bladder prior to treatment with amnioinfusion. Note how much more difficult it is to visualize the fetus when lacking the acoustic window that the amniotic fluid normally provides. This is evident when comparing panels A and B. Note the anechoic vertical "stripe," which is the diaphragm (small white arrow) dividing abdominal contents from the chest. **(B)** In comparison, this image demonstrates normal fluid with fetal diaphragm also visible as an anechoic strip around the abdominal contents (at arrow).

increases in AFV at 15 minutes post hydration/rest. However, after 30 minutes, the AFV increased more rapidly in the hydration group.[15] This was followed by another study examining maternal hydration and pregnancy outcome when employing intravenous (IV) hydration in response to isolated oligohydramnios. The results demonstrated that IV hydration improved the quantity of amniotic fluid in the oligohydramnios group.[16]

Doppler blood flow studies of the fetal–placental pair have further improved obstetric care and antepartum testing, particularly in the growth-restricted fetus. However, concurrent use of color Doppler with assessment of the AFV results in overdiagnosis of oligohydramnios.[17]

Polyhydramnios has been defined as an AFI of greater than 20 (Figure 13–6).[10] Polyhydramnios is associated with numerous congenital anomalies, particularly those involving the GI tract. It is also associated with maternal viral infections.

ASSESSMENT AND SCORING OF THE BPP

The maximum period of time for evaluating the ultrasound parameters of the BPP is 30 minutes, exclusive of the NST. The NST may be performed prior to or following the ultrasound portion of the procedure.

Assessment and scoring of the BPP depends on whether Manning's or Vintzileos' criterion is used. The main difference between the two scoring systems is that with Manning's, the score is 2 or 0: either the behavior is present or it is not. With Vintzileos' system, a partial score of 1 is given with partial demonstration of the behavior. The second difference is that Vintzileos has a sixth parameter, that of placental grading. A mature placenta shows sonographic demarcations of the placental cotyledons, indicating it is mature. The immature placenta has a sonographically smoother appearance (isoechogenic). Once again, it is important that clinicians know which assessment and scoring method is being utilized at the institution performing the BPP.

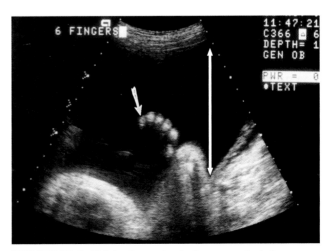

FIGURE 13–6. Polyhydramnios (only one pocket shown, with total fluid measurement of 36 cm). Also note the sixth digit at small arrow.

TABLE 13–3 APPLICATION OF BIOPHYSICAL PROFILE RESULTS

BPP Score	Interpretation	Recommended Management
10	Nonasphyxiated fetus	No intervention. Repeat testing weekly or 2×/week depending on indication
8–10	Normal nonasphyxiated fetus	No fetal indications for intervention. Repeat per protocol
8 or 10 with decreased fluid	Chronic fetal asphyxia suspected	Deliver
6	Possible fetal asphyxia	• Deliver if AFV abnormal. • If normal fluid >36 weeks' gestation with favorable cervix, deliver. • If <36 weeks or immature lungs or cervix unfavorable, repeat × 24 hours. • If repeat test ≤6, deliver. If repeat test >6, observe and repeat per protocol.
4	Probable asphyxia	Repeat testing same day. If repeat is ≤6, deliver.
0–2	Almost certain asphyxia	Deliver

Adapted from Manning et al.[1]

APPLICATION AND MANAGEMENT OF BPP RESULTS

Management recommendations and an example of a management algorithm are described in Table 13–3 and Appendix B. However, the results of all antepartum fetal evaluations should be considered in conjunction with complete maternal–fetal history and clinical circumstances.

The BPP has also been used during labor to assess fetal well-being when the electronic fetal monitor strip was nonreassuring. The BPP has been shown to predict the need for cesarean delivery.[18]

MODIFIED BIOPHYSICAL PROFILE

More recently, the "modified BPP" has been utilized, which consists of an NST in conjunction with AFV assessment using Phelan's four-quadrant AFI method.[18,19] The remaining parameters of the BPP, such as observation of FM and FT, are not used. The rationale is that if accelerations of the FHR are present in response to maternal perception of FM during the NST, then FM exists and does not need to be directly observed by ultrasound. Additionally, the presence of FM indicates that fetal muscle tone is also present.

OTHER INDICATIONS FOR POC AMNIOTIC FLUID ASSESSMENT

Prior to performing external cephalic version, the fetal status is evaluated with some combination of antepartum testing. In most situations, amniotic fluid is assessed prior to the attempt at version. The success rate of the version is directly related to the quantity of amniotic fluid.[20]

In addition, when variable decelerations are present on the reactive NST, an amniotic fluid assessment should be performed to determine if there is oligohydramnios. The reactive NST indicates the absence of fetal metabolic acidemia at the time of testing, but if variable decelerations become recurrent, fetal metabolic acidemia may develop. One of the most common causes of variable decelerations is oligohydramnios; thus the underlying indication to quantify amniotic fluid under these circumstances.

PROCEDURE FOR POC BIOPHYSICAL PROFILE

Nurses and midwives who have obtained the appropriate didactic and clinical education in ultrasound may perform BPPs, fluid assessments, and Doppler studies.[21–23] Preparation with the recommended number of didactic hours and determination of clinical competency must be achieved.

The general technique for performing a BPP is to have the woman positioned in the supine position with some lateral tilt to avoid supine hypotension. The clinician performing the BPP should be in a comfortable position because the test may involve holding the ultrasound transducer somewhat stationary for 30 minutes. The BPP parameters may be obtained in any order.

Once the fetal presentation and lie have been identified, the fetal torso and extremities are observed for movement, flexion, and extension. By holding the transducer in place, fetal movement and tone can be observed by watching the fetal part move in real time. For example, the spine may be visible and then move out of the field of view. This indicates FM. Specific to tone, however, both flexion and extension need to be visualized so as not to confuse it with fetal movement. The flexion/extension may be of the hand opening and closing, or the spine arching and returning to a neutral position. It could also be a leg kicking or toes flexing and extending.

Observing for FBM can be more challenging. Many sonographers will begin by following the fetal spine in the transverse plane. Then, at the level of the heart, the transducer is turned into the sagittal plane, gaining a long axis of the chest and abdomen. It is at this level that the fetal diaphragm will be seen and FBMs observed as the abdominal wall expands and contracts. FBM may also be seen in other planes as well, but the motion should not be mistaken for maternal abdominal wall movements.

At any point during the BPP when FBM is observed, it is advised to focus on the breathing motion until the full 30 seconds have been achieved. Other parameters may also be detected simultaneously; however, since FBM is intermittent and elusive, the sonographer should seize the opportunity.

CONCLUSION

Interpretation and recommended follow-up based on the BPP results are presented in Table 13–3. However, it is imperative that management decisions not be based solely on the NST or BPP score. Such decisions could lead to unnecessary interventions or even adverse outcomes. Management decisions should be made after careful review of the patient's overall clinical picture.

In 2009, the participants at the Eunice Kennedy Shriver National Institute of Child Health and Human Development workshop "Antenatal Testing: A Reevaluation" reviewed the literature on antepartum testing. Their overall conclusion was that there are gaps in the evidence "guiding the clinical application of most antepartum assessments commonly in use today" and that there is a need for further research. However, all antepartum tests that were reviewed (NST, CST, BPP, and modified BPP) showed

very low false-negative rates (0.2% and 0.65%). This means that if the test result were reassuring, it was highly predictive of fetal well-being and the absence of fetal metabolic acidemia. However, if the test result were "positive," indicating possible fetal compromise, it was poorly predictive. Depending on which test was used, between 35% and 90% of the neonates with "positive" test results were born without compromise.[24]

Generally, tests performed in combination (i.e., the NST and BPP) have shown the best results. However, along with these tests comes an associated financial burden. The most common indication for antepartum fetal evaluation is postdates pregnancy, which yields relatively high numbers of women and, therefore, high cost. However, in many "postdates" cases, the dating of the pregnancy is inaccurate. Therefore, one of the most cost-effective methods for reducing the expense of antepartum evaluation of the postdates pregnancy can be accomplished by ensuring accurate dating of the pregnancy. The most predictive methods of pregnancy dating include[25]:

- Ultrasound dating performed at less than 20 weeks' gestation, or
- A minimum of 30 weeks since a positive serum or urine pregnancy test along with documented fetal heart tones for a minimum of 30 weeks by Doppler.

The costs associated with antepartum testing have tremendous societal impact.[26] However, women who have late prenatal care and/or uncertain pregnancy dating must be tested when they reach 41 weeks regardless of how uncertain the dating criteria being utilized.

REFERENCES

1. Manning FA, Baskett TF, Morrison I, Lange, I. Fetal biophysical scoring: A prospective study in 1,184 high risk patients. *Am J Obstet Gynecol.* 1981;140(3):289–294.
2. Manning FA, Morrison MB, Harman CR et al. Fetal assessment based on fetal biophysical profile scoring: Experience in 19,221 referred high-risk pregnancies. *Am J Obstet Gynecol.* 1987;157(4):880–884.
3. Vintzileos AM, Campbell WA, Ingardia CJ, Nochimson, D. The biophysical profile and its predictive value. *Obstet Gynecol.* 1983;62(2):271–278.
4. Finberg HJ, Kurtz AB, Johnson R, Wapner R. The biophysical profile: A literature review and reassessment of its usefulness in the evaluation of fetal well- being. *J Ultrasound Med.* 1990;9(10):583–591.
5. American College of Obstetrics and Gynecology (ACOG). *Antepartum Testing. Antepartum Fetal Surveillance.* Practice Guideline No. 9. ACOG; 1999.

6. Mirghani HM, Weerasinghe DS, Ezimokhai M, Smith JR. The effect of maternal fasting on the fetal biophysical profile. *Int J Gynaecol Obstet.* 2003;81(1):17–21.

7. Jackson JR, Kleeman S, Doerzbacher M, Lambers DS. The effect of glucocorticosteroid administration on fetal movements and biophysical profile scores in normal pregnancies. *J Matern Fetal Neonatal Med.* 2003;13(1): 50–53.

8. Magann EF, Sandlin AT, Ounpraseuth ST. Amniotic fluid volume and the clinical relevance of the sonographically estimated amniotic fluid volume. *J Ultrasound Med.* 2011;1573–1585.

9. Phelan JP, Ahn MO, Smith CV, et al. (1987). Amniotic fluid index measurements during pregnancy. *J. Repro Med.* 1987;32(8):601–604.

10. Magann EF, Doherty DA, Chauhan SP, et al. How well do the amniotic fluid index and single deepest pocket indices predict oligohydramnios and hydramnios? *Am J Obstet Gynecol.* 2004;190(1):164–169.

11. Nabhan AF, Abdelmoula YA. Amniotic fluid index versus single deepest vertical pocket as a screening test for preventing adverse pregnancy outcome. *J Ultrasound Med.* 2012;31(2):239–244.

12. Morris JM, Thompson K, Smithey J, et al. (2004). The usefulness of ultrasound assessment of amniotic fluid in predicting adverse outcome in prolonged pregnancy: A prospective blinded observational study. *Obstet Gynecol Surv.* 2004;59(5):325–326.

13. Driggers RW, Holcroft CJ, Blakemore KJ, Graham EM. (2004). An amniotic fluid index < or =5 cm within 7 days of delivery in the third trimester is not associated with decreasing umbilical arterial pH and base excess. *J Perinatol.* 2004;24(2):72–76.

14. Shanks A, Tuuli M, Schaecher C, et al. Assessing the optimal definition of oligohydramnios associated with adverse neonatal outcomes. *J Ultrasound Med.* 2011; 30:303–307.

15. Kahraman U, Melek C. Effect of maternal hydration on the amniotic fluid volume during maternal rest in the left lateral decubitus position. *J Ultrasound Med.* 2013;32:955–961.

16. Patrelli TS, Gizzo S, Cosmi E, et al. Maternal hydration therapy improves the quantity of amniotic fluid and the pregnancy outcome in third-trimester isolated oligohydramnios: A controlled randomized institutional trial. *J Ultrasound Med.* 2012;31:239.

17. Eden RD, Seifert LS, Kodack LD, et al. A modified biophysical profile for antenatal fetal surveillance. Part 1. *Obstet Gynecol.* 1988;71(3):365–369.

18. Kim SY, Khandelwal M, Gaughan JP, et al. (2003). Is the intrapartum biophysical profile useful? *Obstet Gynecol.* 2003;102(3):471–476.

19. Rutherford SE, Phelan JP, Smith CV, Jacobs N. (1987). The four quadrant assessment of amniotic fluid volume: An adjunct to antepartum fetal heart rate testing. Part 1. *Obstet Gynecol.* 1987;70(3):353–356.

20. Kok M, Cnossen J, Gravendeel L, et al. Ultrasound factors to predict the outcome of external cephalic version: A meta-analysis. *Ultrasound Obstet Gynecol.* 2009;33:76–84.

21. American College of Nurse Midwives (ACNM). (2012). *Position Statement: Ultrasound for Midwives.* Washington, DC: ACNM; 2012.

22. Gegor C, Paine LL, Costigan K, Johnson, TRB. Interpretation of biophysical profiles by nurses and physicians. *JOGNN* 1994;23(5):114–119.

23. Association of Women's Health, Obstetric and Neonatal Nurses (AWHONN). (2010). *Ultrasound examinations performed by nurses in obstetric, gynecologic and reproductive medicine settings.* Washington, DC: AWHONN; 2010.

24. Signore C, Freeman R, Sponge C. Antenatal testing: A reevaluation. *Obstet Gynecol.* 2009;113(3):687–701.

25. American College of Obstetricians and Gynecologists (ACOG). (2009). *Induction of Labor.* Technical Bulletin No. 107. Washington, DC: ACOG; 2009.

26. Fonseca L, Monga M, Silva J. (2003). Postdates pregnancy in an indigent population: The financial burden. *Am J Obstet Gynecol.* 2003;188(5):1214–1216.

Appendices

Example Chain of Command

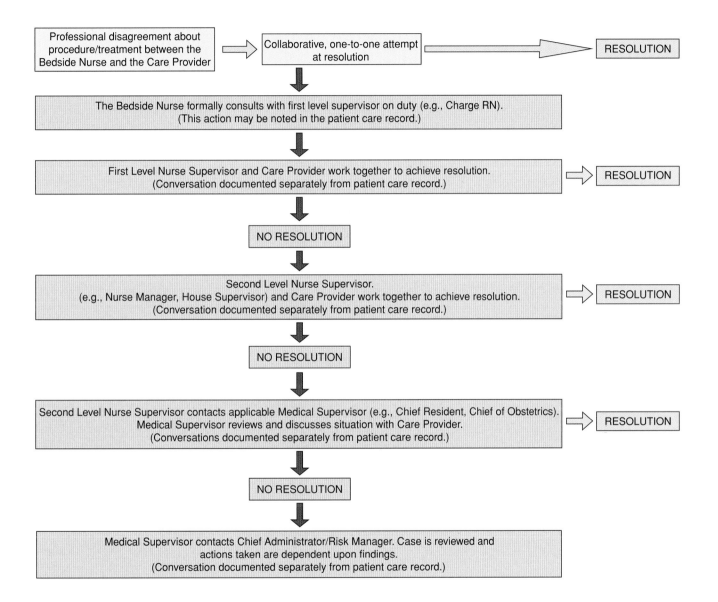

Example of Algorithm for Management of Antepartum Testing

Starting with the NST or CST, this chart outlines options for managing antepartum test results. It is meant to be used as a guide to assist the clinician. Each patient should be evaluated and treated on an individual basis.

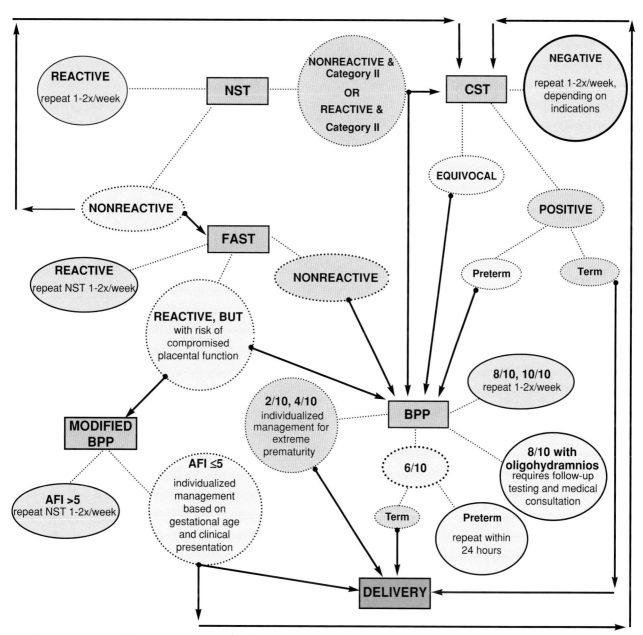

Key: NST, nonstress test; CST, contraction stress test; FAST, fetal acoustic stimulation test (vibra-acoustic stimulation); BPP, biophysical profile; AFI, amniotic fluid index.

Examples of Fetal Heart Rate Baseline Variability

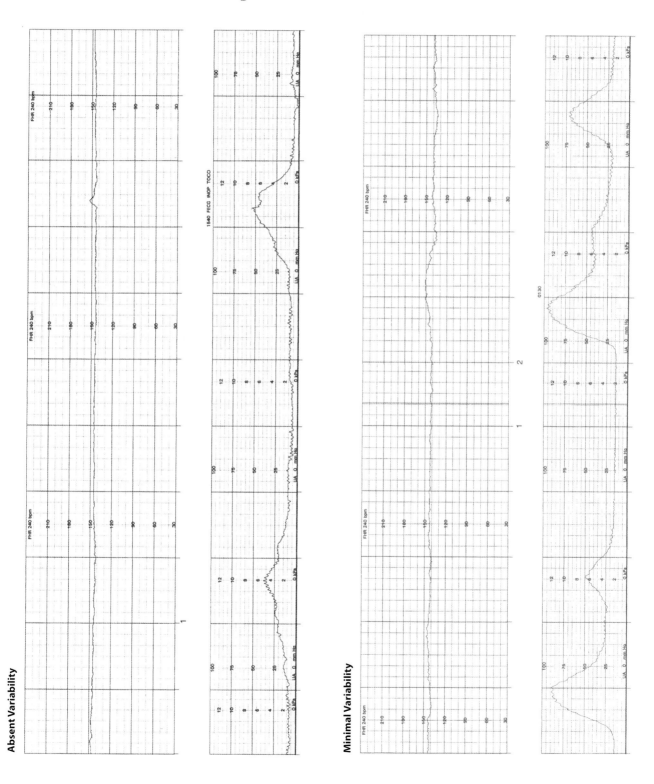

Absent Variability

Minimal Variability

Moderate Variability

Marked Variability

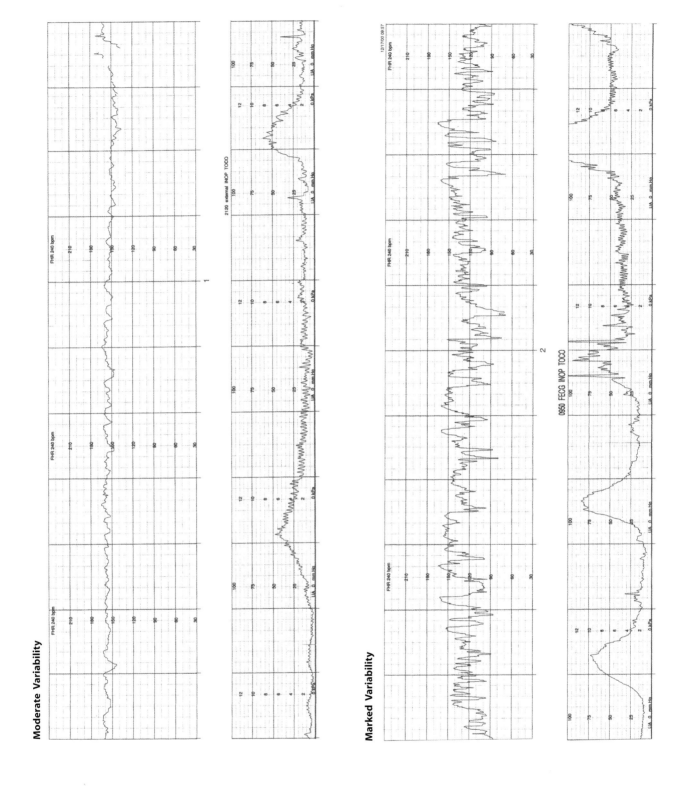

Sample Checklist for Documenting Clinical Proficiency in Sonography

Type of Scan	Date Initials	Date Initials	Date Initials	Date Initials	Date Initials	Date Initials	Completed
Chooses correct transducer for type of exam							
Explains procedure to pt							
Adjusts gains							
Utilizes ALARA principle							
Determines fetal presentation							
Fetal cardiac activity							
AFV AFI							
Placental location							
Fetal breathing							
Fetal flexion/extension							
Fetal gross body movement							
Cervical length							
BPD							
HC							
Abdominal circumference							
Femur length							
EFW							
EGA							

(Note: "Type of Scan" should include any parameter that will be evaluated by the learner and can be specific to what is expected of that learner. But the basics of ultrasound physics and instrumentation should be the same for everyone who is going to be using ultrasound.)

Supervisor's Signature _____ Date: _____

Learner's Signature _____ Date: _____

Glossary of Sonography Terms

Absorption: Decrease or loss of sound wave penetration due to tissues absorbing the sound waves. The energy is deposited in the medium through which it propagates or moves.

Acoustic Enhancement: Opposite of attenuation. Sound is not weakened (attenuated) as it passes through a fluid-filled structure; therefore, the structure behind it appears to have more echoes than the same tissue beside it.

Acoustic Window: An acoustic window is a structure that has no acoustic impedance (no returning ultrasound signals). This lack of impedance allows for passage of sound and enhanced visualization of deeper structures. The full bladder is an example of an acoustic window.

A-Mode Ultrasound: A single dimension display consisting of a horizontal baseline. This baseline represents time and or distance with upward (vertical) deflections (spikes depicting the acoustic interfaces).

Anechoic: Absence of echoes.

Artifact: Artifacts are distortions of the anatomic structures on the image.

Attenuation: Loss of beam amplitude as the sound travels through various tissues. Attenuation may be due to absorption, scattering, or reflection.

Axial Plane: A hypothetical plane parallel to the long axis of an object and is along the ultrasound beam's axis. Also referred to as *horizontal plane.*

Axial Resolution: The minimum required reflector separation along the direction of propagation required to produce separate reflections. The higher the frequency, the better the resolution.

Brightness (B)-Mode: A two-dimensional display of ultrasound. The A-mode spikes are electronically converted into dots and displayed at the correct depth from the transducer. Echoes represented on the display as specific spots that correspond to their point of origin in the body. The brightness of the spot is proportional to the amplitude of the echo.

Coronal Plane: A vertical plane at right angles to a sagittal plane, dividing the body into anterior and posterior portions (front from back). Also called *frontal plane. Coronal* is used when referring to the view obtained by the probe.

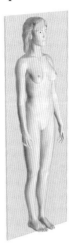

Echo: The returning signal from the interface.

Echogenic: A structure that produces echoes.

Echogenicity: The relative brightness of returning echoes.

Focal Zone: The region of greatest resolution.

Gain: Controls the amount of amplification of the returning echoes.

Homogeneous: Structures that have uniform composition; of uniform appearance and texture.

Hyperechoic: A relative term used to describe a structure which has increased brightness of its echoes in comparison to adjacent structures.

Hypoechoic: A relative term used to describe an area that has decreased brightness of its echoes in comparison to the adjacent structures.

Interface: The boundary between two media (i.e., tissue densities) that produces strong echoes which delineate the boundary of organ.

Isoechoic: A relative term used to describe an area that has an equal distribution of brightness of its echoes.

Lateral Resolution: The ability to separate and define small structures that are perpendicular to the ultrasound beam. It is the minimum reflector separation perpendicular to the direction of propagation required to produce separate reflections. Good lateral resolution is achieved with narrow acoustic beams.

Longitudinal Plane: The plane that runs from head to foot and divides body into right and left halves (also known as median plane). This refers to the position of the probe.

Median Plane: The plane created by an imaginary line dividing the body into right and left halves. Also known as the *sagittal plane.*

Sagittal Plane: The plane that runs from head to foot and divides body into front from back. It is used when referring to the view obtained by the probe. Also known as longitudinal and medial.

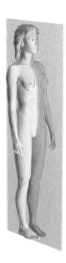

Motion (M) Mode: B-mode trace that is moved as a function of time to demonstrate motion. The motion mode displays moving structures along a single line in the ultrasound beam.

Pulsed Transducers: Consists of one transducer element that functions as both the source and receiving transducers.

Reflection: Loss of sound waves due to inability to penetrate tissues, such as bone.

Resolution: The ability to see two different structures as distinct from one another. The parameter of an ultrasound imaging system that characterizes its ability to detect closely spaced interfaces and displays the echoes from those interfaces as distinct and separate objects. The higher the frequency, the better the resolution, the greater the clarity of an ultrasound image.

Reverberation: An artifact that results from a strong echo returning from a large acoustic interface to the transducer. This echo returns to the tissues again, causing additional echoes parallel and equidistant to the first echo.

Shadowing: Failure of the sound beam to pass through an object (e.g., a bone does not allow any sound to pass through it and there is only shadowing seen behind it).

Sonolucent: Almost devoid of internal echoes or interfaces.

Spectral Flow Doppler: A form of ultrasound image display in which the spectrum of flow velocities is represented graphically on the Y-axis and time on the X-axis; both pulse wave and continuous wave Doppler are displayed in this way.

Time Gain Control (TGC): Employed to correct varying intensities relative to time traveled to avoid losing information from deeper tissues.

Transverse Plane: One passing through the body, at right angles to the sagittal and dorsal planes, and dividing the body into cranial and caudal portions.

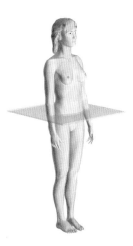

Ultrasound: Sound with a frequency greater than 2 Megahertz or 20,000 Hertz (cycles per second). The higher the transducer frequency, the better the resolution, but with loss of penetration.

Vertical Plane: One perpendicular to a horizontal plane, dividing the body into left and right, or front and back portions.

Terms for Sonography Image Labeling

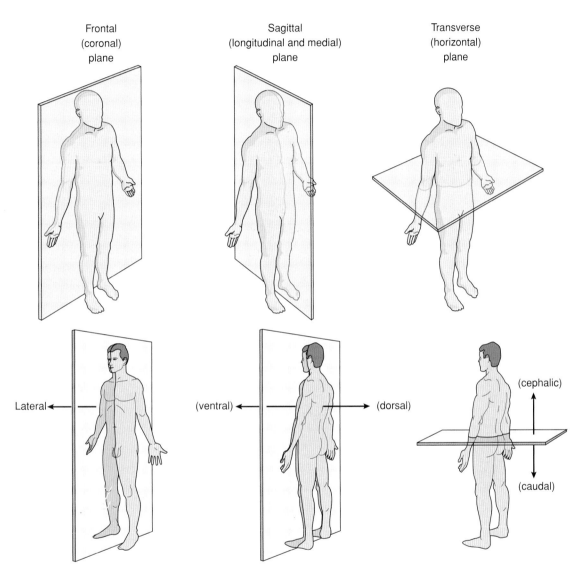

Frontal
(coronal)
plane

Sagittal
(longitudinal and medial)
plane

Transverse
(horizontal)
plane

Lateral ◄

(ventral) ◄ ► (dorsal)

(cephalic)

(caudal)

Coronal: The long axis of a scan performed from the subject's side where the slice divides the anterior from the posterior or the dorsal from the ventral in the long axis

Transverse: A cross-sectional view

Sagittal (Longitudinal): The long axis plane

Superior, Cranial, Cephalad, Rostral: Interchangeable terms indicating the direction toward the head

Inferior or Caudal: Indicating the direction towards the feet

Anterior or Ventral: A structure lying towards the front of the subject

Posterior or Dorsal: A structure ling towards the back of the subject

Medial: Toward the midline

Lateral: Away from the midline

Proximal: Toward the origin

Distal: Away from the origin

Sample Estimated Fetal Weight Charts

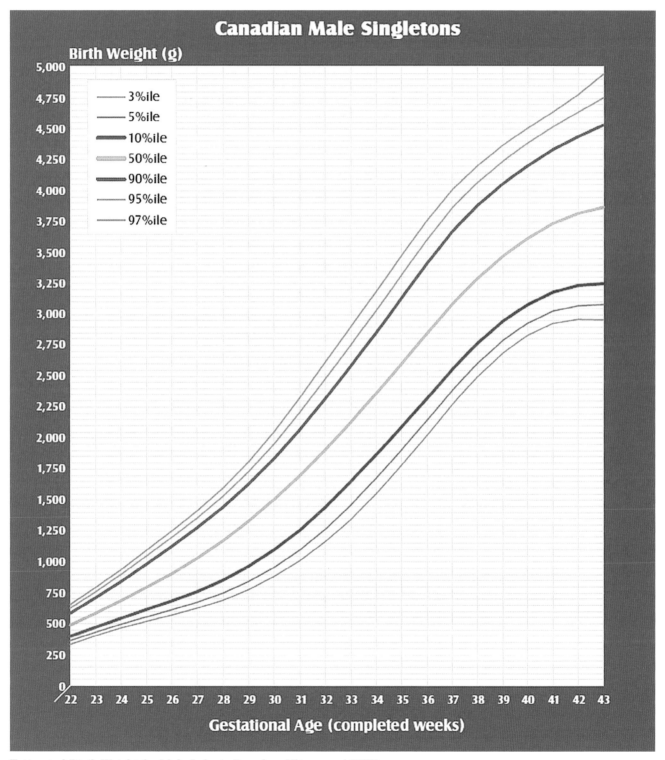

Estimated Birth Weight for Male Infants Based on Ultrasound EFW.

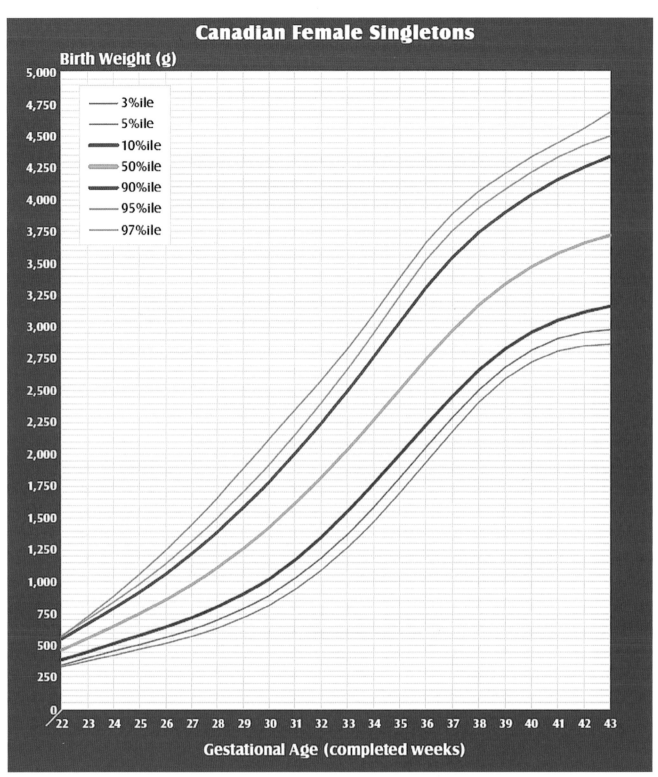

Estimated Birth Weight for Female Infants Based on Ultrasound EFW.

Additional Resources

The American Registry of Diagnostic Medical Sonographers: **www.ardms.org**

The Society for Diagnostic Medical Sonographers: **www.sdms.org**

The American Institute for Ultrasound in Medicine: **www.aium.org**

Art Credits

Chapter 1

Figure 1–1. Adapted from Menihan CA, Kopel E, eds. *Electronic Fetal Monitoring,* 2nd ed. Philadelphia: Lippincott Williams & Wilkins; 2008.

Figure 1–2. Adapted from Menihan CA, Kopel E, eds. *Electronic Fetal Monitoring*, 2nd ed. Philadelphia: Lippincott Williams & Wilkins; 2008.

Chapter 2

Figure 2–1. Menihan CA, Kopel E, eds. *Electronic Fetal Monitoring,* 2nd ed. Philadelphia: Lippincott Williams & Wilkins; 2008.

Figure 2–2. Menihan CA, Kopel E, eds. *Electronic Fetal Monitoring,* 2nd ed. Philadelphia: Lippincott Williams & Wilkins; 2008.

Figure 2–3. Menihan CA, Kopel E, eds. *Electronic Fetal Monitoring,* 2nd ed. Philadelphia: Lippincott Williams & Wilkins; 2008.

Figure 2–4. Menihan CA, Kopel E, eds. *Electronic Fetal Monitoring,* 2nd ed. Philadelphia: Lippincott Williams & Wilkins; 2008.

Figure 2–5. Menihan CA, Kopel E, eds. *Electronic Fetal Monitoring,* 2nd ed. Philadelphia: Lippincott Williams & Wilkins; 2008.

Figure 2–6. Menihan CA, Kopel E, eds. *Electronic Fetal Monitoring,* 2nd ed. Philadelphia: Lippincott Williams & Wilkins; 2008.

Figure 2–7. Menihan CA, Kopel E, eds. *Electronic Fetal Monitoring,* 2nd ed. Philadelphia: Lippincott Williams & Wilkins; 2008.

Figure 2–8. Menihan CA, Kopel E, eds. *Electronic Fetal Monitoring,* 2nd ed. Philadelphia: Lippincott Williams & Wilkins; 2008.

Figure 2–9. Menihan CA, Kopel E, eds. *Electronic Fetal Monitoring,* 2nd ed. Philadelphia: Lippincott Williams & Wilkins; 2008.

Chapter 3

Figure 3–1. Menihan CA, Kopel E, eds. *Electronic Fetal Monitoring,* 2nd ed. Philadelphia: Lippincott Williams & Wilkins; 2008.

Figure 3–2. Menihan CA, Kopel E, eds. *Electronic Fetal Monitoring,* 2nd ed. Philadelphia: Lippincott Williams & Wilkins; 2008.

Figure 3–3. Menihan CA, Kopel E, eds. *Electronic Fetal Monitoring,* 2nd ed. Philadelphia: Lippincott Williams & Wilkins; 2008.

Figure 3–4. Menihan CA, Kopel E, eds. *Electronic Fetal Monitoring,* 2nd ed. Philadelphia: Lippincott Williams & Wilkins; 2008.

Figure 3–5. Menihan CA, Kopel E, eds. *Electronic Fetal Monitoring,* 2nd ed. Philadelphia: Lippincott Williams & Wilkins; 2008.

Figure 3–6. Menihan CA, Kopel E, eds. *Electronic Fetal Monitoring,* 2nd ed. Philadelphia: Lippincott Williams & Wilkins; 2008.

Figure 3–7. Menihan CA, Kopel E, eds. *Electronic Fetal Monitoring,* 2nd ed. Philadelphia: Lippincott Williams & Wilkins; 2008.

Figure 3–8. Menihan CA, Kopel E, eds. *Electronic Fetal Monitoring,* 2nd ed. Philadelphia: Lippincott Williams & Wilkins; 2008.

Figure 3–9. Menihan CA, Kopel E, eds. *Electronic Fetal Monitoring,* 2nd ed. Philadelphia: Lippincott Williams & Wilkins; 2008.

Figure 3–10. Menihan CA, Kopel E, eds. *Electronic Fetal Monitoring,* 2nd ed. Philadelphia: Lippincott Williams & Wilkins; 2008.

Figure 3–11. Menihan CA, Kopel E, eds. *Electronic Fetal Monitoring,* 2nd ed. Philadelphia: Lippincott Williams & Wilkins; 2008.

Figure 3–12. Menihan CA, Kopel E, eds. *Electronic Fetal Monitoring,* 2nd ed. Philadelphia: Lippincott Williams & Wilkins; 2008.

Figure 3–13. Menihan CA, Kopel E, eds. *Electronic Fetal Monitoring,* 2nd ed. Philadelphia: Lippincott Williams & Wilkins; 2008.

Figure 3–14. Menihan CA, Kopel E, eds. *Electronic Fetal Monitoring,* 2nd ed. Philadelphia: Lippincott Williams & Wilkins; 2008.

Figure 3–15. Menihan CA, Kopel E, eds. *Electronic Fetal Monitoring,* 2nd ed. Philadelphia: Lippincott Williams & Wilkins; 2008.

Figure 3–16. Menihan CA, Kopel E, eds. *Electronic Fetal Monitoring,* 2nd ed. Philadelphia: Lippincott Williams & Wilkins; 2008.

Figure 3–17. Menihan CA, Kopel E, eds. *Electronic Fetal Monitoring,* 2nd ed. Philadelphia: Lippincott Williams & Wilkins; 2008.

Figure 3–18. Menihan CA, Kopel E, eds. *Electronic Fetal Monitoring,* 2nd ed. Philadelphia: Lippincott Williams & Wilkins; 2008.

Figure 3–19. Menihan CA, Kopel E, eds. *Electronic Fetal Monitoring,* 2nd ed. Philadelphia: Lippincott Williams & Wilkins; 2008.

Figure 3–20. Menihan CA, Kopel E, eds. *Electronic Fetal Monitoring,* 2nd ed. Philadelphia: Lippincott Williams & Wilkins; 2008.

Figure 3–21. Menihan CA, Kopel E, eds. *Electronic Fetal Monitoring,* 2nd ed. Philadelphia: Lippincott Williams & Wilkins; 2008.

Figure 3–22. American College of Obstetricians and Gynecologists. Management of Intrapartum Fetal Heart Rate Tracings. ACOG Practice Bulletin 116. Washington, DC: ACOG; 2010.

Figure 3–23. American College of Obstetricians and Gynecologists. Management of Intrapartum Fetal Heart Rate Tracings. ACOG Practice Bulletin 116. Washington, DC: ACOG; 2010.

Figure 3–24. Menihan CA, Kopel E, eds. *Electronic Fetal Monitoring,* 2nd ed. Philadelphia: Lippincott Williams & Wilkins; 2008.

Figure 3–25. Menihan CA, Kopel E, eds. *Electronic Fetal Monitoring,* 2nd ed. Philadelphia: Lippincott Williams & Wilkins; 2008.

Figure 3–26. Menihan CA, Kopel E, eds. *Electronic Fetal Monitoring,* 2nd ed. Philadelphia: Lippincott Williams & Wilkins; 2008.

Figure 3–27. Menihan CA, Kopel E, eds. *Electronic Fetal Monitoring,* 2nd ed. Philadelphia: Lippincott Williams & Wilkins; 2008.

Figure 3–28. Menihan CA, Kopel E, eds. *Electronic Fetal Monitoring,* 2nd ed. Philadelphia: Lippincott Williams & Wilkins; 2008.

Figure 3–29. Menihan CA, Kopel E, eds. *Electronic Fetal Monitoring,* 2nd ed. Philadelphia: Lippincott Williams & Wilkins; 2008.

Figure 3–30. Menihan CA, Kopel E, eds. *Electronic Fetal Monitoring,* 2nd ed. Philadelphia: Lippincott Williams & Wilkins; 2008.

Figure 3–31. Clark SL, Nageotte MP, Garite TJ, et al. Intrapartum management of category II fetal heart tracings: toward standardization of care. *Am J Obstet Gynecol.* 2013;2(209):89–97, with permission.

Figure 3–32. American College of Obstetricians and Gynecologists. *Management of Intrapartum Fetal Heart Rate Tracings*. ACOG Practice Bulletin 116. Washington, DC: Author; 2010, with permission.

Figure 3–33. American College of Obstetricians and Gynecologists. *Management of Intrapartum Fetal Heart Rate Tracings*. ACOG Practice Bulletin 116. Washington, DC: Author; 2010, with permission.

Chapter 4

Figure 4–2. Menihan CA, Kopel E, eds. *Electronic Fetal Monitoring,* 2nd ed. Philadelphia: Lippincott Williams & Wilkins; 2008.

Figure 4–3. Menihan CA, Kopel E, eds. *Electronic Fetal Monitoring,* 2nd ed. Philadelphia: Lippincott Williams & Wilkins; 2008.

Figure 4–4. Menihan CA, Kopel E, eds. *Electronic Fetal Monitoring,* 2nd ed. Philadelphia: Lippincott Williams & Wilkins; 2008.

Figure 4–5. Menihan CA, Kopel E, eds. *Electronic Fetal Monitoring,* 2nd ed. Philadelphia: Lippincott Williams & Wilkins; 2008.

Figure 4–6. Menihan CA, Kopel E, eds. *Electronic Fetal Monitoring,* 2nd ed. Philadelphia: Lippincott Williams & Wilkins; 2008.

Figure 4–7. Menihan CA, Kopel E, eds. *Electronic Fetal Monitoring,* 2nd ed. Philadelphia: Lippincott Williams & Wilkins; 2008.

Figure 4–8. Menihan CA, Kopel E, eds. *Electronic Fetal Monitoring,* 2nd ed. Philadelphia: Lippincott Williams & Wilkins; 2008.

Figure 4–9. Menihan CA, Kopel E, eds. *Electronic Fetal Monitoring,* 2nd ed. Philadelphia: Lippincott Williams & Wilkins; 2008.

Chapter 6

Figure 6–1. Menihan CA, Kopel E, eds. *Electronic Fetal Monitoring,* 2nd ed. Philadelphia: Lippincott Williams & Wilkins; 2008.

Figure 6–2. Adapted from Barnes J. Implementing a perinatal clinical information system: A work in progress. *J Obstet Gynecol Neonat Nurs.* 2008;35(1):134–140; and Hunt E, Sproat S, Kitzmiller R. *The Nursing Informatics Implementation Guide.* New York: Springer-Verlag; 2004.

Chapter 9

Figure 9–1A and B. Courtesy of Cydney Menihan.

Figure 9–1C. Menihan CA, ed. *Limited Sonography in Obstetric and Gynecologic Triage.* Philadelphia: Lippincott Williams & Wilkins; 1998.

Figure 9–1G. Menihan CA, ed. *Limited Sonography in Obstetric and Gynecologic Triage.* Philadelphia: Lippincott Williams & Wilkins; 1998.

Figure 9–1D. Pillitteri A. *Maternal and Child Health Nursing: Care of the Childbearing and Childrearing Family,* 4th ed. Philadelphia: Lippincott Williams & Wilkins; 2003.

Figure 9–3. LifeART image copyright © 2014 Lippincott Williams & Wilkins. All rights reserved.

Figure 9–4. Menihan CA, ed. *Limited Sonography in Obstetric and Gynecologic Triage.* Philadelphia: Lippincott Williams & Wilkins; 1998.

Figure 9–5A. From Daffner RH. *Clinical Radiology: The Essentials*, 3rd ed. Philadelphia: Lippincott Williams & Wilkins; 2007.

Figure 9–5B. Menihan CA, ed. *Limited Sonography in Obstetric and Gynecologic Triage.* Philadelphia: Lippincott Williams & Wilkins; 1998.

Figure 9–6. Drawing by Paul Gross, MS.

Figure 9–7C. Menihan CA, ed. *Limited Sonography in Obstetric and Gynecologic Triage.* Philadelphia: Lippincott Williams & Wilkins; 1998.

Figure 9–8. Drawing by Paul Gross, MS.

Figure 9–9. Courtesy of Betty Kay Taylor.

Figure 9–10. Courtesy of Betty Kay Taylor.

Chapter 10

Figure 10–2. From Daffner RH. *Clinical Radiology: The Essentials*, 3rd ed. Philadelphia: Lippincott Williams & Wilkins; 2007.

Figure 10–4. Menihan CA, ed. *Limited Sonography in Obstetric and Gynecologic Triage.* Philadelphia: Lippincott Williams & Wilkins; 1998.

Figure 10–5. MediClip image copyright © 2003 Lippincott Williams & Wilkins. All rights reserved.

Figure 10–6. Menihan CA, ed. *Limited Sonography in Obstetric and Gynecologic Triage.* Philadelphia: Lippincott Williams & Wilkins; 1998.

Figure 10–7. Menihan CA, ed. *Limited Sonography in Obstetric and Gynecologic Triage.* Philadelphia: Lippincott Williams & Wilkins; 1998.

Figure 10–8. Menihan CA, ed. *Limited Sonography in Obstetric and Gynecologic Triage.* Philadelphia: Lippincott Williams & Wilkins; 1998.

Figure 10–10. Menihan CA, ed. *Limited Sonography in Obstetric and Gynecologic Triage.* Philadelphia: Lippincott Williams & Wilkins; 1998.

Figure 10–12. Menihan CA, ed. *Limited Sonography in Obstetric and Gynecologic Triage.* Philadelphia: Lippincott Williams & Wilkins; 1998.

Figure 10–13. Menihan CA, ed. *Limited Sonography in Obstetric and Gynecologic Triage.* Philadelphia: Lippincott Williams & Wilkins; 1998.

Figure 10–14. Drawing by Paul Gross, MS.

Figure 10–15. Drawing by Paul Gross, MS.

Figure 10–16. Menihan CA, ed. *Limited Sonography in Obstetric and Gynecologic Triage.* Philadelphia: Lippincott Williams & Wilkins; 1998.

Figure 10–18. Courtesy of Betty Kay Taylor.

Figure 10–19. Menihan CA, ed. *Limited Sonography in Obstetric and Gynecologic Triage.* Philadelphia: Lippincott Williams & Wilkins; 1998.

Figure 10–20. Menihan CA, ed. *Limited Sonography in Obstetric and Gynecologic Triage.* Philadelphia: Lippincott Williams & Wilkins; 1998.

Figure 10–21. Menihan CA, ed. *Limited Sonography in Obstetric and Gynecologic Triage.* Philadelphia: Lippincott Williams & Wilkins; 1998.

Figure 10–22. Courtesy of Cydney Menihan.

Figure 10–23. Menihan CA, ed. *Limited Sonography in Obstetric and Gynecologic Triage.* Philadelphia: Lippincott Williams & Wilkins; 1998.

Figure 10–24. Courtesy of Diana Dowdy.

Figure 10–25. Courtesy of Diana Dowdy.

Figure 10–27. Menihan CA, ed. *Limited Sonography in Obstetric and Gynecologic Triage.* Philadelphia: Lippincott Williams & Wilkins; 1998.

Figure 10–28. Menihan CA, ed. *Limited Sonography in Obstetric and Gynecologic Triage.* Philadelphia: Lippincott Williams & Wilkins; 1998.

Figure 10–29. Courtesy of Betty Kay Taylor

Figure 10–30. Courtesy of Diana Dowdy.

Chapter 11

Figure 11–1. Menihan CA, ed. *Limited Sonography in Obstetric and Gynecologic Triage.* Philadelphia: Lippincott Williams & Wilkins; 1998.

Figure 11–2. Courtesy of Betty Kay Taylor.

Figure 11–3. Menihan CA, ed. *Limited Sonography in Obstetric and Gynecologic Triage.* Philadelphia: Lippincott Williams & Wilkins; 1998.

Figure 11–4. Courtesy of Betty Kay Taylor.

Figure 11–5. Menihan CA, ed. *Limited Sonography in Obstetric and Gynecologic Triage.* Philadelphia: Lippincott Williams & Wilkins; 1998.

Figure 11–6. Menihan CA, ed. *Limited Sonography in Obstetric and Gynecologic Triage.* Philadelphia: Lippincott Williams & Wilkins; 1998.

Figure 11–7. Menihan CA, ed. *Limited Sonography in Obstetric and Gynecologic Triage.* Philadelphia: Lippincott Williams & Wilkins; 1998.

Figure 11–8. Menihan CA, ed. *Limited Sonography in Obstetric and Gynecologic Triage.* Philadelphia: Lippincott Williams & Wilkins; 1998.

Figure 11–9. Menihan CA, ed. *Limited Sonography in Obstetric and Gynecologic Triage.* Philadelphia: Lippincott Williams & Wilkins; 1998.

Figure 11–10. Menihan CA, ed. *Limited Sonography in Obstetric and Gynecologic Triage.* Philadelphia: Lippincott Williams & Wilkins; 1998.

Figure 11–11. Menihan CA, ed. *Limited Sonography in Obstetric and Gynecologic Triage.* Philadelphia: Lippincott Williams & Wilkins; 1998.

Figure 11–12. Eisenberg RL. *An Atlas of Differential Diagnosis*, 4th ed. Philadelphia: Lippincott Williams & Wilkins; 2003.

Figure 11–13. Eisenberg RL. *An Atlas of Differential Diagnosis,* 4th ed. Philadelphia: Lippincott Williams & Wilkins; 2003.

Figure 11–15. Eisenberg RL. *An Atlas of Differential Diagnosis,* 4th ed. Philadelphia: Lippincott Williams & Wilkins; 2003.

Chapter 12

Figure 12–1A. Menihan CA, ed. *Limited Sonography in Obstetric and Gynecologic Triage.* Philadelphia: Lippincott Williams & Wilkins; 1998.

Figure 12–1B. Courtesy of Betty Kay Taylor.

Figure 12–2. Menihan CA, ed. *Limited Sonography in Obstetric and Gynecologic Triage.* Philadelphia: Lippincott Williams & Wilkins; 1998.

Figure 12–3. Menihan CA, ed. *Limited Sonography in Obstetric and Gynecologic Triage.* Philadelphia: Lippincott Williams & Wilkins; 1998.

Figure 12–4. Courtesy of Betty Kay Taylor.

Figure 12–5. Courtesy of Betty Kay Taylor.

Figure 12–6. Menihan CA, ed. *Limited Sonography in Obstetric and Gynecologic Triage*. Philadelphia: Lippincott Williams & Wilkins; 1998.

Figure 12–7. Courtesy of Betty Kay Taylor.

Figure 12–8. Courtesy of Betty Kay Taylor.

Figure 12–9. Menihan CA, ed. *Limited Sonography in Obstetric and Gynecologic Triage*. Philadelphia: Lippincott Williams & Wilkins; 1998.

Figure 12–10. Ronald L. Eisenberg, an atlas of differential diagnosis Fourth Edition. Philadelphia: Lippincott Williams & Wilkins, 2003.

Figure 12–11. Menihan CA, ed. *Limited Sonography in Obstetric and Gynecologic Triage*. Philadelphia: Lippincott Williams & Wilkins; 1998.

Figure 12–12. Menihan CA, ed. *Limited Sonography in Obstetric and Gynecologic Triage*. Philadelphia: Lippincott Williams & Wilkins; 1998.

Figure 12–13. Menihan CA, ed. *Limited Sonography in Obstetric and Gynecologic Triage*. Philadelphia: Lippincott Williams & Wilkins; 1998.

Figure 12–14. Menihan CA, ed. *Limited Sonography in Obstetric and Gynecologic Triage*. Philadelphia: Lippincott Williams & Wilkins; 1998.

Figure 12–15. Menihan CA, ed. *Limited Sonography in Obstetric and Gynecologic Triage*. Philadelphia: Lippincott Williams & Wilkins; 1998.

Figure 12–16. Menihan CA, ed. *Limited Sonography in Obstetric and Gynecologic Triage*. Philadelphia: Lippincott Williams & Wilkins; 1998.

Figure 12–17. Menihan CA, ed. *Limited Sonography in Obstetric and Gynecologic Triage*. Philadelphia: Lippincott Williams & Wilkins; 1998.

Figure 12–18. Menihan CA, ed. *Limited Sonography in Obstetric and Gynecologic Triage*. Philadelphia: Lippincott Williams & Wilkins; 1998.

Figure 12–19. Menihan CA, ed. *Limited Sonography in Obstetric and Gynecologic Triage*. Philadelphia: Lippincott Williams & Wilkins; 1998.

Figure 12–20. Courtesy of Betty Kay Taylor.

Figure 12–21. Menihan CA, ed. *Limited Sonography in Obstetric and Gynecologic Triage*. Philadelphia: Lippincott Williams & Wilkins; 1998.

Figure 12–22. Menihan CA, ed. *Limited Sonography in Obstetric and Gynecologic Triage*. Philadelphia: Lippincott Williams & Wilkins; 1998.

Figure 12–23. Menihan CA, ed. *Limited Sonography in Obstetric and Gynecologic Triage*. Philadelphia: Lippincott Williams & Wilkins; 1998.

Figure 12–24. Menihan CA, ed. *Limited Sonography in Obstetric and Gynecologic Triage*. Philadelphia: Lippincott Williams & Wilkins; 1998.

Figure 12–25. Menihan CA, ed. *Limited Sonography in Obstetric and Gynecologic Triage*. Philadelphia: Lippincott Williams & Wilkins; 1998.

Figure 12–26. Menihan CA, ed. *Limited Sonography in Obstetric and Gynecologic Triage*. Philadelphia: Lippincott Williams & Wilkins; 1998.

Figure 12–27. Menihan CA, ed. *Limited Sonography in Obstetric and Gynecologic Triage*. Philadelphia: Lippincott Williams & Wilkins; 1998.

Figure 12–28. Menihan CA, ed. *Limited Sonography in Obstetric and Gynecologic Triage*. Philadelphia: Lippincott Williams & Wilkins; 1998.

Figure 12–29. Menihan CA, ed. *Limited Sonography in Obstetric and Gynecologic Triage*. Philadelphia: Lippincott Williams & Wilkins; 1998.

Figure 12–30. Menihan CA, ed. *Limited Sonography in Obstetric and Gynecologic Triage*. Philadelphia: Lippincott Williams & Wilkins; 1998.

Figure 12–31. Menihan CA, ed. *Limited Sonography in Obstetric and Gynecologic Triage*. Philadelphia: Lippincott Williams & Wilkins; 1998.

Figure 12–32. Menihan CA, ed. *Limited Sonography in Obstetric and Gynecologic Triage*. Philadelphia: Lippincott Williams & Wilkins; 1998.

Figure 12–33. Menihan CA, ed. *Limited Sonography in Obstetric and Gynecologic Triage*. Philadelphia: Lippincott Williams & Wilkins; 1998.

Figure 12–34. Menihan CA, ed. *Limited Sonography in Obstetric and Gynecologic Triage*. Philadelphia: Lippincott Williams & Wilkins; 1998.

Figure 12–35. Menihan CA, ed. *Limited Sonography in Obstetric and Gynecologic Triage*. Philadelphia: Lippincott Williams & Wilkins; 1998.

Figure 12–36. Menihan CA, ed. *Limited Sonography in Obstetric and Gynecologic Triage*. Philadelphia: Lippincott Williams & Wilkins; 1998.

Figure 12–37. Menihan CA, ed. *Limited Sonography in Obstetric and Gynecologic Triage*. Philadelphia: Lippincott Williams & Wilkins; 1998.

Figure 12–38. Menihan CA, ed. *Limited Sonography in Obstetric and Gynecologic Triage*. Philadelphia: Lippincott Williams & Wilkins; 1998.

Figure 12–41. Courtesy of Cydney Menihan.

Figure 12–42. Courtesy of Betty Kay Taylor.

Figure 12–43. Courtesy of Betty Kay Taylor.

Figure 12–44. Courtesy of Betty Kay Taylor.

Figure 12–45. Courtesy of Betty Kay Taylor.

Figure 12–46. Courtesy of Betty Kay Taylor.

Figure 12–47. Courtesy of Betty Kay Taylor.

Figure 12–48. Courtesy of Betty Kay Taylor.

Figure 12–49. Courtesy of Betty Kay Taylor.

Figure 12–50. Courtesy of Betty Kay Taylor.

Figure 12–51. Courtesy of Betty Kay Taylor.

Figure 12–52. Courtesy of Betty Kay Taylor.

Chapter 13

Figure 13–3A. Menihan CA, ed. *Limited Sonography in Obstetric and Gynecologic Triage*. Philadelphia: Lippincott Williams & Wilkins; 1998.

Figure 13–3B. Courtesy of Anthony Lathrop.

Figure 13–13C. Courtesy of Betty Kay Taylor.

Figure 13–13D. Courtesy of Betty Kay Taylor.

Figure 13–4B. Courtesy of Betty Kay Taylor.

Figure 13–4C. Courtesy of Betty Kay Taylor.

Figure 13–5. Courtesy of Betty Kay Taylor.

Figure 13–6. Menihan CA, ed. *Limited Sonography in Obstetric and Gynecologic Triage*. Philadelphia: Lippincott Williams & Wilkins; 1998.

Appendices E and F

Cohen BJ, Wood DL. *Memmler's The Human Body in Health and Disease*, 9th ed. Philadelphia: Lippincott Williams & Wilkins; 2000.

Willis MC. *Medical Terminology: A Programmed Learning Approach to the Language of Health Care*. Baltimore: Lippincott Williams & Wilkins; 2002.

Appendix G

© All rights reserved. Michael S. Kramer, et al. A new and improved population-based Canadian reference for birth weight for gestational age. *Pediatrics*, 2001. Reproduced with permission from the Minister of Health, 2013.

Index

Page numbers followed by *b* refer to text in boxes; page numbers followed by *f* refer to figures; page numbers followed by *t* refer to tables.